'A searing condemnation of neglect and [...] services, this is a must-read volume to spur [...] treatment of older people in some of our i[...] as a society, we don't think they matter. If we visited more, challenged more, took ownership more seriously, and gave care staff, often pressurised and underpaid, more respect, things might get better. Michael Mandelstam is to be congratulated for drawing this to our attention. Now it is up to us to find the solution – and that lies partly in valuing those who care for our older people better, paying them better, and regarding care as a serious career choice.'
— *Baroness Julia Neuberger*

'Successive reports on catastrophic failures in the nursing care of desperately sick people in our hospitals have had little effect. They have failed to see the systemic nature of the problem and, worse, have proposed box-ticking solutions to what is often the abandonment of common humanity. Michael Mandelstam's documentation of a continuing scandal that touches on all of us is worth a thousand expensive inquiries. This brilliant and impassioned book should be mandatory reading for policymakers and all of those who care for vulnerable people.'
— *Raymond Tallis FRCP FMedSci, Emeritus Professor of Geriatric Medicine and author of* Hippocratic Oaths: Medicine and its Discontents

'Amidst the striking advances in modern medicine stands the starkly contrasting deterioration in the day to day care of vulnerable patients. Neglect and abuse of elderly and incapacitated patients in our hospitals and nursing homes is not a rare or occasional scandal picked out by the media. The picture painted in this timely book strongly points to a much wider spread of failures of acceptable standards of care. Despite any number of published inquiries little seems to have changed in the last few years. This excellent book now demands action not words from the professions and Government.'
— *Lord Leslie Turnberg*

'*How We Treat the Sick* is a call for action. NHS staff have been smothered and de-motivated by countless targets and controls. Focused regulation and more autonomy for front line staff could transform the experience of patients.'
— *Baroness Molly Meacher*

'Michael Mandelstam has provided a devastating account of some of the more horrifying aspects of the care provided by the National Health Service. As he points out this is not necessarily typical of all care provided, even by those institutions mentioned in the book. It is however a sufficiently alarming book that should be read by everyone concerned with health care in Britain, and demands attention both from the organisations concerned and from those responsible for the management and reorganisation of the NHS.'
— *Tim Yeo MP*

'*How We Treat the Sick* by Michael Mandelstam considers in detail evidence of what has been happening to some hospital patients, particularly older people, over the past 14 years and seeks to explore the moral and legal implications of that record. As a passionate believer in the NHS and what it stands for, and in the prevention of elder abuse, I believe this issue deserves much greater recognition as it has important implications for service provision across the country. Looking forward we must not see the criticisms in the book as a threat to the NHS, but rather as a pathway to better practice.

While the book ends on a pessimistic note, I am more hopeful that matters could change for the better. For as the book tells us the recent past hasn't been a dark experience for everyone and the excellent care and attention provided for most people by the NHS only serves to highlight the fact that, if the will is there, it is perfectly possible to provide good quality care within the current resource limitations.

Going forward we can, and must, do much more to improve, firstly the health and social care of vulnerable people who cannot speak for themselves and secondly, the training and morale of those whose job it is to care for them. A good place to start would be immediately to begin the process of vigorously consigning to history the bad practices so clearly highlighted in this important book.'

— Baroness Sally Greengross OBE

How We Treat the Sick

by the same author

Betraying the NHS
Health Abandoned
ISBN 978 1 84310 482 7

Quick Guide to Community Care Practice and the Law
ISBN 978 1 84905 083 8

Community Care Practice and the Law
4th edition
ISBN 978 1 84310 691 3

Safeguarding Vulnerable Adults and the Law
ISBN 978 1 84310 692 0

Manual Handling in Health and Social Care
An A–Z of Law and Practice
ISBN 978 1 84310 041 6

Michael Mandelstam

Foreword by Lord Justice Munby

HOW WE TREAT THE SICK

Neglect and
Abuse in Our
Health Services

Jessica Kingsley *Publishers*
London and Philadelphia

First published in 2011
by Jessica Kingsley Publishers
116 Pentonville Road
London N1 9JB, UK
and
400 Market Street, Suite 400
Philadelphia, PA 19106, USA

www.jkp.com

Copyright © Michael Mandelstam 2011

Library of Congress Cataloging in Publication Data
A CIP catalog record for this book is available from the Library of Congress

British Library Cataloguing in Publication Data
A CIP catalogue record for this book is available from the British Library

ISBN 978 1 84905 160 6

Printed and bound in Great Britain

This book is written in memory of the staff at the Walnuttree Hospital in Sudbury, Suffolk. For so long they provided skilled, compassionate, dignified inpatient nursing, genuine rehabilitation and palliative care for their patients. It was the very antithesis of the neglect and degrading care described in this book. Until, in October 2010, they were allowed to provide it no longer.

It is surely of interest that they achieved this without outcomes, targets, indicators, priorities, excessive gathering of statistics, unceasing structural change – in fact, without all these hallmarks of the modern health service.

This type of inpatient care was what local people had so appreciated and wanted. They fought for it desperately over a period of six years, during which time it was continually threatened by bureaucrats and accountants. In an age of 'patient choice', it was then taken away.

Acknowledgements

I must thank, above all, Jessica Kingsley for her support and encouragement, and for believing that the book would have something to say. Also her staff, in particular Helen Longmate, Rachel Menzies and Victoria Peters for their unstinting efforts and tolerance. In another quarter altogether, I owe a great debt to Peter Clifford for reading through the draft with such a helpfully critical eye and for finding and digging out some of the raw material.

Contents

Disclaimer

This book mentions the names of many hospitals and some care homes. A number of points should be kept in mind.

Poor, neglectful or abusive hospital care at a particular time in respect of a particular patient, or group of patients, does not necessarily mean that such care was given also to other patients at the same time in the hospital. Although it may do.

Equally, just because such care was afforded at a certain moment or period of time in a particular hospital, this does not necessarily mean that it was present before, and has continued since, any particular reported incident or incidents. Although it may do.

Furthermore, the presence of bad practice in an organisation by no means precludes plenty of good practice in the same organisation. So, in the same hospital, one ward can be as superb in its care as another is atrocious. This book focuses on bad practices because that is what the book is about, not because it is claiming that much good practice does not exist. It is about a particular aspect of our health services only; it is not an all round appraisal.

Some of the book considers legal issues. Nothing in the book should be taken to imply that any individual, not convicted of a criminal offence, is guilty of one. In a similar vein, other than where this is reported as being so, no inference is to be made about any particular individual being in breach of any other (civil) legal duty; about any particular individual being in breach of his or her professional registration requirements; or about whether any particular individual should be barred from working with vulnerable adults by the Independent Safeguarding Authority.

Particularly in the case of Press reports and patient comments on the Internet, the fact that a hospital is mentioned one or more times does not necessarily mean that it provides worse care than other hospitals; conversely, the absence of the name of a particular hospital does not necessarily mean that it provides better care than the hospitals that are mentioned.

Note. A number of quotes from patients are included in this book. Some, particularly those from websites, do not always follow the rules of spelling and grammar. The quotes are reproduced unaltered.

Foreword

by Lord Justice Munby

Michael Mandelstam has written a very important and most timely book. It should be read not merely by everyone who has a professional, managerial, administrative or regulatory involvement in our health services but indeed by every concerned citizen. For the problems which he describes potentially affect every one of us.

The author rightly acknowledges the immense amount of good practice that exists in the health services and the dedication and conscientious commitment of all those staff who seek at all costs to uphold the dignity of their patients. As he says, this is not a book about the health service as a whole, about all the good things in it, nor an attack on the health service.

It is about neglect and abuse.

He quotes my observation that 'One reads too often for comfort accounts of conditions in various institutional settings – hospitals and care homes – which are a disgrace to any country with pretensions to civilisation and which ought to shock the conscience of any decent minded person.' The reader may feel that the material which he piles up for our consideration, relentlessly and remorselessly, and therein lies one of the great strengths and values of the book, more than makes good that bleak assessment, just as it shows that the problems which the author chronicles are indeed, as he says, systemic. Something, he suggests, has gone badly wrong. Can any dispassionate reader of this book disagree?

The author moves on to consider why this may have come about and discusses the responsibilities of administrators, regulators and the professions. Whether or not one agrees with his analysis the questions he raises are important – for surely something needs to be done.

Towards the end the author turns to consider the role of the law. The survey is illuminating but in a sense dispiriting. Why, after all, should the patient or their family and friends even have to contemplate going to law? Surely what we are here concerned with is, or ought to be, nothing more than basic human dignity. And it should not require a lawyer to tell us, least of all to tell the caring professions, what dignity means in this context. Every patient in a hospital is surely entitled to respect as a human being, as a unique individual, requiring understanding, empathy and compassion. It is not very much; but it is fundamental.

In writing this book Michael Mandelstam has performed a most valuable public service. One can only hope that it will bear fruit.

James Munby
February 2011

Preface

> This has been a story of a Trust which has, over a sustained period of time, failed to deliver acceptable standards of care to many of its patients. It is appropriate to echo a statement made by Florence Nightingale 150 years ago: "it may seem a strange principle to enunciate as the very first requirement in a hospital that it should do the sick no harm". (Mid Staffordshire NHS Foundation Trust: Independent Inquiry, 2009)[1]

I have been assailed by doubts about whether I should write this book at all, because of an instinctive doubt or disbelief even that poor and neglectful care is routinely dispensed within our health care system.

What has overcome these doubts is the weight of the evidence, the importance of which my late father conveyed to me. He was a scientist, rationalist and optimist. He emphasised the habit of seeing jars half full rather than half empty, of not being unduly critical or pessimistic but, also, of not shying away from evidence. And the evidence is overwhelming; a problem exists which is not only far more than trivial, but which is systemic. And because its extent is not commonly appreciated, it needs to be put across in all its unedifying detail. I make no apology for doing this. Setting out what should be happening in terms of good practice (which is also included) is simply not enough, much more pleasant though it would be.

As I have got older, I have witnessed, over the last quarter of a century, a number of relatives and close friends deteriorate with illness and die. All but one suffered neglectful care in different hospitals in different geographical locations in England. Statistically, what happened to five particular people in different hospitals might appear insignificant. Equally, though, what are the chances that five out of six of one's nearest and dearest should end up being treated so badly? Even the sixth, with a sudden and aggressive terminal illness, was placed on the wrong ward for her condition. As an 'outlier', she did not receive the support, advice and care that she needed from staff who would have understood her condition. This affected the decisions she made, her ability to cope and added considerably to her distress.

---

1   Francis, R. (Chair) (2010) *Independent Inquiry into care provided by Mid Staffordshire NHS Foundation Trust January 2005–March 2009*. London: The Stationery Office, p.396.

So it occurred to me that perhaps poor and neglectful care is more prevalent than is commonly supposed. Of course, personal experience, no matter how extensive, is insufficient to prove anything; but it has served to dispel my intuitive scepticism that such things *can* go on in our health services. It always helps to have seen with one's own eyes.

ANOTHER DETERMINING FACTOR in writing the book was a conversation held with a National Health Service (NHS) chief executive who, quite matter-of-factly and with refreshing though depressing honesty, commented that there was little point talking to chief executives about health care. This was because their role was political and financial.

It seems to me that, in the light of the care described in this book and which chief executives have overseen, such a comment is extremely telling. It is true that central government, of any hue, is working toward more business-like, market-driven health services. But even on such a model of health care, this is a bit like the founders of Rolls Royce, Charles Rolls and Henry Royce, having no interest in cars. In fact, though very different, one the businessman, the other the engineering wizard, they were both obsessed with motor vehicles.[2] Just as one would have expected.

I am sure that NHS chief executives act in good faith and work extremely hard. But I believe that the political and financial dictates, to which they have become enslaved, are leading us away from the sort of health care system we want; that is, one based on compassion, humanity, transparency and trust.

Amongst other things, the chief executive's comment was a reminder that writing about health care is a sensitive matter; politics are never far behind. I would underline that this book is about poor health care only. The NHS features prominently only because that is where the majority of health care is located in the United Kingdom. But the private sector, too, is afflicted with similar faults, for example, in nursing homes. Thus, the book is not politically or ideologically motivated and is not about whether health care should be public or private or run on free market principles. It is not aiming to supply political grist for anybody's mill, whatever its colour, blue, red or yellow – or its leaning, left, right or centre. New Labour happened to be in power for 13 of the last 14 years and so features prominently; I am in no doubt that an alternative Conservative

2   Marr, A. (2009) *The making of modern Britain: From Queen Victoria to V.E. Day.* London: Pan, pp.91–2.

government during this period would have behaved similarly and presided over the same strain of neglectful care.

In other words, and for the avoidance of all doubt, there is no party political axe being swung here. My relatives and friends have suffered under governments of precisely different hues; in so far as government policy is implicated in neglectful health care, it is a curse on all their houses.

THE THIRD MAIN reason for writing is the reaction of a conscientious and dedicated senior health care professional. I had asked why on earth professionals did not more actively combat the serious erosion of inpatient services for older people, particularly the standards of diagnosis, active treatment, rehabilitation and basic care, some of which undoubtedly led not just to poor but also to neglectful care, The answer was simple and threefold.

Staff were thoroughly demoralised. They would not know where to begin, such was the dead weight of targets, paperwork and under-staffing. And the feeling was that even those managers with a clinical background, and who therefore should have known better, were too often out of their depth. They had compromised, or been forced to compromise, their professional principle; this had fallen victim to a culture of stress, anxiety, politically-based pressures and obedience to clinically ill-informed and sometimes harmful demands made by senior management; an obedience bordering on unthinking servility.

THE HEALTH SERVICE may feature prominently in this book, but it is not about the health service as a whole. I am highlighting but one current, albeit a dark one. To have written a book about all the good things would have been a much greater enterprise. Therefore, it follows that the book is not an attack on the health service. It is a denunciation of poor and neglectful health care and of those responsible for it.

Most of all, therefore, nothing in this book is intended to deny the existence of, or to belittle in any way, the immense amount of good practice that exists in our health services. Nor does it aim to undermine all those staff who dedicatedly and conscientiously provide good care and treatment, seeking at all costs to uphold the dignity of their patients. They do so against all the odds that sometimes are stacked so heavily against them.

I am certain that some readers will approach this book with scepticism. I would hope two things only; that they consider the evidence before coming to judgement and that they do not learn the hard way through their own experience or that of their relatives.

1

Introduction

A decade or so ago we uncovered a quiet outrage, of modern hospitals delivering archaic care, of professional care workers acting in an uncaring and often inhuman way, of sophisticated health services not even delivering on the basics of toileting, mealtimes and communication. Our Dignity on the Ward campaign attracted widespread public support then, for the very significant reason that it rang true to people's experiences. And it led to some change for the better, in the shape of the welcome and well-constructed National Service Framework for Older People in 2001. So now, after ten years of initiatives, reorganisations, plans, targets and frameworks, where do we stand? As the debate turns to how we can exploit the array of modern technologies and opportunities in front of us polypills, remote sensors, shared electronic records and many other such innovations surely we have moved beyond the basics, the mere minimum entitlement in any decent society? Too often the answer is no. (Help the Aged, 2007)[1]

The unwitting reader may wonder what on earth Help the Aged was getting at. Perhaps it was a case of a voluntary organisation getting a little overheated and generating publicity for itself into the bargain? It certainly struck a discordant note against the symphony of boast and bombast orchestrated by both central government and local National Health Service (NHS) bodies. Not only was the NHS supposedly being much revised and doing better than ever before, but in that same year of 2007, the icing on the cake was being spread in the form of a policy of 'world class commissioning' of health services.

A thumbnail sketch may help to explain. For this, it is necessary to return to the start of the decade to which Help the Aged was referring, to 1997. That year marked both an incoming New Labour government that promised to invest in, rescue and modernise the NHS – and also the beginning of what came to be known as the Dignity on the Ward campaign.

---

1   Levenson, R. (2007) *The challenge of dignity in care: Upholding the rights of the individual.* London: Help the Aged, p.4.

In that year, *The Observer* newspaper ran a series of articles about the neglect of older people in hospitals, kick-started by the journalist Martin Bright, outraged at the treatment given to his grandmother.[2] Help the Aged campaigned. Considerable publicity was generated. Politicians were moved, a report was commissioned and a national policy published.[3] And that should have been the end of the story. A fundamental defect in our health care was to be removed in what, after all, is an advanced, relatively wealthy and civilised country. But somehow this didn't happen.

In 2000, the government launched *The NHS Plan*, setting out overarching health care policy. It spoke of supporting and modernising the health service, of patient dignity and of older people. It attracted widespread support; the preface boasts 25 signatures of endorsement from the great and the good in the world of health care.[4]

The beginning of the new millennium saw another intervention in the Press. But this time it was not by a journalist. Martin Bright's lament of 1997 might have reached the ears of the Health Secretary, Frank Dobson, but perhaps not the Prime Minister. This time round the criticism was from a more politically influential source, Lord Robert Winston, a leading fertility expert. Crucially, not only was he an active New Labour supporter but he had also recently been made a peer by the then Prime Minister, Tony Blair. He now went public, accusing the government of overseeing deeply unsatisfactory medical care and of deceiving the voters.

His attack was born not just from professional frustration but from the personal, too. He bemoaned the fate of his diabetic 87-year-old mother admitted to hospital a few weeks before: a 13-hour wait in casualty, admission to a mixed-sex ward, medication not given on time, missed meals, found lying on the floor by the morning staff, contracting an infection and developing an ulcer on her leg. He was quoted as saying there was nothing unusual in this; it was 'normal. The terrifying thing is that we accept it.'[5]

Panic in government reportedly followed. So much so, that Tony Blair announced a few days later, on the David Frost television programme, that health spending would increase significantly.[6] Which it did. But it

---

2   Durham, M. and Bright, M. (1997) 'Join our campaign for the old.' *The Observer*, 5 October. Also: Bright, M. (1997) 'Charity calls for abuse inquiry.' *The Observer*, 26 October.

3   DH (Department of Health) (2001) *National Service Framework for Older People*. London: DH.

4   Secretary of State for Health (2000) *The NHS Plan: A plan for investment, a plan for reform*. Cm 4818-I. London: The Stationery Office, p.6.

5   Riddell, M. (2000) 'The *New Statesman* interview – Robert Winston.' *New Statesman*, 17 January.

6   Marr, A. (2009) *A history of modern Britain*. London: Pan, p.538.

was not spent on those patients such as Lord Winston's mother; she, with respect and figuratively, is still lying on the floor 11 years later.

In 2001, the *National Service Framework for Older People* followed. It had already been in the pipeline and heralded a ten-year plan to ensure that older people were not sidelined, discriminated against and ill treated.[7] The government perhaps expected the *Framework* to have an instant effect and it was in no mood to hear otherwise. Already, in 2002, when allegations were made about the neglectful treatment of an elderly woman, Rose Addis, at the Whittington Hospital in London, the Prime Minister became involved in a furious rebuttal that such a thing could happen.[8]

In fact whether or not she really had been treated badly – and she may not have been – was, in the wider political sense, beside the point and absurd; there was plenty of evidence that lots of other people clearly *were* suffering similar treatment. Assuming charitably that the government's denials were made in good faith, they reveal just how out of touch it was and how determined to shut out the light. Yet such ignorance is entirely believable. A few years later, Julie Bailey, founder of the patients' and relatives' organisation, Cure the NHS, tried to engage a junior health minister, Ben Bradshaw, about the death of her mother at Stafford Hospital. She concluded that he had no grasp of either the hospital or the NHS generally.[9] Her reaction is unsurprising and, in light of what subsequently emerged, apparently entirely justified.

Peter Mandelson, often regarded as an important architect of New Labour, has admitted that, when in government, his party put more emphasis on managing the story about a policy rather than the policy itself. Which is not the way government should work.[10] Perhaps the health service suffered as much as any from this syndrome, fuelled by a combination of nescience, disavowal and political funk.

Indeed by 2006 if not before, the realisation was dawning on others, if not the government, that the goods were not being delivered. In that year, the Healthcare Commission published a report about infection, neglectful care and avoidable death at Stoke Mandeville Hospital.[11]

7   DH (Department of Health) (2001) *National Service Framework for Older People.* London: DH.

8   'Blair rejects patient neglect claim.' BBC News, 23 January 2002. Accessed on 1 October 2010 at: http://news.bbc.co.uk/1/hi/uk_politics/1778546.stm.

9   '"Huge concerns" exist still at Stafford Hospital, inquiry told.' *Birmingham Post,* 24 November 2010.

10   Rawnsley, A. (2010) *The end of the party: The rise and fall of New Labour.* London: Penguin Books, p.9.

11   Healthcare Commission (2006) *Investigation into outbreaks of* Clostridium difficile *at Stoke Mandeville Hospital, Buckinghamshire Hospitals NHS Trust, July 2006.* London: Healthcare Commission.

The following year, worse was reported at Maidstone and Tunbridge Wells NHS Trust, again involving infection, death and extremely poor standards of care.[12]

By now Age Concern England had raised again the spectre of hospital patients being starved, in *Hungry to be heard*.[13] Four years later, in 2010, the same organisation, now in the merged form of Age UK, would be driven to publish *Still hungry to be heard*.[14]

In 2006, too, the journalist Martin Bright, who had previously taken up the cause of his grandmother and of dignity, wrote again. Back in the late 1990s he did not blame the newly elected government for the treatment of older people in hospital; eight years on he did. He argued that it would be judged by the public in terms of whether people's grandmothers were treated with decency and respect in hospital. Which they still weren't.[15]

ROMFORD IN ESSEX. It was here that a specific illustration of the gap between the rhetoric and the experience of some patients stands out. An example only, it nonetheless serves as a parable. In 2006, a new hospital was opened, the Queen's Hospital, now run by Barking, Havering and Redbridge University Hospitals NHS Trust. It cost £261 million to build and was described by the developers as cleverly combining clinical values with aesthetic qualities. In line with current thinking, which tends to view patients as consumers in a health care market place, it was also said to have 'an appearance and an atmosphere…more akin to a hotel than a hospital'. It was to be 'welcoming to patients and visitors alike'. A feature emphasised was also 'quick access to treatment'.[16] In other words, such a hospital was meant to be part of modernised, efficient and dignified health care; seemingly as important was that it looked 'nice'.

In 2009, a coroner passed a verdict of death by natural causes contributed to by neglect at – the Queen's Hospital. The deceased was an 86-year-old man, Mr Walter Gibson, veteran of the Normandy campaign

---

12 Healthcare Commission (2007) *Investigation into outbreaks of* Clostridium difficile *at Maidstone and Tunbridge Wells NHS Trust, October 2007*. London: Healthcare Commission.

13 Age Concern England (2006) *Hungry to be heard: The scandal of malnourished older people in hospital*. London: Age Concern England.

14 Age UK (2010) *Still hungry to be heard: The scandal of people in later life becoming malnourished in hospital*. London: Age UK.

15 Bright, M. (2006) 'The public will judge this government not by how bold it was in challenging left-liberal shibboleths, but whether its grandmothers were treated with respect in hospital.' *New Statesman*, 3 April.

16 Catalyst Lendlease (2010) *Queen's Hospital, Romford, Essex, United Kingdom*. Accessed on 2 September 2010 at: www.catalystlendlease.com/projects/queens-hospital.pdf.

in the Second World War. In early 2008, he died a painful death at the hospital from infected bedsores. These had been caused by his being left on two separate occasions on a hospital trolley for 19 hours, after admission with a chest infection. The hospital, merely three years old, had insufficient beds.

The result of his being on the trolley the second time was to exacerbate the sores that had developed on the first occasion. One of the sores was classed as grade four, sufficiently deep to expose tendon and bone. The wounds were dressed but a further 12 hours elapsed before he was admitted to a ward where a pressure-relief mattress was finally made available. Too late. Mr Gibson died some days afterwards, of septicaemia resulting from open sores. The coroner stated:

> It is quite clear from the evidence I've heard that the length of time Mr Gibson waited at A&E [accident and emergency] both the first and second time – the second time added insult to injury to a man already completely dependent – made a significant contribution to his death... He was at very, very high risk of pressure sores and he should have been provided with appropriate protection against worsening of the pressure sores.

The coroner asked the hospital to increase training for nurses, to improve risk assessment of patients likely to develop pressure sores and to provide more pressure-relieving mattresses.[17]

The moral being how, in all the excitement of the fair – the modernising claims, the visions and the new buildings developed at huge cost by the shiny men and women of the new health service – the patient gets trampled underfoot. And not just any patient. Not, typically, the younger adult patient with a single, discrete condition coming in for elective, predictable treatment, much as a guest books into a hotel. But rather the unglamorous, failing older patient with all sorts of things wrong, promising to take up hospital bed space and to be demanding of staff time and resources. The sort of patient who, as this book shows, hospitals give a good impression of not wanting.

The example is also significant for another reason. In 2006, the NHS Trust running the hospital had announced the cutting of 650 staff and 190 beds in order to tackle its large debt – hospitals built under the private finance initiative (PFI) saddle the relevant NHS trust with large annual debt repayments. But, and in any case, central government has repeatedly defended the closure of tens of thousands of hospital beds

---

17 Schlesinger, F. (2009) 'Coroner's fury as great-grandfather, 86, dies after being dumped on A&E trolley for 19 hours TWICE.' *Daily Mail*, 22 May.

over the last decade. The chief executive, toeing this line, announced that such reductions were 'clinically sustainable'.[18]

Clearly not for Mr Gibson. Nor, in the view of her daughter (a nurse herself), for 81-year-old Mrs Irene Bueggeln. Admitted to the hospital with a fractured hip in 2008, she died after contracting the infection *Clostridium difficile*, and pneumonia. Her daughter pointed to her mother being left for hours sitting in the cold and not being given sufficient nutrition and hydration – and to an insufficient number of nurses.[19]

AND SO ON to 2011, when a public inquiry is due to report on care at Stafford Hospital. In terms of sustained inhumane care and probable associated mortality, what happened there exceeds anything that has taken place – or at least been reported – in the last 14 years. This is known in advance of the public inquiry's conclusions because four other reports have preceded it, including the 850-page account of an independent inquiry.[20]

The Mid Staffordshire scandal is the emblematic nail in the coffin for the ambitions of the ten-year plan of the *National Service Framework for Older People*; it exposed care practices worse than anything the *Framework* had originally in mind.

There are those who will view Stafford Hospital as they might the Titanic: a one-off, colossal and vainglorious aberration. This would be a serious mistake. There are many other substantial mishaps, wrecks and even disasters involving poor and neglectful care for the elderly, even if lesser in scale or not in the public eye. In fact, without a particularly determined group of relatives, Cure the NHS, even Stafford would not have garnered the notoriety which it has – and the disturbing accounts of care provided at the hospital would not have been salvaged and made public.

Stafford Hospital was foreseeable; an all but inevitable progression flowing from a set of conditions, brought about – or at least allowed to develop – by central government. Take Stafford away, suppose it had never happened; this would not change the gravity of the problem within the health service.

---

18 '£24 million debt NHS trust cuts 650 jobs: up to 650 jobs are to be cut and 190 beds closed by an NHS trust that is trying to tackle debts.' BBC News, 28 April 2006. Accessed on 20 July 2010 at: http://news.bbc.co.uk/1/hi/england/london/4954818.stm.

19 'Pensioner death leads to growing concern from MP about care at Queen's.' BBC London, 23 April 2008. Accessed on 20 October 2010 at: www.bbc.co.uk/london/content/articles/2008/04/23/barking_hospital_feature.shtml.

20 Francis, R. (Chair) (2010) *Independent Inquiry into care provided by Mid Staffordshire NHS Foundation Trust January 2005–March 2009*. London: The Stationery Office.

In February 2011, there came a prelude to the Public Inquiry. This was a report to Parliament, called *Care and compassion*, produced by the Health Service Ombudsman, Ann Abraham.[21] It draws on ten complaints from the many hundreds her office receives annually about elderly care and is unequivocal about the failure of the NHS to provide dignity, compassion and basic care.

The report acknowledges the question of extra resources in hospitals but stresses the dismissive attitude and indifference of staff. It then describes neglect. We read of tongues like dried leather, nutrition and hydration ignored, patients squealing with unmanaged pain, pressure sores thriving, call bells out of reach, lack of cleanliness and comfort, multiple unrecorded falls, bathing or showering unavailable, weeping wounds not dressed and an absence of patient monitoring.

On its publication, the media went to town – some for a day, some for several – as is their wont. Equally swift and predictable was the government's downplaying of the report's implications. The NHS Choices website noted that it was not scientific, not a reliable indicator about NHS care – and was selective in highlighting the most serious cases in such 'fine detail'. It quoted the NHS Confederation to the effect that such care was not typical.[22] We should note, in fact, that the Ombudsman included by no means the most serious type of case; whilst the evidence suggests that such care *is* all too typical. It is a characteristic of the NHS. We observe further, given that government proclaims the importance of the patient voice, that the website quoted the NHS Confederation representing NHS organisations – but not, for example, the Patients' Association.

The Care Services Minister, Paul Burstow, did immediately announce a programme of 'spot' inspections of hospitals. But, in effect, he proposes a straw in the wind, conceding that he could not 'flip a switch to turn compassion back on'.[23] Precisely. First, you cannot, through a form of 'policing', inculcate staff with compassion and humanity; such a notion is absurd.[24] Second, inspectors will not easily detect poor care and neglect and, in any case, hospitals are adept at outwitting regulators.

21 Parliamentary and Health Service Ombudsman (2011) *Care and compassion? Report of the Health Service Ombudsman on ten investigations into NHS care of older people.* HC 778. London: The Stationery Office, p.5.

22 NHS Choices. 'NHS failures in elderly care "not typical".' Accessed on 15 February 2011 at: www.nhs.uk/news/2011/02February/Pages/health-service-ombudsman-report-on-care-of-the-elderly.aspx, accessed on 15 February 2011.

23 Johnston, L. (2011) '"Matron's army" to tackle elderly abuse in our hospitals.' *Sunday Express,* 20 February.

24 Tallis, R. (2011) 'More training won't fill a hole in humanity.' *The Times,* 17 February.

Third, it will not work, because the Minister said nothing about tackling government policies, priorities, bed numbers, professional staff (their numbers, competency, training and attitude) and the care of older people; all of which are the crux of the matter.

To understand the government's response to the Ombudsman, we must turn to the seat of power occupied by the chief executive of the whole NHS, Sir David Nicholson. On 15 February 2011, the day of the Ombudsman's report, he sent a letter to NHS trust chairmen. Exhibiting neither urgency nor explicit condemnation, it mentions 'important issues' and urges chairmen to read the report (as a 'learning tool'). It also does refer to the report as a 'reality check' but then, extraordinarily, suggests the answer may lie in consulting an `on-line Patient Experience Network'. The complacency and detachment evident in this letter are arguably indicative of how the elderly, and reports about their neglect, are regarded as a fly in the official ointment, to which lip service must be paid. And its tone gives NHS trust chairmen and chief executives their cue; they will bat few eyelids.

The report, *Care and compassion*, and the reaction it provoked within a period of a few days, form a portrait, effectively a miniature of the broad panorama described in this book. To the story emerging from this wider picture – of repeated patterns of neglect, scandal, indifference and half-hearted promises over a 14-year period – there is, currently, no happy ending in prospect.

IN SHORT, SOMETHING has gone badly wrong. For this reason, the following chapters tease out exactly what. A considerable amount of detail and evidence, though by no means all, is included. Why so much? Because, as a journalist put it, having interviewed Sir Robert Winston 11 years ago:

> I had expected the sort of outspokenness befitting a prophet of gene science and a messiah for the new millennium. Instead I got the reflections of one more disillusioned consultant; one more middle-aged man whose elderly mother was found huddled on the floor of an overcrowded ward. As Winston says, any number of people might offer a similar testimony. But nobody listens to them.[25]

No one listens.

---

25   Riddell, M. (2000) 'The *New Statesman* interview – Robert Winston.' *New Statesman*, 17 January.

2

Health Services:
Public and Private

> At the heart of this Serious Case Review are five people of
> advanced years who died while living in residential care. All those
> involved in this Review wish to express their regret that their
> end of life was marked by unnecessary suffering and avoidable
> physical neglect. We extend our sincere condolences to the
> families who have lost their relatives. (Parkside House Nursing
> Home: Serious Case Review, June 2010)[1]

Poor and neglectful care, particularly, but not only, of older people is to
be found throughout the health services; it is by no means the preserve
of the National Health Service (NHS).

It is true that health services, acute and non-acute, are largely centred
in the NHS. However, non-acute health care in the form of nursing care,
together with palliative care, is provided also within independent nursing
homes. There are in addition private hospitals, but these are responsible
for a relatively small proportion of health care and do not tend to provide
treatment for a particular class of potentially vulnerable patient – older
people with acute needs, underpinned by other complex and chronic
conditions.

Nevertheless, starting with Hinchingbrooke Hospital in 2011,
it appears that the private sector is likely in the future to take over
completely the running of some NHS hospitals; this then will be a true
blend of State and independent sectors. Such a hospital will be used by
health service patients, whose treatment and care will be wholly in the
hands of a private health care company.[2]

This book concentrates on the health service as we know it, the NHS,
for three main reasons. First, overall, the NHS provides by far the majority
of health care in this country – notwithstanding the flow of 'continuing

---

1   Sloper, G. and Seaton, M. (2010) *Serious case review: Parkside House, 49–53 St Matthew's Parade,
    Northampton NN2 7HE: Executive summary*. Northampton: Northamptonshire County Council,
    p.2.
2   Lister, S. (2010) 'Debt-ridden Hinchingbrooke Hospital to be run by a private company.' *The
    Times*, 18 February.

health care' beds away from hospitals and into nursing homes over the last 20 years. That is, beds for patients with serious, chronic, continuing health care problems who are judged sufficiently medically stable to be discharged from an acute hospital bed.

Second, the extent of poor and neglectful care in the NHS has not been acknowledged or believed by many people. It is high time this was set out in some detail. In contrast, it has long been recognised that, whilst some independent nursing homes are very good, there are significant problems in others.

Third, because the NHS is a directly State-run service, the significance of systemic failure within it takes on added political, legal and moral significance.

THUS, TO THE extent that the NHS provides poor care, this is by definition an indictment of a State-run service. But, equally, those with a hankering for the private sector will find similar afflictions in care homes.

Sometimes the argument runs that the private sector operates better or more efficiently than the State and that therefore the latter should commission services from the former. In addition is the notion that, in the case of people paying for themselves privately, the way in which consumer markets operate will see to it that good quality services are provided. Yet the tale of nursing homes does not bear out this thesis. They count amongst their residents both those paid for by the NHS or local councils and those paying purely privately. But poor care and lethal pressure sores, for example, seem not to discriminate by funding source.

So, there is no reason to suppose that, if or when the private sector starts to take over the running of NHS hospitals to any extent, the failings outlined in this book will, as a matter of course, wither away and be a distant bad memory.

In other words, poor standards of basic health care constitute a blight in our society, *wherever* that care is located. And this is the point. It is beyond the scope of this book to analyse this in so far as it manifests itself in the independent sector and especially in care homes. But another book could be written on it.

Some examples from the independent sector are included toward the end of this book, particularly in Chapter 21, which deals with the criminal offences of ill treatment and wilful neglect. In addition, the following examples give a fleeting glance across the last decade or so.

IN 2001, THE journalist Amelia Hill wrote an article for *The Observer* newspaper. It was entitled 'Tide of cruelty sweeps through our care homes'. It talked of 10 per cent of care homes being good. At the other end of the spectrum, it quoted the organisation, Action on Elder Abuse, which stated that there was another 10 per cent of care homes in which you would not want to keep a dead dog. The article focused on one in particular, described as a residential home (which would not normally provide health care), although the resident who died clearly needed it.

Oathurst House Care Home in Oxfordshire was an establishment with which, in 1998, the son of Mr Alec Taylor had been very pleased; he had felt lucky his father was there. It had roses round the door. What he had not realised was that workers at the home would routinely dispel the smell of urine with air freshener and scrape faeces off curtains – when informed that visitors were coming.

Mr Taylor's son also didn't know that his 89-year-old father was 'locked away' in a room upstairs. There, he suffered from pressure sores which had gone right down to the bone. He was unable to move for pain and too confused to call or cry for help. For four months, he was attended only by the owner of the home who would try to manage the sores by hacking with office scissors at the rotten flesh. For hygiene, he wore gloves with which he had just scooped up faeces from the sheets. The staff referred to the 'body in the attic'. Finally, a new manager blew the whistle and informed the local authority. Mr Taylor was taken to hospital where he died a few days later of pneumonia.

The home owner was convicted in 1999 of the criminal offences of ill treatment or wilful neglect. His wife, who also worked at the home, didn't think he had done anything wrong.[3]

At the time this article was written, the government had just introduced a new piece of legislation, the Care Standards Act 2000, and a new inspectorate, precisely to put an end to such goings on. The government put much store in the use of the independent sector, particularly because of the policy, largely unarticulated, of running down NHS hospital beds for many older patients with ongoing health needs.

Flip forward more than a decade, and one might have expected that such stories of literally rotting bodies and gross neglect would have dried up. But if no news is good news, then the picture is not a happy one. And this, it should be emphasised, is on the basis of a few accounts, taken almost at random, a mere skimming of the surface.

In May 2010, a coroner found that Mr Alan Simper, an 84-year-old man, had died because of 'inexcusable failures' and 'for want of care

---

3   Hill, A. (2001) 'Tide of cruelty sweeps through our care homes.' *The Observer*, 18 February.

by those charged with it'. He suffered from Parkinson's disease and dementia, and was also blind and deaf.

This occurred in 2009 at the Swiss Cottage Care Home in Bedfordshire, run by Southern Cross, the largest provider of care homes (730 homes and 37,000 beds) in the United Kingdom. Mr Simper had three bedsores when he had entered the home. These quickly turned into 18 festering wounds covered only with dirty and inadequate dressings. He deteriorated rapidly, was admitted to hospital a month later and died a few days later from infected multiple pressure sores. On readmission he had been in an unkempt state and covered in old faeces. Within a day of his going into the care home, his family reported having found him naked on all fours wearing a nappy, covered in bruises and smeared with congealed blood.[4]

ARE THESE TWO examples but blips, ten years apart? The following are a few examples, picked out from that decade, which suggest not.

In 2009, Mrs Betty Delaney died in hospital, having spent the previous few weeks with agonising bedsores at Oakland Care Home near Rochdale. The condition she eventually died from was unrelated. Whenever the family had visited her, she was crying; the staff at the home had said this was due to her mental deterioration and did not mention the pressure sores. Two of the four sores were stage four, that is, the most serious.

Southern Cross, the company that ran the home, admitted liability when faced with legal action. In particular not only had the home failed to provide a pressure mattress, to turn Mrs Delaney, to check regularly and to conduct a risk assessment – it had not even identified the problem. The north regional director of Southern Cross employed the apparently obligatory under-statement, conceding that the care was not up to the company's usual high standard.[5]

At an inquest in 2009, a coroner criticised the care provided for 54-year-old Mrs Gillian Moore at Forest Manor Care Home in Nottinghamshire. She suffered from Alzheimer's disease. When she died, she had six sores on her legs, mouth ulcers, rotten teeth and filthy matted hair. Her son was advised not to view the body. The coroner concluded that she had been deprived of her dignity before she died. The nursing care was poor, she was given penicillin to which she was allergic and

---

4 'Coroner slams care home after pensioner died of "inexcusable failures" by staff.' *Daily Mail*, 25 May 2010.

5 Devine, P. (2010) 'Care home under fire over pensioner's agony.' *Manchester Evening News*, 11 August.

her case notes had not been transferred with her. The coroner had, the previous year, expressed concerns about the home in relation to the death of another resident.[6]

The neglect visited upon one resident may well be visited on others. Also in 2009, five residents at Parkside House Nursing Home in Northampton died between 22 July and 6 August. Severe pressure sores and lack of food and drink were part of the neglectful care identified. One woman had been admitted to hospital with severe, necrotic grade four ulcers; she was unresponsive, dehydrated and, in the view of the staff, her overall condition was consistent with severe neglect. She died on 22 July. Another resident had similar severe pressure sores but remained at the home and died also on the same day.[7]

Moving backward in time, Mrs Gwendoline Hoar was 91 years old, suffered from dementia and lived at River Court Nursing Home in Watford. In 2007, she died there. The coroner concluded that the care provided for her was 'seriously disturbing'.

Four months after she had gone to live there, concerns had been raised and BUPA asked a skin expert to visit. She found Mrs Hoar frail, undernourished, dehydrated and not being turned in order to relieve pressure on the skin. She found many pressure sores. Some were dressed, some not and so open to infection. A specialist mattress had not been installed properly and provided no benefit. A month later, two district nurses visited and were shocked. They could not even list the sores because there were too many. Some were grade four which had split the skin and underlying tissue down to the bone. Two general practitioners (GPs) were persuaded not to admit her to hospital but to have her treated at the home. The doctors subsequently refused to cooperate with the coroner.

The sores were so painful that they prevented Mrs Hoar moving, this immobility led to pneumonia. However, when asked to provide pain relief, the home resisted installing the necessary equipment until two days before she died.

The company sacked five nursing staff who then faced disciplinary proceedings by the Nursing and Midwifery Council (NMC). The company added insult to injury; it apologised for the fact that the care

---

6   Schofield, B. (2009) 'Coroner hits out at nursing home where Liverpool gran received appalling care.' *Liverpool Echo*, 12 October.

7   Sloper, G. and Seaton, M. (2010) *Serious case review: Parkside House, 49–53 St Matthew's Parade, Northampton NN2 7HE: Executive summary.* Northampton: Northamptonshire County Council, p.4.

was not of the customary 'high standard'. It should perhaps be noted that Mrs Hoar was paying for the 'care' from her own savings.[8]

Mr Charles Hounslow – 85 years old, war veteran and former RAF pilot – was, according to a coroner at the 2007 inquest, treated 'like a parcel' in Miles Court Nursing Home in Brighton. The coroner labelled the care he received as 'lamentable' and said that she feared many other elderly people were being treated in the same way. Mr Hounslow had suffered from vascular dementia and was left in agony for 37 hours, because staff at the home had not noticed that he had a broken hip. He was finally admitted to hospital where he died. The coroner referred to a catalogue of incidents that constituted gross mismanagement. A formal verdict of neglect could not be brought because the injury was not directly the cause of death.[9]

Accidental death, contributed to by neglect including six separate counts of gross failure: this was the verdict of a 2007 inquest into the death of Mrs Brigid O'Callaghan. She had been a resident in 2005 at Amberley Court Nursing Home in Birmingham, run by BUPA. Overnight, she had slipped down in her wheelchair; her neck became caught in the 'posture belt' and she was asphyxiated. She had not been checked since 10.45pm the previous evening. A nurse admitted to this failure, to not changing her incontinence pad and to fabricating the notes so as to suggest that checks had been carried out. The failings were more than individual. None of the staff giving evidence had been trained in the correct use of the belt. There was no care plan. Communication between staff was poor. And staff were poorly supervised and trained.[10]

In 2004, an inquest was held into the deaths of three people – Mrs Edith Glover, Mrs Josie Little and Mr Robert Haines – who had been resident at Roselawns Nursing Home in Reading in 2003. The coroner did not bring in a verdict of neglect, because notwithstanding conditions in the home, they were not the cause of death. In the case of Mrs Little, however, neglect was an exacerbating factor.

A catalogue of faults at the home had previously been identified by the National Care Standards Commission, the regulatory body at the time for care homes. These included out-of-date medication being administered, lack of cleanliness, a smell of urine, unchanged and soaked bandages, call bells not being answered, poor bed linen, inappropriate care, poor record keeping, lack of staff training, no checks made on staff, food kept unhygienically, etc.

---

8   Boniface, S. (2009) 'Gran, 91, left to die in agony in BUPA care home.' *Daily Mirror*, 10 May.
9   'Coroner faults veteran's care at nursing home.' *Daily Telegraph*, 15 December 2007.
10   'Asphyxiated pensioner was left in wheelchair overnight.' *Yorkshire Post*, 11 January 2008.

The Commission had served three statutory notices in 2003 demanding improvement, although none of the residents or their families were aware of this. During this period, the local council had continued to place residents in the home.[11]

Relatives frequently compare the care of their loved ones in hospital or nursing homes with that given to animals. Is this simply loose and careless talk or is there substance to it? 'If a dog was found in the state my father was found in it would have been all over the papers. I felt such disbelief and disgust that the carers didn't care.'[12] So opined the daughter of Mr Payne; in his case, it seemed more than just emotional excess. Two nurses were removed from their professional register in 2006 by the NMC. The reason was their seriously neglectful care of Mr Payne, who died in 2000. He suffered from dementia and had been living in Southover nursing home, Maidenhead. His daughter had often found him wearing other people's clothes including a lady's cardigan; sometimes he had bare feet or was wearing a cardigan without a shirt. He was often wet with urine, and when his pads were changed he was not washed or given a change of clothes.

By April of 2000, he had a sore bottom; he then developed a severe infection. Finding him in a pool of urine, his daughter called the GP; he was then admitted to hospital. He was found to have a massive pressure sore at the base of his spine – it was the size of two fists and through to the bone. His medical notes referred to gas gangrene, septicaemia, cellulitis, dehydration and malnutrition.[13]

IN SEPTEMBER 2010, Jo Williams, chair of the Care Quality Commission, noted that, in terms of independent sector providers of care, the Commission was sometimes dealing in the 'very basics of life', which some providers were failing to supply.[14] A worrying concession, and not one of which the Commission should have been particularly proud; not least because all those failing but still operational care homes were, by definition, registered with the Commission as fit providers.

11 White, H. (2008) 'Tilehurst pensioner died days after leaving nursing home with dirty bedpans and out-of-date medication.' *Newbury Today*, 24 April.

12 McFeran, A. (2006) '"My father looked like he'd just been in the trenches": It's taken seven years for Marilyn Payne to win justice for her father against the care home nurses who neglected him.' *The Sunday Times*, 10 December.

13 McFeran, A. (2006) '"My father looked like he'd just been in the trenches": It's taken seven years for Marilyn Payne to win justice for her father against the care home nurses who neglected him.' *The Sunday Times*, 10 December.

14 Rose, D. (2010) 'Watchdog closes care homes over fears for "the very basics of life".' *The Times*, 29 September.

3

Systemic Nature of Neglect and Abuse within Health Care

Several recent HCC [Healthcare Commission] investigations have shown in detail how senior managers and Boards have failed in their most basic duties as regards patient safety, with disastrous consequences. In each of these cases, patient safety was found to have been crowded out by other priorities... The DH [Department of Health] has been keen to present these as highly exceptional cases of rogue managers and dysfunctional Boards. However, there is evidence of widespread shortcomings in the way that Boards approach patient safety. (House of Commons Health Committee, 2009)[1]

On the 2nd December 2010, the Patients' Association released a report, *Listen to patients, speak up for change.* It simply recorded the accounts of care experienced by 17 inpatients of various hospitals and narrated by relatives or the patients themselves. These were picked from the very many furnished to the Association. The hospitals, too, were a cross section; there is no reason to suppose that they were any different to all those not mentioned. This is a report which, as well as any other single item of evidence, at least suggests – though alone far from establishes – a systemic problem within the health service.

It refers, for instance, to Mrs Peggy May Wood at the Southend University Hospital and the ward stinking of faeces, patients not being helped to eat and drink, and dried food on her clothes. It goes on to note the absence of the recording of turning needed to manage pressure sores, the development in hospital of just such a (serious and ultimately fatal) sore, delay in providing a pressure mattress, lying soiled in faeces and not being changed by nurses – and so on. The 'head of communications and

---

1 House of Commons Health Committee (2009) *Patient safety: Sixth report of Session 2008–09.* HC 151-I. London: The Stationery Office, pp.86–7.

marketing' of the Southend University Hospital NHS Foundation Trust apologised for any distress caused.[2]

And to Mrs Elsie Poague, 99 years old, who was alert and capable when admitted with a fractured femur to St. Helier's Hospital in Carshalton, Surrey. We read of a lack of compassion in the nurses, the call bell constantly being placed beyond her reach even though she was immobile, with drinks also left out of range. Her fingernails grew long and filthy. The chief executive of the Epsom and St. Helier University Hospitals NHS Trust expressed regret for the unhappiness felt by Mrs Poague's niece about her aunt's care, and offered to meet with her.[3]

To Mrs Brigid Wainwright, a younger patient in her sixties at Derriford Hospital, who observed other patients on the ward. She recounts how one frail, confused, bewildered and frightened woman next to her would flop against the bed side rails, calling for help, thinking she was on her farm with her arm trapped in a gate. The nurses didn't come and didn't answer the call bell. Mrs Wainwright would help the woman herself. Special drinks and snacks left in the woman's locker by her daughter were forgotten about or ignored by staff. Another elderly woman was left, in acute embarrassment, for a long period, having soiled herself. And a third patient, whose waste bag needed changing; no nurse came and it burst. The responsible Plymouth Hospitals NHS Trust was sorry that Mrs Wainwright did not raise these issues at the time and suggested she do so formally now.[4]

The report details also the experience of Mr David Perkins, admitted for a bladder and prostate operation to Southend Hospital in 2009. On one occasion, his pyjama bottoms were on so tight that the surgical bag had ruptured; his wife found him lying in urine and faeces. On another occasion, she found him falling out of his chair and calling for help. He was given clinically-prohibited food and would suffer cuts when he was shaved. Staff did not always wear gloves. He was allowed to fall out of a hoist twice. A manager told his wife to stop complaining, otherwise the nurses and he wouldn't want the patient on their ward. He was moved from ward to ward at 3am. The family had to buy several pillows when he needed propping up in hospital; the ward didn't have any. Two days

2 Patients' Association (2010) *Listen to patients, speak up for change.* London: Patients' Association, pp.11–18, 99.

3 Patients' Association (2010) *Listen to patients, speak up for change.* London: Patients' Association, pp.26–28, 99.

4 Patients' Association (2010) *Listen to patients, speak up for change.* London: Patients' Association, pp.29–31, 99.

before he died, he was covered in dried vomit, which must have been there for some time.[5]

And, as a last example, at Ipswich Hospital, 96-year-old Mrs Muriel Browning died. But not before she had been allowed to fall, after a hip operation, because of the delay in assessing the need for side rails. She was not helped with food and drink, which was left out of her reach; she suffered from thirst. Then, increasingly, she had diarrhoea and was being left in soaked pads, with fingers and nails covered in excrement. Her lower body was covered in a red raw rash as a result, leading to pain and distress. The hospital rejected the complaint made to it, referring to different perspectives.[6]

SUGGESTIVE PERHAPS OF a serious issue, but then again only one report; is it in any sense representative? We have to attempt to answer this question because ascertaining whether neglect and abuse in the National Health Service (NHS) is systemic, as this book maintains, is pivotal.

This is so for three main reasons. First, were it piecemeal and occasional, it would still be of concern, but not of an order of magnitude. Second, so long as there remains a denial or at least ambivalence about its extent, it will not command sufficient priority for effective remedial action to be taken. Third, if it is systemic, the finger of accountability and blame begins to point upward through the hierarchical, pyramidal, command and control structure of the NHS – ultimately to government ministers. After all, the overall legal duty to provide health services in England lies within sections 1 and 3 of the *National Health Service Act 2006*. It is placed on the Secretary of Health, who is effectively the head of the business, the ultimate chief executive.

In which case, the possibilities seem to be as follows. Neglectful care is either deliberately perpetrated from the centre. Or it is tolerated and quietly accepted as the unfortunate but necessary collateral damage caused by health care policy. Or it is simply the fruit of a gross, reckless omission to acknowledge and do anything seriously about it.

Whichever the explanation, central government bears a heavy responsibility; the evidence collated in this book attests to a systemic, rather than sporadic and opportunistic, affliction within our health services.

---

5   Patients' Association (2010) *Listen to patients, speak up for change*. London: Patients' Association, pp.37–40, 100.

6   Patients' Association (2010) *Listen to patients, speak up for change*. London: Patients' Association, pp.44–48, 101.

THERE IS A great deal of fuzzy thinking when it comes to consideration of the evidence.

Often one hears, not least from central government, that the 'majority' of patients receive good care or that only a 'few' people suffer bad. And that, because of this, we should not get too upset about isolated instances. Promulgation of a bit of guidance here, appointment of a 'dignity champion' there, and a 'national dignity day' will sort it all out.

Furthermore, in this, the age of the consumer and of voracious and ubiquitous media, patients and relatives sometimes get unduly, ignorantly and irrationally upset – and garner into the bargain a disproportionate degree of publicity. In some circumstances, this can skew public perception and unfairly heap opprobrium on government, health managers and clinicians. As Raymond Tallis has pointed out generally, this can be a real concern; angry or grieving relatives, as a class, are not *necessarily* expert, balanced or conducive to medical progress and to the public good.[7]

So are accounts of poor and neglectful care no more than a storm in the proverbial teacup; a choppy but essentially superficial agitation? The response must be no. There is sufficient evidence, independent of outraged relatives, to suggest that, far from being over reported, poor and neglectful care is in fact downplayed. Far from being disproportionately amplified, it has arguably been far too muted.

For example, a statement that the majority of patients receive good care is ludicrous. Such a claim would, after all, be true even if 49 per cent of people received poor care; this could scarcely be cause for celebration even within the strange corridors of Whitehall. But let us not take the statement too literally and accept that the 'vast majority' receive adequate care as the Department of Health maintains – and that the minority receiving poor care comprises few people.[8] But even this will not do. The Patients' Association has pointed out that it requires only a small percentage of patients treated to suffer from substandard care – as little as 2 per cent – for a great many people to be affected. Given the number of treatment episodes provided by the NHS each year, it believes that perhaps as many as a million patients have been subjected to poor care over a period of a few years.[9]

7   Tallis, R. (2004) *Hippocratic oaths: Medicine and its discontents.* London: Atlantic Books, Chapters 6 and 7.

8   Smith, R. (2009) '"Cruel and neglectful" care of one million NHS patients exposed.' *Daily Telegraph*, 27 August.

9   Patients' Association (2010) *Listen to patients, speak up for change.* London: Patients' Association, p.3.

The Association bases this 2 per cent figure on the results of patient responses to something called the National Inpatient Survey.[10] Even this may be conservative and indeed unnecessarily deferential to the Department of Health's claims. As the Association points out, many patients who may have suffered poor care would be unable to participate in such a survey, for the good reason that they have died soon after or lack the ability or capacity to participate.[11] It suggests, therefore, turning to the views of relatives instead, as the Alzheimer's Society did when trying to gain insight into the hospital treatment of 1000 people with dementia. Its findings cast a different light altogether: only 23 per cent were satisfied with the help given to patients with food and drink, 30 per cent with bowel and bladder care, and 32 per cent with assistance with personal hygiene.[12]

So any meaningful statistical claims, one way or another, should certainly not be made in the context of all NHS patient episodes. Instead they need to focus as well on a particular class, such as older hospital inpatients, or be narrowed still more. A further example of such an approach is the work carried out by the National Confidential Inquiry into Patient Outcome and Death. It looked at 800 older people who had received surgery and died within 30 days. Its conclusion was that only *36 per cent* of those patients had received acceptable care.[13]

In addition, in order to gauge seriousness, we have to factor in not just the incidence of poor care but also the consequences. As Ken Jarrold, a former chief executive of several health authorities, asked: how many times is it acceptable to leave patients in urine or faeces – ten times a month or twenty? Likewise, how often is it alright for staff to squeal, giggle and ignore confused and semi-naked patients wandering the corridors at night? He accepted that a health service could be forgiven for erroneous diagnosis in a difficult case – but not forgiven for allowing things that should *never* happen: wilful neglect relating to basic cleanliness and dignity.[14]

---

10 Garratt, E. (2009) *The key findings report for the 2008 inpatient survey.* London: Picker Institute.

11 Patients' Association (2010) *Listen to patients, speak up for change.* London: Patients' Association, p.4.

12 Alzheimer's Society (2009) *Counting the cost; caring for people with dementia on hospital wards.* London: Alzheimer's Society.

13 Wilkinson, K., Martin, I.C., Gough, M.J. *et al.* (2010) *An age old problem: A review of the care received by elderly patients undergoing surgery.* London: National Confidential Enquiry into Patient Outcome and Death, p.5.

14 Quoted in: Patients' Association (2010) *Listen to patients, speak up for change.* London: Patients' Association, p.3.

In other words, let us consider your relative or mine, on a general ward, humiliated, starved, dehydrated, pressure sores developing from scratch, fluid and nutrition not monitored, bowel movement and serious constipation likewise unmonitored, regularly naked in front of other patients, left wet in urine, unbathed, smelly, falling regularly with a thump on the ward floor, dressed in clothes intended for the opposite sex – and attacked in the middle of the night by another patient wielding a walking aid. Do we – and does the Department of Health – really want to maintain that it is of no real matter because this sort of thing happens only to 10 per cent, 5 per cent or even just 2 per cent of patients in that hospital during their stay?

THE WORD 'SYSTEMIC' denotes something universal in the sense of affecting, or tending to affect, an entire system. But importantly a systemic issue does not negate the existence of good practice. At Mid Staffordshire NHS Foundation Trust, the Board believed that the Healthcare Commission investigation was unfair because it had not taken into account the good practice that existed at the hospital. The subsequent independent inquiry pointed out that the existence of good practice does not preclude systemic defects:

> Unhappily, the view of nearly the whole Board can be characterised as one of denial. Board members have shared a fallacy common among many witnesses from the hospital in considering that the HCC [Healthcare Commission] was unfair because it did not recognise good practice where it occurred. No one has denied that there has been good practice… Further, good practice in one part of a hospital does not mean that there are no systemic failings in another.[15]

The Inquiry knocked clean away the crutch that bad practice can be explained away by referring to the good:

> Those that say there is good practice in Stafford are correct. Witnesses have singled out various areas and individuals for praise, and rightly so in my view. For example, it appeared to me that the critical care unit was particularly well run. Various nurses have been praised for their dedication in some of the evidence that has been cited. However, no amount of good practice can disguise or excuse the deficiencies in service provision that have been identified. These cannot be brushed off as isolated incidents

---

15 Francis, R. (Chair) (2010) *Independent Inquiry into care provided by Mid Staffordshire NHS Foundation Trust January 2005–March 2009.* London: The Stationery Office, p.338.

> attributable to the sort of lapse that can occur in any well run hospital.[16]

The gist of these comments, in the context of one hospital, could be applied equally well to the health service as a whole; a fair prospect being marred by conspicuous blotches in the landscape.

In any case, to deny poor practice, because of the existence of admirable practice, is a *non sequitur* and a diversionary ploy. It is a bit like telling Little Red Riding Hood, confronted with the wolf in the forest, not to worry because in the next glade there are deer at rest and butterflies fluttering. A simplistic analogy maybe, but no more crude than the irrationality deployed to explain away the bad by virtue of the good. Little consolation is it for patients who, saved by superb nursing on the intensive care ward, are immediately ignored, starved and allowed to develop pressure sores on the general ward to which they are subsequently transferred.

WITHIN ANY INDIVIDUAL hospital, poor practices have a tendency to run together and to indicate systemic issues at local level.

All of a piece, within a single hospital, may be the following: not taking people to the toilet, not responding to call bells, lack of continence care more generally, not ensuring people receive appropriate (or indeed any) food and drink, not communicating with patients, not respecting their dignity, fatal lapses in infection control, moving patients from ward to ward for non-clinical reasons, allowing patients to fall, poor pressure sore care, inadequate staffing in terms of numbers and competence – and so on. And, as was revealed at Mid Staffordshire NHS Foundation Trust, such neglectful omissions may be associated not just with suffering, misery and pain, but also with high mortality rates.[17]

Apart from this magnetic clustering together of shortcomings in single hospitals, reported by regulatory commissions, many individual accounts reported in the Press and elsewhere refer to multiple aspects of neglect visited upon individual, vulnerable patients. This is not surprising; if staff lack the time to give people food and drink, they will also not have the time to provide other basic care.

The hounds of neglect therefore hunt in packs, closing in, for example, on Mrs Elizabeth Cavanagh, 88 years old and admitted in November 2009

---

16 Francis, R. (Chair) (2010) *Independent Inquiry into care provided by Mid Staffordshire NHS Foundation Trust January 2005–March 2009.* London: The Stationery Office, p.180.

17 Healthcare Commission (2009) *Investigation into Mid Staffordshire NHS Foundation Trust, March 2009.* London: Healthcare Commission, p.35.

to the flagship hospital in Romford, the Queen's – already highlighted in the Introduction to this book. Her daughter recorded how, during her stay, she was not helped to eat and drink but the family was still told not to visit at mealtimes. Her nutritional state was not monitored. Food was left out for her to which she was recorded as being allergic. Call bells were placed consistently out of reach. Medication was not given, nor pain relief, despite her screams of pain.

She was sometimes left exposed from the waist down. Nurses would laugh and joke at the nursing station whilst she was in distress. A sink would be left full of bloody water and gauze, bedding saturated with blood, and a bedside table with needles, dirty water, blood and gauze. Serious pressure sores developed on her feet during the stay in hospital, unobserved and unrecorded by staff. They caused immense pain and were discovered only by her daughter when she removed her mother's bed socks. Charts and records of tissue viability and breakdown had not been kept; a pressure mattress had not been supplied.[18]

Mrs Cavanagh's daughter referred to the mentally 'dark place' she was cast back into by Barking, Havering and Redbridge Hospitals NHS Trust's response to her complaint:

> When I received their final report I was sent back to that dark place again as every time I read it I want to scream out in pain. My mother, my poor defenceless lovely mother went through so much pain and neglect in a place where she should have received the best possible treatment. My mother was let down by the NHS, when she needed them the most. She was let down by something that she believed in and supported all her life.[19]

The Trust owned up to inadequate nursing care, and a 'safeguarding' investigation concluded that the hospital had been neglectful.

AS ALREADY NOTED, the nature of the NHS makes it less likely that a pattern of ongoing failure at local level will be down to purely local factors, and probable that the way the overall 'business' is run makes a significant contribution.

Priorities, financial imperatives and targets are set and enforced at central level. Strategic health authorities (SHAs) at regional level have, to date (they are due to be abolished), been the middle men, conveying

---

18 Patients' Association (2010) *Listen to patients, speak up for change.* London: Patients' Association, pp.62–75.

19 Patients' Association (2010) *Listen to patients, speak up for change.* London: Patients' Association, p.75.

messages from central government to local NHS bodies. Constituting a shadowy bureaucracy, protesting an innocent role when caught in the spotlight, they have been deeply implicated in forcing, at the Department of Health's bidding, policies and decisions on to primary care trusts (PCTs) and NHS trusts at local level.

The PCTs presently commission local services, although they, too, are due to be replaced – by general practitioner (GP) commissioning bodies. NHS trusts then deliver hospital services as do NHS foundation trusts. The latter are under the oversight of a separate organisation called Monitor. All trusts are in principle regulated by the Care Quality Commission (CQC). At the very top, in the Department of Health, sits the chief executive of the NHS, and above him or her, the politicians.

In other words, the centre bears a heavy responsibility for what occurs on the periphery. Some call it micro management; Aneurin Bevan, founder of the NHS, is much quoted as saying: 'If the bedpan lands on the floor in the hospital in Tredegar, it should be clanging in Whitehall.'[20] In more recent years the equivalent has been the ring of the till, the hitting of a target and the dread word 'breach' when the four-hour accident and emergency (A&E) target has been exceeded.

We do not have to rely on logical inference that widespread and repeating local problems constitute more than just random occurrences. The Healthcare Commission was blunt, in some of its investigations into individual NHS trusts, that there were wider lessons to be learnt by the whole of the NHS. This was because the pressures facing those particular trusts were in fact common to all. They were significant, arguably principal, factors in what went wrong in places such as Stoke Mandeville, Maidstone and Tunbridge Wells, and Mid Staffordshire. Had those failures truly been outlying anomalies, it would have been unnecessary to sound repeated warning bells for the rest of the health service.

Pressing this point home in 2007, the Commission reported that significant numbers of NHS trusts were struggling to reconcile the management of health care-associated infection with targets. In fact, 45 per cent of trusts struggled in relation to A&E targets, 29 per cent in respect of waiting times and lists for inpatient treatments, and 36 per cent in relation to financial targets. Furthermore, the Commission noted that minimising the movement of patients in hospital was associated with

---

20 Quoted in: Benjamin, A. (2009) 'Beyond the limits.' *The Guardian*, 18 February.

lower infection rates. Yet only half of NHS trusts monitored compliance with policies for the management of beds.[21]

Thus, at Stoke Mandeville, the Commission had noted tensions facing all acute NHS trusts:

> There is much in this report to suggest that there may be continuing tensions between the control of infection in hospitals and other national priorities. Whereas the trust had a particularly strong focus on the achievement of the Government's targets, there is no doubt that the potential conflict between these targets and the control of infection is an issue that faces all acute trusts.[22]

Likewise at Mid Staffordshire, the Commission emphasised that a number of its findings were of potential relevance to the whole of the NHS. These related to various matters including reliable information about patient care and mortality, ensuring that a focus on finances and objectives does not lead to insufficient focus on care, and that systems of governance that look good on paper actually work in practice.[23]

The cross-party House of Commons Health Committee has expressed no doubts about the contributory role of government policy to 'appalling care':

> Government policy has too often given the impression that there are priorities, notably hitting targets (particularly for waiting lists, and Accident and Emergency waiting), achieving financial balance and attaining Foundation Trust status, which are more important than patient safety. This has undoubtedly, in a number of well documented cases, been a contributory factor in making services unsafe.[24]

It is not only that government policy has been implicated, but that safeguards in the wider system – designed to stop NHS trusts veering off the rails – are also perceived to have failed.

For instance, the commissioning bodies, the PCTs, have arguably encouraged NHS trusts to put politics and finance before patients. One of the Department of Health's own reports about events at Mid Staffordshire

---

21 Healthcare Commission (2007) *Health care associated infection: What else can the NHS do?* London: Healthcare Commission, pp.7, 17.

22 Healthcare Commission (2006) *Investigation into outbreaks of* Clostridium difficile *at Stoke Mandeville Hospital, Buckinghamshire Hospitals NHS Trust, July 2006.* London: Healthcare Commission, p.88.

23 Healthcare Commission (2009) *Investigation into Mid Staffordshire NHS Foundation* Trust, March 2009. London: Healthcare Commission, p.12.

24 House of Commons Health Committee (2009) *Patient safety: Sixth report of Session 2008–09.* HC 151-I. London: The Stationery Office, pp.7, 10.

also pointed to a wider failure. Professor Sir George Alberti significantly implicated the local PCT, responsible for commissioning services out to the foundation trust hospital. Even following the Healthcare Commission report, the Professor expressed disappointment that the PCT's focus remained more on patient throughput and business than on patient care.[25]

At Mid Staffordshire, likewise, the Healthcare Commission noted that the PCT, which had commissioned hospital services from the NHS trust, had not enquired into the quality of care being provided.[26] In Cornwall, where people with learning disabilities were abused, the investigating commissions implicated not just the NHS trust, but also the PCT for commissioning inappropriate services, and the SHA for not adequately monitoring what was going on.[27]

In 2009, too, the House of Commons Health Committee picked out a deficiency in safeguards and regulation. It referred to a lack of clarity of role between commissioning, performance managing and regulating bodies. There were:

> ...as Baroness Young put it, "a lot of players on the pitch" and we are concerned that too often they are not an effective team. There is evidence of overlapping functions and multiple submission of information to different regulators... What all the complex panoply of organisations has actually achieved is called into question by the fact that these systems have been shown recently to have failed in several instances promptly to expose and address major instances of unsafe care.[28]

In June 2010, a new Secretary of State for Health conceded that the failure at Mid Staffordshire went beyond the local; it was 'a national failure of the regulatory and supervisory system, which should have secured the quality and safety of patient care'. Instead it had only been exposed by a determined group of families.[29]

---

25 Alberti, G. (Professor Sir) (2009) *Mid Staffordshire NHS Foundation Trust: A review of the procedures for emergency admissions and treatment, and progress against the recommendation of the March Healthcare Commission report.* London: Department of Health, pp.15–16.

26 Healthcare Commission (2009) *Investigation into Mid Staffordshire NHS Foundation Trust, March 2009.* London: Healthcare Commission, p.118.

27 Healthcare Commission and CSCI (Commission for Social Care Inspection) (2006) *Joint investigation into the provision of services for people with learning disabilities at Cornwall Partnership NHS Trust, July 2006.* London: Healthcare Commission and CSCI, p.60.

28 House of Commons Health Committee (2009) *Patient safety: Sixth report of Session 2008–09.* HC 151-I. London: The Stationery Office, p.84.

29 Lansley, A. (Secretary of State for Health) (2010) *Hansard.* House of Commons Debates, 9 June, col. 333.

In sum, a blight of poor and neglectful care in the health service is insidious and far reaching. Horizontally, it takes hold within individual hospitals affecting multiple aspects of basic care, and is found replicated in almost identical form across different hospitals. And, vertically, causes for it – both in terms of perpetration and omission – are to be espied all the way up the health service hierarchy.

NOT NOW, BERNARD is a very simple, illustrated children's book written by David McKee. In it a small boy sees a monster in the garden. He tells his parents but they are too busy to take notice, preoccupied in a humdrum world of their own. Eventually, the monster eats Bernard, enters the house and trashes his bedroom. The monster then takes Bernard's place. The final scene is of the mother taking up a drink to the monster who is sitting up in bed. Her eyes are closed, she switches off the light, still not realising what has occurred.[30]

This book for the very young can be read on many levels, including the amusing, the sad and the disturbing. The last sums up well *our* subject matter. There is a monster on the loose in the health service; the supposed custodians of the NHS need to recognise and to stop it. To the extent they have dimly acknowledged that something is not quite right, their timid corrective actions seem to be saying: not yet, not quite now.

---

30   McKee, D. (1980) *Not Now, Bernard.* London: Red Fox Books.

4

Assessing the Evidence for Neglectful and Abusive Health Care

> The truth is that we know about this in our hearts. Look at the fear, the terror in the eyes of some older people in hospital wards, in care homes, in nursing homes. Listen to what they say in code. Listen to how their carers speak about them. It is not universal, by any means, but it is common. And one of the terrifying things is that we have known about it, subliminally perhaps, for many years. (Baroness Julia Neuberger: on the abuse of elderly people, 2005)[1]

In order to outline and then colour in a plausible picture, it is important to know what we are looking for and where the evidence is.

There is a spectrum. Within it we find poor care, neglect and abuse in that sequence. Where they shade one into another is a moot point; for the purpose of the book it really doesn't matter; and the meaning of the word neglect is in any case wide enough to cover what we might call substantially poor care. But it is important to see the continuum; it is only an increasingly widespread seed bed of poor care that allows dense patches of neglect and sometimes abuse to grow.

THE WORDS 'NEGLECT' and 'abuse' are used generally in a fairly broad way. We do not need to be too precise when applying these words in their everyday sense; we know them when we see them. Indeed, at one edge they shade simply into poor care. At another, they take on the garb of criminal offences, in which case much greater precision is required; these are considered, in the form of ill treatment and wilful neglect, in Chapter 21.

Or at least we think we know them when we see them. A relative's perception of outrageous neglect of a patient may, for a health service

---

1   Neuberger, J. (2005) *The moral state we are in: A manifesto for a 21st century society.* London: HarperCollins, p.44.

manager, be no more than another incident of 'sub-optimal care'.[2] In any event and in any parlance, everyday or legal, they are emotive words. Abuse is defined in the dictionary as maltreatment or as using a person or thing to bad effect or for a bad purpose. Neglect means lack of care or a failure to care for.[3]

Further help comes in the form of guidance from central government. In 2000, local councils responsible for providing social services were alerted by it to the need to safeguard vulnerable adults from abuse. Called *No secrets*, the guidance defined abuse to include, amongst other things, neglect and omissions.[4]

Following suit ten years later, legal regulations, enforceable by the Care Quality Commission (CQC) against health and social care providers, define abuse. It encompasses physical or psychological ill treatment and also 'neglect and acts of omission which cause harm or place [service users] at risk of harm'.[5] In the specific context of nursing, the Nursing and Midwifery Council (NMC) is more expansive, with an advice note aimed at registrants. Taken at face value, it would seem to implicate significant numbers of nurses associated with the poor care identified in this book:

> Neglect is the refusal or failure on the part of the registered nurse, midwife or health visitor to meet the essential care needs of a client. Examples include failure to attend to the personal hygiene of a client, failure to communicate adequately with the client and the inappropriate withholding of food, fluids, clothing, medication, medical aids, assistance or equipment.[6]

Certainly in everyday language, abuse sometimes tends to indicate greater ill intent than the word neglect. A well intentioned, kind but struggling or inadequate relative may be neglectful but scarcely abusive. Nonetheless, according to Department of Health guidance and these health care regulations, neglect and omissions all fall under the umbrella of the term 'abuse'.

---

2   Phair, L. (2010) 'The Vetting and Barring Scheme and its role in safeguarding.' Presentation notes at 'Safeguarding vulnerable adults: empowerment through implementation of "No secrets"' Conference held on 17 March 2010 at 4 Hamilton Place, London.

3   *Concise Oxford Dictionary of Current English.* 8th ed. Oxford: Clarendon Press, 1990.

4   DH (Department of Health) (2000) *No secrets: Guidance on developing and implementing multi-agency policies and procedures to protect vulnerable adults from abuse.* London: DH, para. 2.7.

5   SI 2010/781. *The Health and Social Care Act 2008 (Regulated Activities) Regulations 2010,* r.11.

6   NMC (Nursing and Midwifery Council) (2006) *Registrant/client relationships and the prevention of abuse.* London: NMC, p.3.

THE EVIDENCE OF abuse and neglect in our health services comes broadly from three main sources. These are: reports from regulatory bodies established by statute, other formal reports produced by a variety of organisations and finally incidents and events reported in the Press (and some other sources) more widely. The question that needs answering is twofold: how serious, and how widespread, is the poor and neglectful care depicted within this body of evidence? The seriousness of what occurs is not in dispute; the sticking point is the prevalence. The rest of the answer seems to be that, taken on their own, none of these sources would be enough to point conclusively to a systemic issue. Taken together, however, they make a powerful argument, not least because they corroborate one another. It is a bit like verifying an observation, by making it from more than one angle and using different instruments.

FIRST UP ARE the reports of regulatory bodies. The Commission for Health Improvement (CHI) functioned as a regulatory body for the health service between 1999 and 2004. It was then superseded by the Healthcare Commission, which in turn gave way to the CQC in April 2009. Between them, the first two of these bodies published a number of prominent and disquieting reports about health services in acute and sometimes non-acute settings. In addition, during this period, the Mental Health Act Commission highlighted instances of completely unacceptable care for mental health patients in some hospitals. This Commission was finally absorbed also into the CQC.

Of these reports a number stand out. Neglectful care of mainly older people was uncovered at Mid Cheshire National Health Service (NHS) Hospitals Trust,[7] East Kent Hospitals NHS Trust,[8] Stoke Mandeville Hospital (Buckinghamshire Hospitals NHS Trust),[9] Maidstone and Tunbridge Wells NHS Trust[10] and Mid Staffordshire NHS Foundation Trust.[11]

---

7   Healthcare Commission (2006) *Investigation into Mid Cheshire Hospitals NHS Trust, January 2006*. London: Healthcare Commission.

8   CHI (Commission for Health Improvement) (2002) *Clinical performance review: East Kent Hospitals NHS Trust*. London: CHI.

9   Healthcare Commission (2006) *Investigation into outbreaks of* Clostridium difficile *at Stoke Mandeville Hospital, Buckinghamshire Hospitals NHS Trust, July 2006*. London: Healthcare Commission.

10 Healthcare Commission (2007) *Investigation into outbreaks of* Clostridium difficile *at Maidstone and Tunbridge Wells NHS Trust, October 2007*. London: Healthcare Commission.

11 Healthcare Commission (2009) *Investigation into Mid Staffordshire NHS Foundation Trust, March 2009*. London: Healthcare Commission.

A report about Gosport War Memorial Hospital found similar failings in care, but also identified serious flaws in the prescribing of drugs for people with dementia,[12] the ramifications of which are still playing out nearly a decade after the original events.

At Stoke Mandeville and at Maidstone and Tunbridge Wells NHS Trust, poor care practices were in particular associated with uncontrolled and lethal outbreaks of *Clostridium difficile* and scores of deaths. This infection was also a problem in Mid Staffordshire. Notably in these reports, the Healthcare Commission found abundant evidence that NHS trust boards were preoccupied with matters other than basic patient care, in particular finance and government-set priorities.

Reports were issued of investigations into what the CHI termed the abuse of older people with mental health problems in non-acute settings. This occurred in the North Lakeland NHS Trust[13] and on Rowan Ward at the Manchester Mental Health and Social Care Trust.[14] Abusive non-acute care of people with learning disabilities was subsequently uncovered by the Healthcare Commission at the Cornwall Partnership NHS Trust[15] and at the Sutton and Merton Primary Care Trust (PCT).[16]

At the end of 2009, the CQC reported on significant lapses in infection control at Basildon and Thurrock University Hospitals NHS Foundation Trust, where unusually high mortality rates had been identified.[17]

These are the well-publicised examples. But the regulatory commissions have also made findings of lack of dignity of care in local reports that have not received widespread, if any, publicity. To give but one instance: the CHI reported in 2002 about care at the acute hospital in Bury St Edmunds, Suffolk; it referred to complaints about the treatment of older patients on the wards and the lack of basic nursing care available to them.[18] Concerns were also raised about the lack of attention to patients'

---

12   CHI (Commission for Health Improvement) (2002) *Investigation into the Portsmouth Healthcare NHS Trust: Gosport War Memorial Hospital, July 2002*. London: CHI.

13   CHI (Commission for Health Improvement) (2000) *Investigation into the North Lakeland NHS Trust, November*. London: CHI.

14   CHI (Commission for Health Improvement) (2003) *Investigation into matters arising from care on Rowan Ward, Manchester Mental Health and Social Care Trust, September 2003*. London: CHI.

15   Healthcare Commission and CSCI (Commission for Social Care Inspection) *Joint investigation into the provision of services for people with learning disabilities at Cornwall Partnership NHS Trust, July 2006*. London: Healthcare Commission and CSCI.

16   Healthcare Commission (2007) *Investigation into the service for people with learning disabilities provided by Sutton and Merton Primary Care Trust*. London: Healthcare Commission.

17   CQC (Care Quality Commission) (2009) *Inspection report: The prevention and control of infections, Basildon and Thurrock University Hospitals NHS Foundation Trust*. London: CQC.

18   CHI (Commission for Health Improvement) (2002) *West Suffolk Hospitals NHS Trust*. London: CHI.

basic needs in terms of accessing the toilets and help with eating and drinking.[19]

Eight years later, the hospital resurfaced in a Patients' Association report about Mrs Anne Robson. She was admitted to the West Suffolk Hospital in January 2010, having fallen out of bed. Conflicting and confusing judgements were made by different staff, made worse by a delay in obtaining previous X-rays of her hip. It turned out not to be broken; but the apparently avoidable delay, including the misreading of notes by staff, meant she stayed in hospital longer than necessary. This effectively seems to have contributed to her death.

She was admitted to a ward on which norovirus was present, which meant the family was not at liberty to visit normally, if at all. Indeed, her youngest daughter never saw her mother alive again after she had passed into that 'closed ward'. Her mother then developed diarrhoea. She did speak to her again on the telephone, when her mother explained that she was very thirsty, was expected to eat her lunch in a urine-soaked bed, but was in any case not being assisted to eat and drink.

Another sister did visit the closed ward. She found her mother with her night dress soaked in urine up to her arm pits; the nurses, dubiously, claimed they had only just changed her clothes. Her teeth had not been cleaned for a week. A third sister also visited, finding her mother, again, very thirsty and unable to eat and drink for herself. No fluid balance chart or record was kept. Pill cups, containing pills, were on her table; she had not taken them. She could not move her hand or pick anything up with it.

The hospital then unexpectedly said she could be discharged; she returned to her nursing home by private ambulance arranged by the family where she died within a few hours of arrival. She had been in hospital for just a week. Her general practitioners had not expected her to die. The hospital's recorded response was circumspect, stating that it had investigated and fed the results back to Mrs Robson's family.[20]

Many hospitals have thus passed largely under the radar when it comes to adverse publicity about poor and neglectful care. But this does not mean that there are not persistent undercurrents of such care, undetected.

Apart from such investigations into individual NHS trusts, the Healthcare Commission also produced *overview* reports and surveys

19 CHI (Commission for Health Improvement) (2002) *West Suffolk Hospitals NHS Trust*. London: CHI.
20 Patients' Association (2010) *Listen to patients, speak up for change*. London: Patients' Association, pp.19–25.

indicating a less than wholesome picture, in particular the failure to uphold people's dignity sufficiently:

> We found that some older people experienced poor standards of care on general hospital wards, including poorly managed discharges from hospitals, being repeatedly moved from one ward to another for non-clinical reasons, being cared for in mixed-sex bays or wards and having their meals taken away before they could eat them due to a lack of support at meal times. All users of health and social care services need to be treated with dignity and respect. However, some older people can be particularly vulnerable and it is essential that extra attention is given to making sure that givers of care treat them with dignity at all times and in all situations. To fail to do this is an infringement of their human rights.[21]

It referred to the lessons to be learnt generally, across the NHS – from its findings in high profile reports such as Stoke Mandeville, Maidstone and Tunbridge Wells NHS Trust and Mid Staffordshire NHS Foundation Trust. In effect, the Commission was alluding to the sentiment, discreetly prevalent within NHS trusts that have not hitherto been caught out, 'there but for the grace of God go I'.[22]

The picture that builds up is that when things go wrong, they have done so precisely *not* because of outlying, maverick behaviour. Instead the failures appear to be an obvious, if not inevitable, consequence of pressures in the system. Therefore, the chances of similar problems – on a greater or lesser scale – existing elsewhere, unknown, are arguably substantial.

AMIDST THIS EVIDENCE from the regulatory commissions, the Mid Staffordshire NHS Foundation Trust warrants special mention. The Healthcare Commission was attracted initially to investigate because of unusually high mortality rates at the hospital. It went on to publish a highly critical report.[23] Such was the concern generated by the Commission's findings that the Department of Health commissioned the

---

21 Health Commission, CSCI (Commission for Social Care Inspection) and Audit Commission (2006) *Living well in later life: A review of progress against the National Service Framework for Older People: Summary report.* London: Healthcare Commission, p.9.

22 The variant of a quote commonly attributed to the Protestant martyr, John Bradford, uttered when he saw criminals being led to execution. He was subsequently burned as a heretic in 1555. Quoted in: Partington, A. (ed.) (1992) *The Oxford Dictionary of Quotations.* 4th ed. Oxford: Oxford University Press, p.139.

23 Healthcare Commission (2009) *Investigation into Mid Staffordshire NHS Foundation Trust, March 2009.* London: Healthcare Commission.

Thomé and Alberti reports. The former referred to 'appalling' standards of care.[24] The government was then effectively forced, though only under threat of legal action from patients' relatives, to appoint an independent inquiry.

And it is this last inquiry that is so telling, albeit that – or perhaps precisely because – it was not conducted by a regulatory body.[25] The preceding three reports about what happened (including that of the Healthcare Commission) concentrated more on process and mechanism; they glossed over the extent and detail of what patients actually went through. The independent inquiry fathomed the iniquities and suffering inflicted upon patients.

For this reason the Mid Staffordshire independent inquiry report is cited as evidence throughout this book; it covers in detail what other reports from regulatory commissions have referred to more fleetingly. There is no reason to suppose that the experience, for instance, of not being taken to the toilet and being left in one's own urine and faeces, was different in Mid Staffordshire from at other NHS trusts reported to have treated patients in the same way. Therefore, the graphic descriptions from the Mid Staffordshire inquiry serve to indicate patient experiences elsewhere and on a much broader scale.

DESPITE THE REVEALING nature of some of their reports, it cannot be maintained with confidence that the regulatory commissions have identified every hospital afflicted with poor and neglectful care practices.

It was only the whistleblowing of student nurses, highlighting the abuse of older patients in North Lakeland, that led to a formal investigation.[26] What if they had not piped up? Likewise, it was only the leaking to the national Press, of information about uncontrolled and lethal infection at Stoke Mandeville Hospital, that led to a full-scale Healthcare Commission investigation.[27] Suppose there had been no

---

24 Thomé, D.C. (Dr) (2009) *Mid Staffordshire NHS Foundation Trust: A review of lessons learnt for commissioners and performance managers following the Healthcare Commission investigation*. London: Department of Health, p.3; Alberti, G. (Professor Sir) (2009) *Mid Staffordshire NHS Foundation Trust: A review of the procedures for emergency admissions and treatment, and progress against the recommendation of the March Healthcare Commission report*. London: Department of Health.

25 Francis, R. (Chair) (2010) *Independent Inquiry into care provided by Mid Staffordshire NHS Foundation Trust January 2005–March 2009*. London: The Stationery Office.

26 CHI (Commission for Health Improvement) (2000) *Investigation into the North Lakeland NHS Trust, November*. London: CHI, p.9.

27 Healthcare Commission (2006) *Investigation into outbreaks of* Clostridium difficile *at Stoke Mandeville Hospital, Buckinghamshire Hospitals NHS Trust, July 2006*. London: Healthcare Commission, p.28.

leak? Even the nature of events at Stafford Hospital might have remained largely unknown, had it not been for the exceptional efforts of Cure the NHS to highlight what happened there.

AT MID STAFFORDSHIRE, apparently high mortality rates drew the Healthcare Commission to investigate. Its draft report had suggested anything between 400 and 1200 excess deaths as a result of the standard of care on offer at the hospital. These figures were removed from the final publication.[28] This removal did not prevent widespread coverage in the Press – of the upper figure.[29]

The Independent Inquiry at Mid Staffordshire hedged its bets on a causal link between the bad care provided and the mortality rate at the hospital. It acknowledged that the methodology for measuring standard mortality rates (and their significance) was attended with uncertainty and controversy. Thence came the difficulty of inferring particular numbers of avoidable or unnecessary deaths. Nonetheless, the Inquiry concluded that there was 'strong evidence to suggest that these figures mandated a serious investigation of the standards of care being delivered'.[30] For example, at one NHS Trust, it turned out that mortality rates for emergency admissions rose on certain days of the week; the very days when insufficient senior staff were on call.[31]

This is a view held generally by Professor Brian Jarman, Emeritus Professor at Imperial College's School of Medicine. In March 2010, he identified 25 NHS trusts at which, in the year 2007–08, the number of patients who had died – over and above the expected statistical rate – amounted to 4600. He did not claim that this meant the NHS trusts were necessarily doing things wrong, but that they at least merited investigation in order to identify wider issues.[32]

Quite so. It was indeed rising death counts at the three hospitals referred to immediately above that drew down regulatory reports, independent inquiries and opprobrium all round. But the death rates, to the point in one way, were quite beside it in another. Even without higher

28 Francis, R. (Chair) (2010) *Independent Inquiry into care provided by Mid Staffordshire NHS Foundation Trust January 2005–March 2009*. London: The Stationery Office, pp.360–2.

29 See: Boseley, S. (2010) 'Mid Staffordshire NHS trust left patients humiliated and in pain.' *The Guardian*, 24 February.

30 Francis, R. (Chair) (2010) *Independent Inquiry into care provided by Mid Staffordshire NHS Foundation Trust January 2005–March 2009*. London: The Stationery Office, p.23.

31 Vincent, C. (2010) *Patient safety in the UK National Health Service: The events in Mid Staffordshire in context*, p.23. Accessed on 20 December 2010 at: www.midstaffspublicinquiry.com/hearings/s/120/week-two-15-18-nov-2010.

32 Boseley, S. (2010) 'Death rates in hospitals too high, says professor.' *The Guardian*, 25 March.

mortality rates, the care being provided was appalling. If those hospitals had provided degrading care, but managed to keep a few more people alive or reported the mortality statistics in a different way, they might well have remained below the parapet. But plainly this would not have ameliorated the degrading care being visited upon vulnerable patients.

In other words, for every one NHS trust formally investigated, there may be another behaving similarly but shunning the limelight.

There is yet one more ingredient to add to this pot. In a number of conspicuous cases, regulatory bodies have accepted that an NHS trust is performing well, only hurriedly to revise their opinion when the error of that judgement has been exposed by other means. The outstanding instance of this was that prior to becoming a foundation trust, the Mid Staffordshire NHS Trust was judged to be 'fair' and then 'provisionally good'; and when it was given foundation status, the regulatory body, Monitor, officially accepted that the hospital was providing a high quality of care for its patients.

Other such examples are given towards the end of this book in Chapter 24, which outlines the legal framework for regulation. They suggest strongly that, as evidence of the extent and prevalence of poor and neglectful care, the reports of regulatory bodies are not the full ticket.

COMPLEMENTING, AND CONSISTENT with, the findings of regulatory organisations are reports and other publications by a range of bodies such as the Patients' Association, Help the Aged and Age Concern England (now merged to form Age UK), MENCAP, the Nutrition Action Plan Delivery Board, the House of Commons Health Committee, the Joint Parliamentary Committee on Human Rights and the National Audit Office. And occasionally, even, reports produced by the Department of Health itself. These reports add convincingly to the evidence; the following give a flavour.

As already mentioned, in 1997 *The Observer* newspaper ran a series of articles called 'Dignity on the Ward', highly critical about the care of older people in acute hospitals.[33] The then Secretary of State for Health, Frank Dobson, took the matter seriously. He commissioned a piece of work, published in 2000, by the Health Advisory Service, part of the Department of Health.

33 Durham, M. and Bright, M. (1997) 'Join our campaign for the old.' *The Observer*, 5 October. Also: Bright, M. (1997) 'Charity calls for abuse inquiry.' *The Observer*, 26 October.

Called *Not because they are old*, it highlighted a string of failings in the hospital care of older people.[34] These comprised deficiencies in the physical fabric of wards, shortage of basic supplies and technical equipment, staff shortages, lack of assistance in helping people to eat and drink, diminution of dignity (related to personal hygiene and dressing) because of the physical environment but also staff attitudes, inadequate communication with patients and relatives because of time pressures on staff – and so on.[35]

In 2004, the National Audit Office issued a report on patient safety and infection. It accurately drew attention to the fact that NHS trusts had taken their eye off the ball, and in effect anticipated precisely the scandals to come at Stoke Mandeville Hospital and at Maidstone and Tunbridge Wells NHS Trust.[36]

Age Concern England published *Hungry to be heard* in 2006, highlighting the fact that significant numbers of older people were suffering from malnourishment and dehydration in NHS hospitals.[37]

In 2009, the Patients' Association published *Patients not numbers, people not statistics*, containing a number of detailed accounts of highly neglectful care – stories drawn from the experiences of the many patients and relatives regularly contacting the Association.[38] In that same year, the Nutrition Action Plan Delivery Board produced its annual and final report. It advised that there was a significant and continuing problem of malnutrition and help with eating – and that official figures underestimated the prevalence of malnutrition in hospitals and care settings.[39]

That same year saw the publication of a House of Commons Health Committee report on patient safety, drawing attention to what it considered to be widespread defects in the approach to patient safety and welfare in NHS trusts.[40] In 2010, Age UK followed up Age Concern's 2006 report on malnutrition in hospitals with *Still hungry to be heard*.[41]

---

34 HAS (Health Advisory Service) (2000) *Not because they are old: An independent inquiry into the care of older people on acute wards in general hospitals.* London: HAS, pp.iii–iv.

35 Black, D. (2004) 'Not because they are old – revisited.' *Age and Ageing 5*, 33, 430–2.

36 NAO (National Audit Office) (2004) *Improving patient care by reducing the risk of hospital acquired infection: A progress report.* London: NAO.

37 Age Concern England (2006) *Hungry to be heard: The scandal of malnourished older people in hospital.* London: Age Concern England.

38 Patients' Association (2009) *Patients not numbers, people not statistics.* London: Patients' Association.

39 Lishman, G. (Chair) (2009) *Nutrition Action Plan Delivery Board end of year progress report.* London: Department of Health, p.5.

40 House of Commons Health Committee (2009) *Patient safety: Sixth report of Session 2008–09.* HC 151-I. London: The Stationery Office, p.87.

41 Age UK (2010) *Still hungry to be heard: The scandal of people in later life becoming malnourished in hospital.* London: Age UK.

And likewise, late in 2010, the Patients' Association added to its 2009 report with a further publication called *Listen to patients, speak up for change*, containing more individual accounts of poor and neglectful hospital care.[42]

IF THESE FORMAL reports are the knights on chargers, in the vanguard and heavy armour, then the supporting infantry come in the form of individual incidents and occurrences as reported by the Press and, increasingly, on the Internet as related by patients and relatives. The infantry in this sense is sizeable and, perhaps, decisive in winning the battle to expose a systemic problem within the health service.

Many Press accounts are included in this book and many are not – for reasons of space but also because they are greatly dispersed and not so easy to find. Only some seams have been explored by the author, and even they have not been played out, whilst other seams remain untapped.

Stories in the Press can of course be dismissed by the sceptic as mere anecdote and unreliable; after all, so what if a family makes claims which a newspaper chooses to play up into sensationalist, and sometimes politically motivated, headlines? Especially as relatives naturally do get upset; illness, suffering, death and grief make for an unstable mix.

Nevertheless, several factors make such accounts more compelling than might be supposed. There are many of them, and there is no reason to suppose that collectively they form a body of colourful fiction. Even were a significant proportion fanciful, ill motivated or based on genuine misunderstanding or misperception, this would still leave many unsettling descriptions of shocking care. The veracity of a substantial proportion of these individual stories could anyway be inferred from the more formal reports of regulatory bodies and other organisations; the former corroborate the latter. They all tie up. It is implausible to suggest that such consistency is the result of a grand, coordinated conspiracy or, alternatively, an infectious hysteria.

Besides, whilst one should beware of exaggerated and one-sided accounts, equally one must be mindful of the degree of denial and euphemism sometimes emanating from NHS trusts in order to deflect criticism. This is discussed in Chapter 16. Accordingly, we should not naturally assume that the word of a hospital – or of the public relations firm speaking on its behalf, or at least coordinating its response – is inherently more reliable than that of an aggrieved patient or relative.

---

42   Patients' Association (2010) *Listen to patients, speak up for change.* London: Patients' Association.

The accounts of individual incidents substantially extend the number of NHS trusts implicated in poor standards of care closely linked to the neglect and abuse of patients. Furthermore, if one patient is accurately reported as having been treated badly in a hospital – not because of an unusual event or a villainous member of staff, but rather as a function of the system (e.g. under-staffing, lack of beds, skewed priorities) – then it is probable that other patients will have been treated in the same way. After all, the Press do not pick up all incidents of poor patient care; and many patients are unable or unwilling to make a fuss, likewise their relatives. They suffer in unreported silence. In any case, in a number of individual accounts, relatives frequently report that they observed similar poor treatment being provided for other patients as well as for their own family member.

Finally, Press accounts are lent greater force and reliability when, for instance, a coroner has been involved and expressed concern – or when an NHS hospital trust has either publicly apologised and admitted blame, or has settled a legal compensation claim out of court. Many of the individual stories cited in this book lay claim to this more compelling status.

Even then, one must remember the limitations of relying on coroners' inquests to identify the extent of poor care. After all, it is potentially unexplained or unexpected deaths which draw the attention of coroners, not neglectful care *per se*. A coroner's verdict essentially aims to ascertain the cause of death. Certainly, poor and neglectful care surfaces in inquests but, primarily, the coroner is not investigating whether patients are being neglected. If the neglect did not cause death, it is of limited relevance to the inquest verdict. This is easily illustrated.

'The verdict is to a large extent irrelevant'; so said the family, following the inquest into the death of their 83 year old mother, Mrs Mary Healey, at Leeds General Infirmary. She was admitted with a broken hip. She had died from pneumonia after having been given drugs, over a period of six days, for epilepsy, schizophrenia and insomnia – drugs that had been prescribed for another patient. Twelve different doctors apparently failed to pick up the error. The coroner confirmed, however, that these drugs were not the cause of death. The family had a point; the coroner's verdict took nothing away from the inadequacy of their mother's care. The Leeds Teaching Hospitals NHS Trust stated that it had identified improvements to make.[43]

---

43   Lavery, M. (2010) 'Leeds pensioner drugs mix up verdict.' *Yorkshire Post*, 15 October.

Likewise, a serious case review into the deaths of five residents at a care home in Northampton took issue with the coroner. The latter had given a verdict of death from natural causes; the review noted that a number of professionals were clear that there was serious neglect.[44] The point being, of course, that a person can be subject to horrendous neglect and still die of something else.

This means that falling back on death as an indicator – whether investigated by a coroner (or by the CQC) – of failings in basic care, is crude in the extreme. By itself, this is not a reassuring way of tackling things; many terrible things can happen short of death and it is anyway all too late for those who have already died.

CERTAIN INTERNET WEBSITES act as additional sources of evidence. A number exist, containing comments about, and criticism of, the health service. One example is NHS Exposed.[45] This book has in general not used these sites, although this particular site has provided the odd lead for substantiation elsewhere. In addition are the many 'blog' comments one finds attached to Press reports accessed on the Internet.

Two sites that have been used, however, are NHS Choices[46] and Patient Opinion,[47] both of which record comments by patients. The former is run by the government. The latter is a not-for-profit social enterprise set up by Paul Hodgkin, a general practitioner (GP), and in fact partly funded by contributions from NHS trusts and PCTs. Even the Care Quality Commission, arch regulator of health care, has been reported – possibly in some desperation – to be considering the use of a computer software tool that can 'crawl' over social networks such as Facebook. The purpose would be to pick up on comments about standards of care in hospital and elsewhere.[48]

Plainly, care has to be taken when judging the reliability of these comments, but some judgements can be made on the basis of tone and plausibility – particularly if the NHS trust has posted a reply, conceding a problem and apologising – or if there is corroboration from another source about issues at a particular hospital. In any case, more or less true, more or less reasonable, they reflect the patient voice which,

---

44 Sloper, G. and Seaton, M. (2010) *Serious case review: Parkside House, 49–53 St Matthew's Parade, Northampton NN2 7HE: Executive summary.* Northampton: Northamptonshire County Council, p.8.

45 www.nhsexposed.com/index.shtml (from October 2010, 'closed for fun at the beach').

46 www.nhs.uk/Pages/HomePage.aspx.

47 www.patientopinion.org.uk.

48 Clover, B. (2010) 'CQC to trawl online networks to find complaints.' *Nursing Times,* 6 December.

central government protests, is all important. This voice can be blunt, as illustrated by the relative of a patient in 2009, at North Manchester General Hospital:

> ...the person was my mum they left her with the runs for days she got CDT she got so weak she had to be tube fed when the tube came out she was left without fluid for 2 days and food for 4 days they let her bottom get that sore she was screaming in pain then gave her drugs to shut her up she was a mess by the time she died and thats not all of it ttey [sic] treat old people worse than animals.[49]

Such statements contrast strikingly with the well-manicured statements of health service chief executives, chairmen or others spokespersons. A trawl through the comments of patients and relatives on the two websites suggests recurring neglectful and undignified care within our hospitals. It also throws up many favourable comments. The combination accords with the thesis of this book; there is plenty of good care provided in our health services, as well as an unacceptable and substantial stratum of bad.

LAST, INFERENCE CAN be made from one further source of evidence. Paradoxically, this source does not describe bad practice at all, but good. It comprises a large quantity of good practice guidance (including standards) and policy statements from central government, regulatory bodies, voluntary organisations and professional bodies. It is referred to in detail in the next chapter, and in various other chapters as well.

This guidance covers treating patients with dignity, making sure they eat and drink, taking them to the toilet, talking and communicating with them properly, not discharging them from hospital prematurely and avoiding or at least managing pressure sores, etc.

These are all very basic matters; so basic, one might have assumed they would have been taken for granted and barely mentioned. The position is quite the opposite. There is so much advice on these matters that four observations can be made.

First, if standards of hospital care equated to what was on paper, there would, as they say these days, be 'no worries'. Second, the very quantity of guidance suggests strongly that a systemic problem exists. If there were not an endemic corrosion of basic care why, for the past decade, talk and exhort so much about it?

---

49 Patient Opinion. Accessed on 20 October 2010 at: www.patientopinion.org.uk/opinions/14164.

Third, and in any event, it is disconcerting that so much guidance is required to convince staff and managers of the importance of the most basic and humane requirements imaginable – like helping people to eat and drink, taking them to the toilet and not leaving them in soiled bedding and clothes for hours. And observing basic hygiene measures to avoid patients dying of infection.

Last, is the question of what it is in health care policy, systems and practice that undermines such basic care, makes the guidance necessary in the first place, and then continues to undermine and render it, all too often, ineffective.

IN SUMMARY, THIS is about joining up the dots. They are scattered, as evidence, all over the sheet of paper. As always, care must be taken not to link them in the wrong way and end up with a misleading image. But there are so many points, forming such a salient pattern, that the picture emerging is only too clear.

5

Dignity in Care: All the Good Guidance

> The NHS will treat patients as individuals, with respect for their
> dignity. (*The NHS Plan*: on what should be happening, 2000)[1]

> In the next room you could hear the buzzers sounding. After
> about 20 minutes you could hear the men shouting for the nurse,
> "Nurse, nurse", and it just went on and on. And then very often
> it would be two people calling at the same time and then you
> would hear them crying, like shouting "Nurse" louder, and then
> you would hear them just crying, just sobbing, they would just
> sob and you just presumed that they had had to wet the bed. And
> then after they would sob, they seemed to then shout again for
> the nurse and then it would go quiet… (Mid Staffordshire NHS
> Foundation Trust: evidence to the Independent Inquiry, 2009)[2]

Dignity is something we put great store by in daily life. Erosion of it is
therefore something we do not spontaneously associate with hospital
health care; indeed one might be forgiven for assuming that the precise
opposite would be the case. When typically an older person (but indeed
somebody of any age) is acutely ill in hospital, fearful, anxious, maybe
mentally confused, frail, physically helpless – and may be dying – dignity
is sometimes all that remains. For it to be stripped away in hospital, at the
hands of caring professions, is unthinkable and unspeakable. But think
and talk about it we must.

Like the relative in March 2010, who praised the care on the intensive
care unit at Hinchingbrooke Hospital but told a different story about the
subsequent ward:

> The call bells not being answered. Would arrive to find my
> relative weeping because he was bedbound, and saying I'm so
> sorry, I've been ringing for ages but I've had to wet the bed.
> Where's the dignity in that? We helped ourselves to bottles

1 Secretary of State for Health (2000) *The NHS Plan: A plan for investment, a plan for reform.* Cm
4818-I. London: The Stationery Office, p.4.
2 Francis, R. (Chair) (2010) *Independent Inquiry into care provided by Mid Staffordshire NHS Foundation
Trust January 2005–March 2009.* London: The Stationery Office, p.53.

from the sluice because "I'll get you one in a minute" generally translates as never. If he had a bottle within reach he would not wet the bed and not have to be changed so his skin didn't break down… It also seemed common sense to me that if you take a full bottle away, if you spend thirty seconds bringing an empty one back you might even not have to answer the buzzer. The washing bowl, as he could not get to the bathroom, had faeces in the bottom. My relative was told to drink more, again, we did point out that as he was bed-ridden, and his jug and glass were on a table across the room, that could present a problem. We encouraged him to drink, and asked for more water, and like the bottles none forthcoming. We asked for permission to go into the kitchen and get water, and were told off limits. We the family had to FIGHT for everything for a decent standard of care for my relative. We are not a family from hell, we just wanted our relative dealt with, with a modicum of dignity.[3]

This chapter considers what we mean by dignity and then goes on to outline numerous statements of good practice, emanating both from central government and the health care professions themselves. These utterances tend to give the impression of a much recited mantra. Although repetitious, a selection is outlined below. This is in order to indicate its nature but also to make starker the gap that can open up between obligatory incantation and what actually goes on in practice.

It is hard to avoid the conclusion that much of the guidance is, on the whole, ignored. Those many health care professionals who understand about dignity on a human level, without bureaucratic direction, get on with the business of proper care, if they are allowed adequate time and resources to do so. Those staff and managers who cannot, or choose not to, comprehend what it is all about, simply carry on regardless with policies and practices that are demeaning to patients and incompatible with dignity.

So WHAT IS dignity? It is defined in the dictionary as a sense of pride in oneself, self-respect – or the state or quality of being worthy of honour or respect.[4]

Like neglect and abuse, we might think that we recognise it, and its absence, when we see it. This is probably so to a large extent, but not always. For instance, some may be tempted to take such a definition

---

3   NHS Choices. Accessed on 20 September 2010 at: www.nhs.uk/Services/Hospitals/ PatientFeedback/DefaultView.aspx?pid=RQQ31&id=1429.

4   *Concise Oxford Dictionary of Current English.* 8th ed. Oxford: Clarendon Press, 1990.

too literally. They maintain that if people lack mental capacity – to the extent that they are unaware of the degrading and undignified treatment to which they are being subjected – then in fact the care or treatment is by definition not demeaning or undignified. Self evidently, such a belief is tantamount to saying that the more vulnerable a person, the more can dignity be dispensed with.

The law courts have reacted against such a view, stating that it is not just the 'sentient or self-conscious who have dignity interests protected by the law'.[5] This extends even to unconsciousness, never mind to a conscious but mentally incapacitated person; it is 'demeaning to the human spirit to say that, being unconscious, he can have no interest in his personal privacy and dignity, in how he lives or dies'.[6]

A 2007 report prepared for the organisation, Help the Aged, attempted to divine the key elements of dignity required, if people are to maintain self-respect. These included communication (without which patients may feel unworthy and uncared for), privacy (including modesty and confidentiality), self-determination and autonomy, food and nutrition, pain and symptom control, personal hygiene (bathing, using the toilet) and death with dignity.[7]

Adding in another concept to the mix, Niall Dickson, the former chief executive of the King's Fund, referred in 2008 to a need for compassion on the part of health care staff. He maintained that it was diminishing in the National Health Service (NHS), but that without it, the system would fail.[8] For instance, in the following case, a patient reflected that a cleaner had more compassion in her little finger than all the nurses put together:

> We had more compassion from the cleaner... Yes, she was wonderful. She found us a fan because he was so hot; she found us pillows, didn't she, when his own had been pinched. She found him a little white one of those cotton blankets. Just to put over him. She was wonderful. We said to her, we were both together, and I said to her: you know, they ought to be doing the cleaning and you ought to be doing their job because you have

5   *R (Burke) v General Medical Council* [2004] EWHC 1879 (Admin), High Court (overall decision overturned by the Court of Appeal but not on this point).

6   *Airedale NHS Trust v Bland* [1993] AC 789, House of Lords.

7   Levenson, R. (2007) *The challenge of dignity in care: Upholding the rights of the individual.* London: Help the Aged. See also: Help the Aged (2008) *The challenge of assessing dignity in care.* London: Help the Aged.

8   'NHS fast losing its compassion.' BBC News, 30 December 2008. Accessed on 30 August 2010 at: http://news.bbc.co.uk/1/hi/health/7797868.stm.

> more compassion in your one little finger than there is in the whole – in the rest. And that was true, it really was.[9]

Another way of coming at dignity is to say what it is not. And two things it definitely isn't are neglect and abuse. Without these two unwanted guests, one should at least be well on the path to dignity, if not all the way there.

WHATEVER ITS PRECISE definition in the context of health care, the term 'dignity' – in policy and good practice statements – is not in short supply. Theoretically, this means there is no excuse for NHS executives, boards, senior management and staff to plead ignorance of what they should be doing, even supposing it were not naturally obvious.

The practical obstacle has been that dignity remains outside the inner sanctum. That is, it is not counted amongst the principal forces driving the Department of Health, strategic health authorities (SHAs) and NHS boards at local level. Performance, financial and ideological priorities are the currents in which politicians, senior civil servants and chief executives swim; dignity and compassion the mere surf high above their heads, to which they seem profoundly oblivious.

Nonetheless, if spray it is, then there is plenty of it. This is what is so troubling. At work is apparently a law of inverse proportions; the more the guidance about dignity, the greater the departure from it.

AT A VERY general level, *The NHS Plan* – the overarching government policy for health care between 2000 and 2010 – stated very simply:

> The NHS will treat patients as individuals, with respect for their dignity.[10]

Within a year, the Department of Health had published good practice guidance about the nursing care of older people. Its Standing Nursing and Midwifery Advisory Committee laid down the gauntlet:

> During the acute phase of illness, older people [should] receive services and care, which ensure their dignity and privacy.[11]

---

9   Francis, R. (Chair) (2010) *Independent Inquiry into care provided by Mid Staffordshire NHS Foundation Trust January 2005–March 2009.* London: The Stationery Office, p.129.

10 Secretary of State for Health (2000) *The NHS Plan: A plan for investment, a plan for reform.* Cm 4818-I. London: The Stationery Office, p.4.

11 Standing Nursing and Midwifery Advisory Committee (2001) *Caring for older people, a nursing priority, practice guidance: Principles, standards and indicators, a resource tool.* London: Department of Health, p.3.

It went on to stipulate that personal hygiene and appearance should be maintained according to the older person's wishes and care should not be carried out in public view.[12]

In 2001 also, the *National Service Framework for Older People* heralded a ten-year plan to ensure 'that all older people and their carers are always treated with respect, dignity and fairness'.[13]

Nonetheless, even back in the early 2000s, sober elements at the Department of Health must have quietly doubted easy success; at the very least it was going to be a long haul. The Department produced detailed guidance in the form of a 'tool' for practitioners. It was called *Essence of Care* and was about 'getting the basics right'. Though issued by the NHS Modernisation Agency (part of the Department of Health), it was a reminder that change did not mean throwing out the fundamentals of care with the bath water.

This guidance concentrated on continence and bladder and bowel care, personal and oral hygiene, food and nutrition, pressure ulcers, privacy and dignity, record keeping – and safety of clients with mental health needs in acute mental health and general hospital settings.[14] In particular, the *Essence of Care* stated that patients should benefit from care focused upon respect for the individual. This would include privacy, dignity and modesty.[15]

The decade wore on, but further reminders were required. In 2006, the Department of Health published standards about better health care, to be used by the Healthcare Commission in its regulatory role. The guidance, at heart, repeated what had already been said: health care organisations should ensure that 'staff treat patients, their relatives and carers with dignity and respect'.[16]

Two years later, Lord Darzi, a clinician and leading surgeon, produced a much trumpeted report for the Department of Health. Called *High quality care for all*, it too invoked the watchwords of dignity and respect.

12 Standing Nursing and Midwifery Advisory Committee (2001) *Caring for older people, a nursing priority, practice guidance: Principles, standards and indicators, a resource tool.* London: Department of Health, p.3.

13 DH (Department of Health) (2001) *National Service Framework for Older People.* London: DH, Foreword.

14 NHS Modernisation Agency (2003) *Essence of Care: Patient focused benchmarks for clinical governance.* London: Department of Health, p.1. (Original edition published in 2001; revised again in 2010 as DH (Department of Health) (2010) *Essence of Care: Benchmarks for the fundamental aspects of care.* London: DH.)

15 NHS Modernisation Agency (2003) *Essence of Care: Benchmarks for privacy and dignity.* London: Department of Health, p.1. (Revised from 2001 edition.)

16 DH (Department of Health) (2006) *Standards for better health.* London: DH, p.14.

> It is the quality of that care that really matters. People want to know they will receive effective treatment. They want care that is personal to them, and to be shown compassion, dignity and respect by those caring for them. People want to be reassured that they will be safe in the care of the NHS.[17]

As for undignified and neglectful care, the report failed to spell out just what the problem really was, wheeling out rather general, strategic and ideological statements. Fine, maybe, as far as they went, but more vision than concrete solution. Little help to those suffering on the wards.

The previous year, the Healthcare Commission had stated in a national report that dignity was a human rights issue. It entreated NHS trusts to ensure that people were not subject to inhumane and degrading treatment – such as being left in soiled clothes, being provided with inadequate nutrition, being given no help with eating, or being placed in situations that patients found embarrassing.[18] The Commission was doing its best within its limits, but the report gives the impression of a cry for help from an organisation that was up against it. It was a substitute for what the Commission should have been doing but had failed to: putting a firm stop to undignified care.

In 2009, a newly formed Care Quality Commission (CQC), the current health care regulator, weighed in. Guidance now states that health care providers should uphold and maintain the privacy, dignity and independence of people who use services.[19] A second set of guidance from the Commission states that the environment should allow for privacy in relation to the intimate care, treatment and support needs of people.[20]

A DECADE OF imploration has passed but evidence of progress is thin on the ground. In 2010, the outgoing Labour government made one last broad, electoral gesture in the form of *The NHS Constitution*. This duly refers to 'guaranteed' rights including a 'professional standard of care', to services being provided in a 'clean and safe environment' and to patients

17 Secretary of State for Health (2008) *High quality care for all: NHS next stage review final report.* Cm 7432. London: The Stationery Office, p.33.

18 Healthcare Commission (2007) *Caring for dignity: A national report on dignity in care for older people while in hospital.* London: Healthcare Commission, p.9.

19 CQC (Care Quality Commission) (2009) *Guidance about compliance: Summary of regulations, outcomes and judgement framework.* London: CQC, p.8.

20 CQC (Care Quality Commission) (2009) *Guidance about compliance: Essential standards of quality and safety.* London: CQC, p.46.

being 'treated with dignity and respect' in accordance with their human rights.[21]

It can be argued that repetition, even if ineffective, is at least harmless. Nevertheless, it takes some *chutzpah*, for a government of any political hue that has been implicated in such dreadful care for so long, to continue to wheel out such misleading statements. This is especially so, when there is no easy or new way to enforce the 'guarantee'. For this *Constitution* creates no new legal rights. Any remedy for 'breach' of it relies on the same well-worn channels of complaints procedure or legal remedy, which hitherto have so staggeringly failed to protect vulnerable patients. It is very hard to avoid the conclusion that the *Constitution* was and is empty, gesticulation only.

If guidance and entreaty from central government have had little effect, nonetheless there remains another source, namely, ethical codes, overseen and legally enforceable by regulatory bodies for the health care professions. From them help should be at hand; if detached bureaucrats in government departments can't get their guidance and good practice to stick, surely the caring professions can.

HOSPITAL PATIENTS ARE treated and cared for by health care professionals, who also have oversight of non-professionally qualified health care assistants. Thus, when people are neglected, this takes place at the hands of trained individuals who are bound by ethical codes and guidance. The codes are not over long, are readable and, as one would expect, explicit about the upholding of patient dignity. If all professionals followed the codes to the letter, there would be no undignified treatment in health care. At its most basic level, this proposition holds true even if one accepts that there are sometimes real obstacles – such as under-staffing, lack of resources and management priorities inimical to good patient care   to professionals achieving this.

It sounds so straightforward. General Medical Council (GMC) guidance states that, amongst other things, doctors should (a) be polite, considerate and honest, (b) treat patients with dignity, (c) treat each patient as an individual, and (d) respect patients' privacy and right to confidentiality.[22] The Nursing and Midwifery Council's (NMC) *Code* states that:

---

21   DH (Department of Health) (2010) *The NHS Constitution.* London: DH, p.6.
22   GMC (General Medical Council) (2006) *Good medical care.* London: GMC, p.15.

> You must treat people as individuals and respect their dignity. You
> must not discriminate in any way against those in your care. You
> must treat people kindly and considerately.[23]

The Health Professions Council (HPC) regulates various health
professionals other than doctors, nurses and midwives. These are
arts therapists, biomedical scientists, chiropodists and podiatrists,
clinical scientists, dieticians, hearing aid dispensers, occupational
therapists, operating department practitioners, orthoptists, paramedics,
physiotherapists, practitioner psychologists, prosthetists and orthotists,
radiographers, and speech and language therapists. A lot of professionals
but bound by a simple rule: 'You must treat service users with respect and
dignity.'[24]

There is in addition a *Code of conduct for NHS managers*, which states:

> I will respect and treat with dignity and fairness, the public,
> patients, relatives, carers, NHS staff and partners in other
> agencies.[25]

This last code sounds fine but lacks teeth. There is no formal, legal
mechanism for sanctions against managers who breach it. This contrasts
with the legally based sanctions that lie against medical doctors, nurses
and allied health professionals for over-stepping the mark.

Notwithstanding these codes and the protestations made by the
professional bodies that enforce them, the evidence suggests that many
health care professionals are more or less active, or at least complicit,
in poor and sometimes shocking health care. Many others are passive
observers; some have spoken out, many have not. It seems then that
in the face of systematic neglectful care, as opposed to the individual
misdemeanours, the codes lie relatively dormant.

PERHAPS THEN, AFTER all, there is some harm in endless repetition of
'all the good guidance'. That is, if its track record is one of limited
effectiveness and, as already pointed out above, if it is often ignored. It
can degenerate into overkill; the 2003 edition of *Essence of Care* ran to

---

23 NMC (Nursing and Midwifery Council) (2008) *The Code: Standards of conduct, performance and ethics for nurses and midwives.* London: NMC, p.2.

24 HPC (Health Professions Council) (2008) *Standards of conduct, performance and ethics.* London: HPC, p.8.

25 DH (Department of Health) (2002) *Code of conduct for NHS managers.* London: DH, p.4.

175 pages;[26] its successor in 2010 to 322 pages.[27] It is arguable that the latest version has even further obscured – by its bulk and repetitious, formulaic and vague instructions – matters of basic care. It is almost as if the Department of Health believes that, by issuing more and voluminous guidance, the world will at some point transmute from base metal into the gold of decent care. In fact, it appears that the size of such guidance is in direct proportion to the Department's self-induced impotence on the matter.

Not only do people stop taking any notice, but the guidance may also come to play a more damaging role. It is plain that central government, as well as the NHS bodies at local level echoing their essentially political masters, fall too often into the trap of believing what they say and write.

They announce a new policy, issue guidance and believe the job is done. The promise made is enough; of central government at the turn of the millennium, it could be said: 'if they promised something no doubt it would happen. If they said something of course it was true.'[28] When reality starts to break in, they need a further quick fix to blot it out once more; so more guidance gets issued. In this sense, the guidance acts as a drug that first seduces and then hooks policymakers. It takes the edge off reality, insulates them from the consequences of their decisions and fuels their incredulity about accounts of poor care.

CENTRAL GOVERNMENT AND NHS trusts spend a lot of time telling us how they provide modern, efficient and dignified health care, world class, in fact. There is a striking incongruity between these statements and some of the care now dispensed, as well as corresponding lack of insight. An apparently unshakeable complacency precludes contemplation of the fact that for some patients we are still at an elementary stage in achieving dignity; a stage that policymakers and senior management assume we have long since left behind in the great march of progress.

A corrective to this comes in the form of an essay written by George Orwell, called 'How the poor die'. It recalled his experience in 1929 of a French hospital in Paris. Some of what he writes corresponds with descriptions in this book; most ironically he is also emphatic how what he observed and experienced could not happen in English hospitals. In

---

26 NHS Modernisation Agency (2003) *Essence of Care: Patient focused benchmarks for clinical governance.* London: Department of Health.

27 DH (Department of Health) (2010) *Essence of Care: Benchmarks for the fundamental aspects of care.* London: DH.

28 Marr, A. (2009) *A history of modern Britain.* London: Pan, p.514.

particular, he refers amongst other things to faecal smell, beds excessively close together, patients having to help themselves or go without, lack of privacy, staff who don't talk to the patients, people dying with nobody caring much, unwashed constipated patients on unmade beds, and dirt:

> In the year 1929 I spent several weeks in the Hôpital X, in... Paris... It was a long, rather low, ill-lit room, full of murmuring voices and with three rows of beds surprisingly close together. There was a foul smell, faecal and yet sweetish. As I lay down I saw on a bed nearly opposite me a small, round-shouldered, sandy-haired man sitting half naked while a doctor and a student performed some strange operation on him...it was my first experience of doctors who handle you without speaking to you or, in a human sense, taking any notice of you...
>
> At five in the morning the nurses came round, woke the patients and took their temperatures, but did not wash them. If you were well enough you washed yourself, otherwise you depended on the kindness of some walking patient. It was generally patients, too, who carried the bed bottles and the grim bedpan, nicknamed la casserole... And the sordid publicity of dying in such a place! In the Hôpital X the beds were very close together and there were no screens...
>
> But it is a fact that you would not in any English hospitals see some of the things I saw in the Hôpital X. This business of people just dying like animals, for instance, with nobody standing by, nobody interested, the death not even noticed till the morning – this happened more than once... You certainly would not see that in England... A thing we perhaps underrate in England is the advantage we enjoy in having large numbers of well-trained and rigidly-disciplined nurses...they don't let you lie unwashed and constipated on an unmade bed... You wouldn't, either, see in England such dirt as existed in the Hôpital X...[29]

As with other historical comparisons made in this book, circumspection is called for. But, equally, it is surely folly not to recognise the salutary nature of such recollections from the recent past. In fact in at least one respect, the hospital described did better than we sometimes hear happens now.

For instance, in 21st-century England, there are many reports of vulnerable patients not being assisted with bowel and bladder function in a dignified manner. They are left to wet their bed or worse, and then

29 Orwell, G. (2003) 'How the poor die.' In G. Orwell. *Shooting an elephant and other essays.* London: Penguin Books, pp.277–90. (Essay first published in 1946.)

to lie in it; compare George Orwell's description of the nurse who stood beside his neighbour's bed for a long time with a bed bottle:

> My right-hand neighbour was a little red-haired cobbler with one leg shorter than the other... His worst suffering was when he urinated, which he did with the greatest difficulty. A nurse would bring him the bed bottle and then for a long time stand beside his bed, whistling, as grooms are said to do with horses, until at last with an agonized shriek of "Je Pisse!" he would get started...[30]

30 Orwell, G. (2003) 'How the poor die.' In G. Orwell. *Shooting an elephant and other essays.* London: Penguin Books, p.281. (Essay first published in 1946.)

6

Dignity in Care: All the Bad Practice

We respond with humanity and kindness to each person's pain, distress, anxiety or need. We search for things we can do, however small, to give comfort and relieve suffering… We do not wait to be asked because we care. (NHS Constitution: pledge by the NHS, 2010)[1]

We got there about 10 o'clock and I could not believe my eyes. The door was wide open. There were people walking past. Mum was in bed with the cot sides up and she hadn't got a stitch of clothing on. I mean, she would have been horrified. She was completely naked and if I said covered in faeces, she was. It was everywhere. It was in her hair, her eyes, her nails, her hands and on all the cot side, so she had obviously been trying to lift herself up or move about, because the bed was covered and it was literally everywhere and it was dried. It would have been there a long time, it wasn't new. (Mid Staffordshire NHS Foundation Trust: evidence to the Independent Inquiry, 2009)[2]

The contrast between these two quotes casts a harsh light into what is sometimes a chasm between the official line and the real world. Thus, whilst the previous chapter outlined a glut of good practice guidance and statements about dignity, this one illustrates the other, grubbier, side of the coin. The chapters, after this one, are also about dignity but focus on more specific aspects of it.

A chart needs plotting from 1997 onwards, of how the dignity of hospital patients has been, and continues to be, undermined. Before doing so, the plight and death of Mrs Clara Stokes in 2010, former Land Army girl during the Second World War, sets the dismal scene.

IN MAY 2010, Luton and Dunstable Hospital apologised to the daughter of Mrs Stokes who had taken photographs and kept notes during daily

---

1   DH (Department of Health) (2010) *The NHS Constitution*. London: DH, p.12.
2   Quoted in: Francis, R. (Chair) (2010) *Independent Inquiry into care provided by Mid Staffordshire NHS Foundation Trust January 2005–March 2009*. London: The Stationery Office, p.55.

visits. Her daughter recounted how her 84-year-old mother had been admitted in December 2009 to hospital, where she subsequently died, helpless and confused after a stroke. She was left dehydrated, hungry and lying in her own faeces for six hours, as she was ignored by overworked nurses. Her water was left out of reach, and she had not been helped to drink for 16 hours.

The daughter and granddaughter were so appalled at what they observed on the ward that they tried to help other patients with their food – but were forbidden by nurses on health and safety grounds. They took to visiting and remaining in the stroke ward daily, between midday and 8pm, changing, washing and feeding Mrs Stokes. At one point, they were excluded from the ward because of an outbreak of a stomach bug. When they were allowed back on the ward, they related how:

> We finally walked in and my daughter said what is that under her arm? We lifted it up and she was covered in her own diarrhoea. She was paralysed and couldn't call for help. This was after 3pm in the afternoon and the last time she had been checked was at 9am.

The daughter's account continued of how, a day later, the family found her foot trapped between bed posts, caused by a faulty bed pump. She had to be freed by the matron. The daughter recalled how the nurses were so overworked they had no time to be compassionate:

> They gave out food but left it out of reach of patients. You are lying there, hungry, you can't move because you've had a stroke and there is food just out of reach. We were warned not to feed them but you can't just sit there and watch.

On another occasion, a nurse misread Mrs Stokes' notes and forced crushed tablets down her throat, almost causing her to choke to death.

The hospital's immediate response to the complaint was to deny everything; it referred to 'compelling evidence' from detailed documentation that Mrs Stokes had received attentive, good nursing care.[3] Within a month the tune had changed. Having actually now investigated the complaint, the hospital conceded that under-staffing on the stroke ward had led to unacceptable mistakes in the care of Mrs Stokes, including leaving her lying in diarrhoea for so long.[4]

---

3   Wilkes, D. (2010) 'How could this happen? Former Land Girl honoured by Brown dies after she is left to "wallow in her own filth" on NHS ward.' *Daily Mail*, 28 April.

4   'Daughter whose Land Girl mother was left to die in filth on NHS ward wins apology from hospital chief.' *Daily Mail*, 25 May 2010.

The aftermath saw the irony, the anger and the political ramifications emerge. In July 2008, in recognition of her war-time contribution, Mrs Stokes had been awarded a medal and certificate at a ceremony in Bedford by the then Prime Minister, Gordon Brown. Now, in 2010, her daughter had written to him to complain; he had referred the matter to the Department of Health. The latter almost certainly leant on the National Health Service (NHS) Trust to resolve the matter and to give way with reasonable grace, given the ample, adverse Press coverage. The daughter's view was that the Prime Minister would not be making claims about how good the NHS was if it had been his own mother treated in such an inhumane way, namely, left in her own filth and treated worse than a dog.[5]

A footnote. Luton and Dunstable Hospital was an NHS foundation trust, which meant it was one of the designated elite of NHS hospitals. Yet three months before Mrs Stokes' admission in December 2009, inspectors from the Care Quality Commission (CQC) had warned the hospital about squalid conditions on the stroke ward, including soiled curtains, sticky medical equipment and contaminated commodes.[6] This suggests that the care of Mrs Stokes was no mere eccentricity on an otherwise spick, span and caring ward. By September 2010, the CQC had removed the final condition, relating to infection, which the Trust had been ordered to meet by the Commission – and the NHS Trust was, for the time being, in the clear. The removal of this condition was on the basis that the Trust had provided 'sufficient assurance of compliance'.[7]

THIRTEEN YEARS PRIOR to these events in Luton, Martin Bright, as already noted, had been telling of the ordeal suffered by his 88-year-old grandmother. Rushed to hospital following a stroke, she had been left for hours on a trolley in a corridor. Eventually put on a mixed ward, she was given neither a drip to help control her diabetes nor drops for her glaucoma. For five days she was left without food or drink because no speech therapist was available to test her swallowing reflex. Transferred to a female geriatric ward, she was then found with her head on a pillow soaked from a leaking drip and on another occasion lying in her own faeces. Without speech, she left notes by her bedside about the neglect

---

5   Wilkes, D. (2010) 'How could this happen? Former Land Girl honoured by Brown dies after she is left to "wallow in her own filth" on NHS ward.' *Daily Mail*, 28 April.

6   Rayner, G. (2010) 'Former Land Girl honoured by Gordon Brown dies after "inhumane" NHS treatment.' *Daily Telegraph*, 28 April.

7   CQC (Care Quality Commission) (2010) *Review of compliance: Luton and Dunstable NHS Foundation Trust*. London: CQC.

she had endured, including telephone calls to her not being put through by staff – and attempts to force feed her through her nose, without her consent. In addition, without her knowledge, the doctors had written that she was not to be resuscitated.[8] This story became associated with Help the Aged's Dignity on the Ward campaign.

In that same year of 1997, Help the Aged had surveyed complaints received by community health councils about the care of older people in hospital. The most common complaints included inadequate (or lack of) care, lack of respect shown by nurses, poor communication, lack of privacy and dignity, inappropriate discharges from hospital, lack of assistance with eating and dressing and washing, neglect of personal hygiene, lack of staff time and staff shortages.[9]

By 2001 the Department of Health's Standing Nursing and Midwifery Advisory Committee advised that a 'large critical literature has been amassed which shows that current standards of care often fail to preserve older people's dignity, privacy, autonomy and independence'.[10]

The Committee went on to point out that hospital nurses had in principle to attend to not just acute symptoms but also to the needs of the whole person including nutrition, tissue viability and promotion of independent activity. Yet it reported that the nursing care of older people was in practice deficient in such very fundamental aspects including the need for food, fluid, rest, activity and elimination – and recognition of people's psychological, mental health and rehabilitation needs. The Committee identified an ominous list of recurring areas of concern to be found in practice:

- respect for older people's dignity
- promotion of choice, involvement and independence
- communication with older people and their carers
- individualised care and its management
- continence
- dementia
- mental health

8   As recounted in: Bright, M. (2006) 'The public will judge this government not by how bold it was in challenging left-liberal shibboleths, but whether its grandmothers were treated with respect in hospital.' *New Statesman*, 3 April.

9   Willcock, K. (1997) *The tip of the iceberg: A survey of complaints registered by community health councils concerning the care of older people in NHS hospitals.* London: Help the Aged.

10 Standing Nursing and Midwifery Advisory Committee (2001) *Caring for older people: A nursing priority integrating knowledge, practice and values: A report.* London: Department of Health, p.3.

- mobility
- nutrition and hydration
- pain management
- palliative care
- pressure damage prevention and management.

The Commission spoke of loss of privacy and dignity on mixed-sex wards and of toilet doors not locking. This would then mean that people might not use the toilet at all, becoming more dependent through using a commode or bedpan instead.[11]

Ominous, because the Committee's warning of what was happening went essentially unheeded by central government, a few lightweight measures excepted, because the list it had compiled anticipated accurately all that was to go wrong in the coming decade.

Alan Milburn, Secretary of State for Health in 2001, responded to the Committee's findings with an airy statement, to the effect that the government had the matter in hand and that a radical blueprint – the *National Service Framework for Older People* – would root out age discrimination.[12] The *Framework* was legally weak, less than a biting priority, and grafted on to numerous incompatibilities beneath. This made the minister's statement unconvincing at the time and, in hindsight, fatuous.

TAMESIDE GENERAL HOSPITAL has not been at the centre of a highly publicised major scandal of the order of some other hospitals. Equally, it has cultivated a degree of notoriety of its own. Highlighting this here is not necessarily to suggest that it is any worse or better than many other hospitals, though it may be. It may also have received more publicity because of an effective patient action group and an incisive coroner. In any event, it suffices as an illustration.

In 2007, an independent review of care at Tameside was published. It accentuated a long list of failings, which had been collated by the Tameside Hospital Action Group. Ten years on from the inception of *The Observer* campaign, it represented the very antithesis of all the good practice guidance, the easy words of politicians, the smooth reassurance of

---

11 Standing Nursing and Midwifery Advisory Committee (2001) *Caring for older people: A nursing priority integrating knowledge, practice and values: A report.* London: Department of Health, pp. 17–18, 29.

12 Laurance, J. (2001) 'Routine abuse of elderly in NHS care.' *The Independent*, 28 March.

NHS trust chief executives and chairmen – and the hopes of campaigners. The roll call is lengthy and dispiriting and so warrants reproduction here:

- basic nursing care of older people with regard to nutrition, hydration, continence, personal hygiene and pressure area care
- lack of confidence in medical management
- management of infections such as MRSA and *Clostridium difficile*
- lack of proactive communication between nurses and relatives, doctors and relatives, doctors and nurses
- responsiveness of the complaints procedure
- lack of nurses' knowledge regarding patients' deterioration
- staff intimidation
- alteration of notes
- dirty wards
- poor décor
- poor hygiene practices, lack of basic washing and bathing
- staffing shortages
- uncaring attitude of nurses
- poor nursing assessments of patient needs
- rudeness and aggression from doctors
- lack of responsiveness to patients' needs
- poor information giving from doctors and nurses
- failure to inform relatives about falls or deterioration in a patient's condition
- relatives not involved in plans for discharge
- development of pressure sores
- lack of help regarding feeding and drinking
- poor documentation of fluid balance especially in vulnerable patients
- dependence on relatives to provide basic care
- call bells left out of reach
- patients left in wet beds, being told to wet the bed
- lack of investigations and treatment

- mixed-sex wards and toilets
- management of MRSA and *Clostridium difficile* Toxin.[13]

The review unsurprisingly stated that the 'quality of care experienced by some patients over a number of years had been seriously deficient'; it also recorded that the Trust was trying to improve things.

The review had been set up following a coroner's severe criticism of the hospital in 2006, after the death of four older people.[14] He condemned the treatment it had offered them. 'Absolutely despicable' was the treatment of an 84-year-old war veteran, Mr Watkins Davies, for whom a verdict of accidental death was given. He had entered hospital with a fractured hip, contracted MRSA and then been subjected to a catalogue of nursing failures. This included his falling out of a chair when washing and then receiving no X-ray, being left to lie in his own waste and in severe pain for hours, and having his meals left six feet beyond his reach.

Another patient, Mrs Hilda Douglas (a 75-year-old voluntary worker), had died from a heart attack at the hospital after fracturing her pelvis following a fall from a hospital trolley; no record of the fall had been made. Her medication had been left on the floor, a chaotic situation in the view of the coroner. A third person, Mr Raymond Lees, died with MRSA after a knee operation. During his hospital stay, his waist had shrunk by 14 inches. And Mr James Kelly, recovering from surgery, contracted pneumonia after being left sitting in a dressing gown in a draught.

The coroner said he would contact the chief executive about the basic nursing care provided and would scrutinise carefully future deaths at the hospital. Asked for comment at the time about the coroner's findings, the Health Minister's reply was a *non sequitur*: it was his understanding that the hospital had a system to ensure that patients received 'high quality care'.[15]

Moving forward three years, in March 2010, the CQC visited the hospital and imposed an improvement plan on the responsible trust, the Tameside and Glossop Acute Services NHS Trust. This was part of its registration requirements as a health care provider under the *Health and Social Care Act 2008*. Three months later, the Commission removed the

13 Fielding, F. (Professor Dame) (2007) *Independent review of older people's care at Tameside General Hospital.* Manchester: NHS North West, p.5.

14 Fielding, F. (Professor Dame) (2007) *Independent review of older people's care at Tameside General Hospital.* Manchester: NHS North West, p.2.

15 Jenkins, R. (2006) 'Hospital under attack over "painful, degrading deaths".' *The Times*, 29 September.

compliance conditions, though recorded that patient safety and welfare remained a 'moderate concern'.[16]

Plainly, three years on, the hospital had made progress but it was less than overwhelming; the Commission's general approval in 2010 does not mean that the local patient action group had been imagining things.

In early 2009, for example, a family kept a diary of what had happened to their 79-year-old relative, Mrs Betty Dunn. She had been admitted to Tameside General Hospital with a routine stomach problem but deteriorated over a six-week period and then died after contracting *Clostridium difficile*. The diary referred to her being forced to sleep on a bare mattress, having to wait 40 minutes for a bedpan, being treated by staff who could barely speak English and being made to eat a food substitute against medical advice. The family even called the police at one point, so concerned were they.

On one occasion, her saline drip had come out and was leaking all over the floor. Her arm was bleeding, her feet were blue with cold and her catheter had come out. On another, her daughter noticed that the antibiotic drip was blocked; the nurse said that it needed flushing, but there was no way she was going to do that and it would have to wait. As a result Mrs Dunn missed her medication. Despite wearing a wristband indicating allergy to penicillin, she was given it. A doctor finally stopped this, but the nurses then mistakenly discontinued all the other antibiotics she was receiving as well. The hospital seemed to accept the substance of the complaint; it apologised for shortcomings in the care of Mrs Dunn.[17]

Notwithstanding this background of practical issues facing patients, the nature of a report commissioned by the regulatory body for the elite foundation trusts, Monitor, is telling. It is about governance at the Trust.[18] Although the Press characterised it as 'slamming' the Trust,[19] it is in fact a report which can more or less be read without realising just what the Trust's business was, far less that it was with patients, their safety and their dignity – all of which had been consistently reported as compromised over the last few years. The report's concentration on the management process, and indeed management speak, seems to reflect the

---

16 CQC (Care Quality Commission) (2010) *Review of compliance: Tameside Hospital NHS Foundation Trust, Tameside General Hospital*. London: CQC, pp.6–7.

17 Tozer, J. (2009) 'Diary of despair of pensioner who died in "zoo" hospital after "catalogue of blunders by staff".' *Daily Mail*, 7 July.

18 Korn Ferry Whitehead Mann (2010) *Review of integrated governance: Tameside NHS Foundation Trust, June 2010*. London: KFWHM.

19 Crook, A. (2010) 'Tameside Hospital bosses slammed in new report.' *Manchester Evening News*, 30 June.

inward looking and detached way in which NHS boards work. Reading a report such as this, it is little wonder that the patient ends up at the bottom of the pile.

In June 2010 also, NHS North West published its own report into Tameside, pointing to difficulties in finding out just what was going on in the hospital, and about complaints and patient experience.[20] This report, in turn, had followed a rating by the Dr Foster 2009 hospital guide, which indicated high mortality rates at the hospital and gave a score of 4.79 per cent for patient safety.[21]

BY THE MIDDLE of the decade, concerned onlookers were weighing in with reports of poor care from around the country and with corresponding calls for dignity. The tempo needed to be raised, once it had become clear that the white magic of the *National Service Framework for Older People* was not so potent in the more desolate wastes of health care. In 2006, the British Geriatrics Society and Age Concern England, together with a number of other organisations, noted the following practices that were continuing to undermine people's dignity and privacy:

- visiting at ward rounds
- split-back nightdresses
- inappropriate hoists
- mixed-sex wards on medical admissions units
- patients wearing pads without underwear
- ward curtains or nightdresses or smocks which did not fit properly, exposing patients or allowing 'mooning'
- hoisting patients without covers.[22]

And it was in 2007 that Help the Aged marked the 10th anniversary of its Dignity on the Ward campaign. The message was not cheerful; it was 'clear that dignity is denied to many of our citizens at a perilously low point in their lives'.[23]

20 NHS North West (2010) *NHS Tameside and Glossop Review: Commissioning for quality and safety.* Manchester: NHS North West.

21 Dr Foster Health. *Tameside Hospital NHS Foundation Trust: Quality account for 2008/09.* Accessed on 20 October 2010 at: www.drfosterhealth.co.uk/quality-accounts/trust.aspx?otype=2&id=118.

22 British Geriatrics Society, Age Concern England, Department of Geriatric Medicine (Cardiff University), Carers UK, Continence Foundation, Help the Aged, InContact and Royal College of Nursing (2006) *Behind closed doors: Using the toilet in private.* London: British Geriatrics Society.

23 Levenson, R. (2007) *The challenge of dignity in care: Upholding the rights of the individual.* London: Help the Aged, p.4.

But another year on and the Mental Health Act Commission was making a veiled reference to the war between the forces of light and dark being waged in our hospitals. Certainly evil is not a word that regulatory bodies tend to use these days, but in 2008, in its biennial report, the Commission used the term, albeit vicariously. It harked back to the *Parliamentary Inquiry into madhouses of 1815/6* that had identified a number of 'basic evils'. The Commission asked what possible comparisons could be made between care at the beginning of the 19th century and care in the early 21st century. This was especially in the light of the enormous differences in medical knowledge, treatment and social structure.

In fact, its report found a number of uncomfortable parallels, dishing up a reminder that hospitals were in some instances failing patients badly; the Commission had come across a slew of unacceptable practices undermining people's dignity, privacy and safety.[24]

These included, for instance, restrictions on bathing because of staff shortages, inappropriate restraint, a dying man being nursed in the dining room while other patients were having lunch (again, because of lack of staff), vulnerable women housed with predatory men, blinds to patients' rooms being kept open permanently for staff convenience, seclusion rooms with no privacy to use the toilet, new acute wards being run at *135 per cent* bed occupancy with patients sleeping in day rooms and staff run off their feet, inappropriate use of closed circuit television – and a woman in seclusion deprived of sanitary protection whilst menstruating.[25]

MUCH HAS BEEN made of the continuation of mixed-sex wards, and many the political promises to end the affront to dignity that they are perceived to represent. However, mixed sex or not, it would help not to leave patients totally exposed.

At the age of 86, the Reverend John Brindle was not only healthy but had never been to hospital in his life. However, he suffered a knock to his head and was admitted for tests to the University Hospitals of Morecambe Bay NHS Trust. His daughter recounted how she visited and found him completely naked, save for an incontinence pad; his feet were blue with cold. She dressed him, only to be reprimanded by a nurse for doing so; it constituted a breach of health and safety rules. When the nurse was asked why he was in incontinence pads and not being helped to the toilet, she

---

24 Mental Health Act Commission (2008) *Risk, rights, recovery: Twelfth biennial report, 2005–2007.* London: Mental Health Act Commission, pp.10–11.

25 Mental Health Act Commission (2008) *Risk, rights, recovery: Twelfth biennial report, 2005–2007.* London: Mental Health Act Commission, pp.17–29.

replied that he was incontinent. The daughter pointed out that he had been continent before admission to the ward. She reflected: 'He seemed to have given up completely. This man, who was proud and private, was treated like a child, like a no-hoper.' His family tried to move him to a private hospital, but he died before this could be organised. The Trust stated it was investigating.[26]

Naked to the ward. A man who had worked in the NHS for over 20 years told of how his stepfather, having suffered a series of strokes, was admitted to Rotherham General Hospital. Cure and rehabilitation were out of the question, but he had assumed that his stepfather's suffering would be minimised and his dignity preserved. Of the catalogue of undignified care, one item concerned a visit when the family came on to the ward, to find the stepfather naked on his bed, with no surrounding screens and no staff to be seen. He was in and out of consciousness and could not move. A senior nurse apologised but had no explanation as to how it had been allowed to happen.[27]

Joyce Brassam was 90 years old and blind. She related how she had been training a new blind dog, but tripped and broke her knee cap. She was admitted to hospital. One morning, she was helped out of bed by a nurse, who took off her nightdress, and then sat her down in a chair. A shout for a break was heard; the nurse went away leaving her naked in the chair. She sat there until coffee time, when somebody looked in through the curtain and saw her still there, still naked.[28]

A relative told of her visit to Stafford Hospital and of an elderly man with a hospital gown half on, covered in faeces, with no help from nurses forthcoming. The account uses forthright and earthy language, and merits reproducing in detail:

> I will never forget him, a tall elderly man. He was covered all the way down in faeces, he was showing all of his genitals, and I said to [my son]: it is a good job your Nan can't see. I just shut the blinds... Nurses were down on the nursing station towards the bottom of the door, and this poor guy was shouting... I went and got to the nearest bed which I thought was his bed... I got this duvet and I said: come on, sweetheart, and I talked to him and got him back and sat him down on his chair, covered him over. And I pulled the blinds round and I went down to the

---

26   Revill, J. (2007) 'The dirty truth on the wards.' *The Observer*, 14 October.
27   Patient Opinion (2008) 'Concern about poor nursing care on Rotherham hospital ward.' Accessed on 20 September 2010 at: www.patientopinion.org.uk/opinions/7826.
28   'Sharing experiences of care.' BBC News, 20 July 2005. Accessed on 20 September 2010 at: http://news.bbc.co.uk/1/hi/programmes/panorama/4701329.stm.

nurses' station. I said: can somebody please come and help this poor guy? And this nurse turned round and said: who? I said in the bay opposite where my Mum is. Oh: that is Mr […], he has lost it. I says: no, he has not lost it. I says: that man is crying for, I think it is his wife. That man is somebody's husband, he is somebody's Dad, I says, he was somebody's son. I says: now get your arse from that desk and get up there and see to that man. He is caked from head to foot in crap. I said: now get up there and wash that man down and give him some dignity. That man was left 25 minutes and no one came to that man while me and my son were on that ward and I was thoroughly disgusted. I thought a dog at a vet's would not be left like that, and this guy, he has probably fought in two World Wars, has been left.[29]

IF, IN THE future, a turning point is ever identified, when the tide imperceptibly turned and flowed toward dignity in care, then the Mid Staffordshire NHS Foundation Trust may turn out to be that juncture. The Healthcare Commission made ripples when it reported in March 2009 but it was the waves of the Independent Inquiry a year later that rocked the boat. And the Public Inquiry, due to be published in 2011, carries the potential for upset and capsize.

The Commission reported multiple failures in care that compromised the dignity of patients. These included *not* doing the following things: answering call bells, assisting people to the toilet or commode, respecting privacy and dignity, giving medication promptly and appropriately and making sure it was taken, helping with food and drink, completing charts accurately, paying attention to skin and avoiding pressure sores.[30]

The subsequent Independent Inquiry focused explicitly at the outset on the headings in the Department of Health's document, *Essence of Care*,[31] nine years after the latter's original publication date and seven since its revision. It found deficiencies in continence and bladder and bowel care, safety, personal and oral hygiene, nutrition and hydration, pressure area care, cleanliness and infection control, privacy and dignity, record keeping, diagnosis and treatment, communication, and the management

29 Francis, R. (Chair) (2010) *Independent Inquiry into care provided by Mid Staffordshire NHS Foundation Trust January 2005–March 2009*. London: The Stationery Office, p.110.
30 Healthcare Commission (2009) *Investigation into Mid Staffordshire NHS Foundation Trust, March 2009*. London: Healthcare Commission, p.35.
31 NHS Modernisation Agency (2003) *Essence of Care: Benchmarks for privacy and dignity*. London: Department of Health. (Revised again in 2010: DH (Department of Health) (2010) *Essence of Care: Benchmarks for the fundamental aspects of care*. London: DH.)

of discharge from hospital.[32] These were the very types of defect that the Standing Nursing and Midwifery Advisory Committee had so aptly stressed no fewer than nine years before.

Under the heading 'privacy and dignity' in particular, the Inquiry referred to incontinent patients left in degrading conditions; patients left inadequately dressed in full view of passers-by; patients moved and handled in unsympathetic and unskilled ways, causing pain and distress; failures to talk to patients by name, or by their preferred name; and rudeness or hostility. The Inquiry stated that there could be no excuse for such treatment and that respect for dignity should be a priority.[33]

This is such a veritable and comprehensive catalogue that it is difficult to think what else could be added and also reasonable to ask whether 'health care' was being provided at all for some patients. But none of it should have come as a surprise; the Healthcare Commission had long since been revealing similar concerns elsewhere, even if on a seemingly lesser scale, not to mention reports throughout the decade from other sources. In other words, Mid Staffordshire was merely a foreseeable progression in the undercutting of patient dignity.

IN 2007, THE Commission had published a document that drew attention to the absence of dignified health care for older people in a significant proportion of NHS trusts.[34] In 2009, it was still worrying away at the same bone, conceding that dignity is difficult to define but perhaps best understood by highlighting situations in which it is compromised. Based on complaints it had received, the Commission alluded to (in paraphrase):

- patients addressed in an inappropriate manner or being spoken about as if they were not there
- patients not given proper information
- patients' consent not sought or their wishes considered
- patients left in soiled clothes or exposed in an embarrassing manner
- patients not given appropriate food or help with eating or drinking

---

32 Francis, R. (Chair) (2010) *Independent Inquiry into care provided by Mid Staffordshire NHS Foundation Trust January 2005–March 2009.* London: The Stationery Office, p.10.

33 Francis, R. (Chair) (2010) *Independent Inquiry into care provided by Mid Staffordshire NHS Foundation Trust January 2005–March 2009.* London: The Stationery Office, p.13.

34 Healthcare Commission (2007) *Caring for dignity: A national report on dignity in care for older people while in hospital.* London: Healthcare Commission, Executive Summary.

- patients placed in mixed-sex accommodation
- patients left in pain
- a noisy environment at night causing a lack of sleep
- wards and toilets unclean and smelly
- lack of protection of personal property including hearing or sight aids
- patients subjected to abuse and violent behaviour.

The Commission noted that, encouragingly, dignity, nutrition and privacy were moving up the agenda.[35] But how could it, or should it, ever have been otherwise? This rather tame and matter-of-fact comment suggests both the entrenched status of undignified care, but also how accepting of this the Commission had – for all its hand wringing – in effect become.

In 2009 also, Claire Rayner, President of the Patients' Association and a former nurse, was predictably and justifiably much blunter about what was going on:

> For far too long now, the Patients' Association has been receiving calls on our Helpline from people wanting to talk about the dreadful, neglectful, demeaning, painful and sometimes downright cruel treatment their elderly relatives had experienced at the hands of NHS nurses.[36]

An example given by the Association in its report of that year illustrates how dignity is so simply removed. A woman reported that her mother, Mrs Alice Flower, and other patients in Barnet General Hospital would be left on commodes for up to half an hour at a time; on one occasion the daughter returned to the ward to find, slumped on the commode, her 94-year-old mother, with end-stage heart failure, left like a 'sack of potatoes, with no means of calling for help'. When blood was taken from her mother and some spilled on the floor, it was the daughter who had to clean it up, after requests for staff to do so had been in vain. Her mother's embolism stockings were not changed for more than three weeks, and only then only when the daughter had pointed out how filthy they were.[37]

---

35   Healthcare Commission (2008) *State of healthcare 2008*. London: Healthcare Commission, p.107.

36   Patients' Association (2009) *Patients not numbers, people not statistics*. London: Patients' Association, p.3.

37   Patients' Association (2009) *Patients not numbers, people not statistics*. London: Patients' Association, p.58.

The Association had been touching on just a few cases, merely illustrative of many more being reported elsewhere. For instance, on the Patient Opinion website in 2009, a relative related of the Northern General Hospital:

> My mother, aged 85 was in Northern General Hospital from February until May this year, following a fall at home, and also having a urinary infection, which was causing her to hallucinate. I feel she did not receive the care that she deserved, she was left to sit in a chair all day with nothing at all to do. It seemed as if it was too much for the staff to even give her the necessary care she needed. She was incontinent and was left in wet and soiled clothing, even though we complained to the staff. Her washing was supposed to be done by the hospital, but numerous times they left a bag of soiled and wet clothing at the side of her bed and every time we visited it absolutely stunk round her bed. She was transferred to a care home in May, and the ambulance men that took her went into the home and asked the staff to look at my mother, her hair had never been washed and she was wearing soiled clothing. They said it was a disgrace the state the hospital had allowed her to go to the home.[38]

LOSS OF DIGNITY through poor and neglectful care may, at an extreme, lapse into what would more commonly be termed abusive care. This is not to say that it is not within the same spectrum; it is just rather far along it. For instance, it was revealed in 2003 that staff had strayed far from the path of good care on Rowan Ward, part of the Manchester Mental Health and Social Care NHS Trust. Initial inquiries suggested that abuse of elderly people with dementia, over a period of several years, included hitting, slapping, stamping on feet, thumb twisting, intimidatory language and emotional abuse in the form of restricting food and playing on known anxieties of patients. The Commission for Health Improvement (CHI) was called in and confirmed that such practices had been taking place.[39]

In another, subsequent report about mental health trusts generally, the Commission pointed to what it considered to be predictors of neglect or abuse. Referring back to Rowan Ward, it highlighted a poor and institutionalised environment, low staffing levels, high use of bank and agency staff, little staff development, poor supervision, lack of knowledge

---

38 Patient Opinion. Accessed on 20 September 2010 at: www.patientopinion.org.uk/opinions/21486.

39 CHI (Commission for Health Improvement) (2003) *Investigation into matters arising from care on Rowan Ward, Manchester Mental Health and Social Care Trust, September 2003*. London: CHI, p.8.

about incident reporting, a closed and inward-looking culture – and weak management at ward and locality levels.[40]

At North Lakeland NHS Trust, practices reported on by the same Commission, three years earlier in 2000, included the following: a patient being restrained by being tied to a commode, patients being denied ordinary food, patients being fed while sitting on commodes and patients being deliberately deprived of clothing and blankets.[41] An external review had already concluded that the occupational therapy department had made a wooden board and harness for use as a restraint device.[42]

There have also been reports about the non-acute care of people with learning disabilities by the health service and a systematic undermining of dignity. Important though the issue is as a whole, and these particular reports are, it is beyond the scope of this book to give them detailed consideration. In short, significant defects were identified by the Healthcare Commission at Bromley Primary Care Trust (PCT),[43] Cornwall Partnership NHS Trust[44] and Sutton and Merton PCT.[45] To give but an idea, in Cornwall, the Healthcare Commission investigated a catalogue of poor and abusive care. The NHS Trust had itself previously ascertained this from members of staff who reported having witnessed 64 incidents over a five-year period. They included:

> ...staff hitting, pushing, shoving, dragging, kicking, secluding, belittling, mocking and goading people who used the trust's services, withholding food, giving cold showers, over zealous or premature use of restraint, poor attitude towards people who used services, poor atmosphere, roughness, care not being provided, a lack of dignity and respect, and no privacy.[46]

40 CHI (Commission for Health Improvement) (2004) *What CHI has found in mental health trusts: Sector reports.* London: CHI, p.22.

41 CHI (Commission for Health Improvement) (2000) *Investigation into the North Lakeland NHS Trust, November.* London: CHI, p.5.

42 CHI (Commission for Health Improvement) (2000) *Investigation into the North Lakeland NHS Trust, November.* London: CHI, p.29.

43 Healthcare Commission (2007) *Summary of intervention at Bromley Primary Care Trust.* London: Healthcare Commission, p.7.

44 Healthcare Commission and CSCI (Commission for Social Care Inspection) (2006) *Joint investigation into the provision of services for people with learning disabilities at Cornwall Partnership NHS Trust, July 2006.* London: Healthcare Commission and CSCI.

45 Healthcare Commission (2007) *Investigation into the service for people with learning disabilities provided by Sutton and Merton Primary Care Trust.* London: Healthcare Commission.

46 Healthcare Commission and CSCI (Commission for Social Care Inspection) (2006) *Joint investigation into the provision of services for people with learning disabilities at Cornwall Partnership NHS Trust, July 2006.* London: Healthcare Commission and CSCI, p.31.

DIGNITY MAY BE eroded in less obvious ways, as recounted by the government-appointed National Dignity Ambassador, Sir Michael Parkinson:

> It was during my mother's illness that Mary, my wife, and I gained some understanding of what being in care meant, the good and the bad, which included my mother being patted on the head and called "ducky", "dear" and "love". Normally, she would have broken the arm of anyone who talked to her like that. At other times, we visited and my mother was dressed in some-one else's clothes. One day, her face had been painted garishly, like Bette Davis in "Whatever Happened to Baby Jane?" She looked like a clown, a figure of fun, and far from the woman who brought me up; a woman who took great pride in her appearance and who had never before been seen in public looking anything other than perfect.[47]

More generally, baths, showers, oral hygiene, wearing one's own clothes, nails, hair, being in a tidy state – these matters go not just to hygiene but also to a person's dignity, sense of well-being, personality and to their spirit and morale. Not only are these intrinsic goods, but they are also important to recovery from illness. On this very point is the following account:

> What a transformation in care there was once she was at Walnuttree. It became obvious that she was in the best possible place she could be. The nursing staff were caring, they made time to talk to the patients and relatives. They are giving the patients some dignity in their lives by simple acts such as combing their hair, manicuring fingernails and most of all, smiling and being happy and cheerful in their work. We cannot thank those staff enough... It is going to be a very, very sad day for Sudbury if we lose such a wonderful, caring hospital.[48]

Many years before, Florence Nightingale had something to say precisely about this sort of care, including washing:

> The amount of relief and comfort experienced by the sick after the skin has been carefully washed and dried, is one of the commonest observations made at a sick bed. But it must not be forgotten that the comfort and relief so obtained are not all. They are, in fact, nothing more than a sign that the vital powers have been relieved by removing something that was oppressing them.

47 Parkinson, M. (2010) *My year as National Dignity Ambassador*. London: Department of Health, p.4.

48 Quoted in: Mandelstam, M. (2006) *Betraying the NHS*. London: Jessica Kingsley Publishers, p.263. ('Schwenk family, "Our caring local hospital".' Letter. *Suffolk Free Press*, 12 January 2006.)

> The nurse, therefore, must never put off attending to the personal cleanliness of her patient under the plea that all that is to be gained is a little relief, which can be quite as well given later. In all well-regulated hospitals this ought to be, and generally is, attended to.[49]

She may have written this all those years ago, but few health care professionals would disagree in principle with what she said. However, the care described above was forged at a traditional community hospital and the sands have been slipping away for such care.

The priorities that count, measured and linked to finance, are blind to such matters. Hair washing and brushing, fingernails, smiles – and nurses who have time to be compassionate – have not been known to figure prominently, if at all, at NHS trust board meetings. And the specialist elderly care beds, the rehabilitation beds and the community hospital beds – perhaps the last, mainly reliable, outpost of this sort of inpatient health care – have ebbed away, as they have been closed in their tens, hundreds and thousands. Where units and wards have not closed then, under resourced and their purpose diluted, many are but a shadow of what they once were.

Some hospitals have travelled far from Florence Nightingale's edict. In 2010, it was reported that patients at Hinchingbrooke Hospital cheered and clapped when they received help with oral care, with blankets, with washing and with bathing. They referred to the person who had been helping them as a guardian angel. However, their deliverer was not a nurse; she was another inpatient, 74-year-old Mrs Janet Halsall. She had found nurses repeatedly ignoring requests for help from patients (who were left to fend for themselves), a dirty pantry, a patient cold and left without a blanket, a patient not being taken to the toilet and patients needing washes and baths. She helped them all. Mrs Halsall put it down to shortage of staff: 'Never before have I seen so many people rushing around, working so hard but achieving nothing.'[50]

THE STANDING NURSING and Midwifery Advisory Committee had in 2001 referred to a lack of essential resources with which to care for older people on hospital wards, the absence of which would undermine dignity. The scarcities identified included linen and pillows, continence

---

49 Nightingale, F. (1860) *Notes on nursing: What it is, and what it is not.* New York: Appleton (1st American ed.), p.93.
50 'Grandmother disgusted at filthy hospital nursed and bathed other patients on her ward.' *Daily Mail*, 30 January 2010.

pads, spare clothing, aids for mobility (and also for eating, dressing and bathing), hospital mattresses and other pressure-relief equipment – and personal items such as toothbrushes, toothpaste, soap, razors, combs and hairbrushes.[51]

For instance, seven years later, at the supposedly state of the art Queen's Hospital, Romford, a relative found pillow slips being used to dry patients, including her mother:

> My 88 year old mother was admitted to your hospital after a serious fall. We were very pleased with her treatment and the aftercare she received. Unfortunately she had a second fall two weeks ago and this resulted in a broken hip, Whilst we are pleased with the treatment she has received we were most disappointed to be asked by members of staff to bring in towels for her as they were having to use pillowslips to dry patients with. On arriving at the hospital it is most impressive and very much state of the art so the above issue seems quite pathetic.[52]

At Gosport War Memorial Hospital, relatives reported distress that patients were not dressed in their own clothes – even when families had specifically provided labelled clothing. They also pointed out possible cross-infection risks of wearing other people's clothes.[53]

In Mid Staffordshire, it was relatives rather than staff who had to spend significant time attending to the hygiene needs of patients. This included help with getting to and from the bathroom, with washing, with personal care needs and cleaning up patients who had soiled themselves. Families believed that if they did not do these things, they would not get done by staff.

When staff did attend patients, bad practice was observed by relatives. The same razor might be used on more than one patient, likewise the same wash bowl. Mouthwash might not be provided for patients with ulcers, teeth not be cleaned and mouths not rinsed out. Hair was not washed and brushed.[54] An elderly woman was in hospital for four weeks; during that time she was not washed; she smelled badly. The staff said they did not have time; she was due to have a bath on the day she died.[55]

---

51 Standing Nursing and Midwifery Advisory Committee (2001) *Caring for older people: A nursing priority integrating knowledge, practice and values: A report.* London: Department of Health, p.29.

52 Patient Opinion. Accessed on 20 October 2010 at: www.patientopinion.org.uk/opinions/10006.

53 CHI (Commission for Health Improvement) (2002) *Investigation into the Portsmouth Healthcare NHS Trust: Gosport War Memorial Hospital, July 2002.* London: CHI, p.23.

54 Francis, R. (Chair) (2010) *Independent Inquiry into care provided by Mid Staffordshire NHS Foundation Trust January 2005–March 2009.* London: The Stationery Office, p.75.

55 Francis, R. (Chair) (2010) *Independent Inquiry into care provided by Mid Staffordshire NHS Foundation Trust January 2005–March 2009.* London: The Stationery Office, p.75.

One woman, whose husband was dying in the hospital, related how he not only received inadequate pain relief but also how he was not given any oral care; she recalled that his mouth was in a 'dreadful mess'. She herself had to ask for oral packs and provide the care herself; at the time it was 'extremely distressing and difficult to do this for him'.[56] In conclusion, the Mid Staffordshire Independent Inquiry stated that failure to ensure personal cleanliness and hygiene:

> …degrades patients, aggravating the feelings of illness, disability and separation from home and familiar surroundings. A wholly unacceptable standard was tolerated on some of the Trust's wards for a significant number of patients.[57]

Altogether disturbing, but Mid Staffordshire does not represent a novel characteristic of hospital care. It was just that a thorough and compassionate inquiry chairman was pulling out, from under the proverbial carpet, the filth and dirty laundry (sometimes literally) which had been swept there for far too long. One doesn't need to turn up the edges too far to find it.

A RELATIVE DESCRIBED what happened at the Royal Cornwall Hospital (Treliske) in Cornwall, to which her 82-year-old father had been admitted in 2007, suffering from terminal throat and lung cancer but remaining unwashed, in dirty sheets, mouth uncared for, unemptied commode, unmanaged diarrhoea and no nursing in sight:

> The medical side of his care appears to be good, however… Elderly, frail, terminal, undernourished and dehydrated – these five factors to me say vulnerable and at risk of developing pressure sores… He has not been offered a wash, he has not had his pressure areas checked, he has had a soiled sheet on his bed for two days. I have had to ask for a commode to be emptied, for toilet roll for mouth care, and for pads since he has developed diarrhoea. This is not rocket science it is very basic nursing care. The side room he is in has no bowl and no plug in the sink. I have been providing all the basic nursing care for my father including washing diarrhoea off his legs and I return to work on Monday which concerns me greatly.[58]

56 Francis, R. (Chair) (2010) *Independent Inquiry into care provided by Mid Staffordshire NHS Foundation Trust January 2005–March 2009*. London: The Stationery Office, p.394.
57 Francis, R. (Chair) (2010) *Independent Inquiry into care provided by Mid Staffordshire NHS Foundation Trust January 2005–March 2009*. London: The Stationery Office, p.12.
58 Patient Opinion. Accessed on 20 September 2010 at: www.patientopinion.org.uk/opinions/1888.

Thus, Help the Aged had in 2007 drawn attention to too many austere cold, smelly and poorly maintained hospital bathrooms. Continuing problems included absent locks and signs, inadequate heating, poor privacy, insufficient bath aids, wet floors and inappropriate use of bathrooms as store rooms.[59]

Another survey, also published in 2007 by the Health and Social Care Advisory Service, reported that patients, particularly on acute rather than rehabilitation wards, might go without a full wash or bath for days. Hair washing was generally unavailable with the consequence that patients would feel that their hair was dank and dirty. Likewise, dust or articles might be left for days under hospital beds. The old fashioned approach of making beds every day and changing soiled or crumpled linen might no longer be followed and stained bedding remain in place for the length of the patient's stay. This was distressing to patients who were normally fastidious but, in their vulnerable hospitalised state, powerless to do anything about the situation.[60]

More specifically, in 2010, Leicester General Hospital was accused by the daughter of Mrs Brenda Barnett of not providing proper care for her 77-year-old mother before she died. She allegedly did not receive help with eating, even though she could not hold a knife and fork and had a red tray maker to indicate she required help. Other patients had to step in to help her. In addition, her mother's hearing aids were either left in at night or not put back in during the day, and her hands were never washed; they were covered in faeces. The daughter felt that the nurses spent time laughing and joking while her mother died in squalor under their noses.[61] Nor was this an isolated occurrence; a few weeks earlier, a coroner had condemned the hospital for denying another dying patient her dignity.[62]

The lack of dignity may be shown both to the living and the dead at the same time. It was reported in March 2010 by a patient at the Heartlands Hospital in Birmingham that she had lain next to a dead patient for eight hours, divided by a thin curtain only, and that two other

59 Levenson, R. (2007) *The challenge of dignity in care: Upholding the rights of the individual.* London: Help the Aged, p.25. And see: Monro, A. and Mulley, P. (2004) 'Hospital bathrooms and showers: a continuing saga of inadequacy.' *Journal of the Royal Society of Medicine 97,* 5, 235–7.

60 Health and Social Care Advisory Service (2007) *Quality of inpatient care for older people: A Department of Health funded section 64 project, 2003–2006, Final report.* London: Health and Social Care Advisory Service, pp.14, 19.

61 Schlesinger, F. (2010) 'Left unwashed and fed by fellow patients...yet another life ends without dignity.' *Daily Mail,* 5 May.

62 Schlesinger, F. (2010) 'Grandmother "gave up on life" in hospital that stripped her of all dignity.' *Daily Mail,* 15 April.

patients who died on the same day on the same ward were also left for hours – until all three bodies were removed during visiting hours. The hospital denied the length of time but did concede delays.[63]

THEY SAY IT IS all about money.

A woman, aged 93 and hitherto of ironclad constitution, was in hospital, following heart failure. She had been there for two weeks, without a bath, shower or proper wash (including her hair). She was getting grubby and smelly; this was made worse by drug-induced frequency of urine, her immobility and the lack of help to get to the toilet. This depressed her; cleanliness was for her next to, or part of, godliness. A doctor then appeared out of the blue. Astonishingly, given her age, he offered a surgical heart procedure. This was because of how remarkably physically and mentally tough she was. The woman replied to the effect: 'Don't be silly young man. I have had a marvellous life and I don't want to be messed around with now. But what I would really like is a bath.'[64] The doctor turned away but she didn't get a bath. Perhaps, having only just missed out on being born a baby of the Victorian rather than the Edwardian age, she really did belong to another era, that of Florence Nightingale:

> It cannot be necessary to tell a nurse that she should be clean, or that she should keep her patient clean, seeing that the greater part of nursing consists in preserving cleanliness.[65]

In any case, never mind the demeaning care, concentrate on the money: what price heart surgery and what price a bath?

63 Schlesinger, F. (2010) 'Dead body was left on bed next to me for eight hours: patient tells of horror on packed ward.' *Daily Mail*, 10 March.

64 Personal communication: from a patient, and relatives' observations, at a South London hospital, 1995.

65 Nightingale, F. (1860) *Notes on nursing: What it is, and what it is not.* New York: Appleton (1st American ed.), p.87.

7

Getting to the Toilet and Management of Continence

Nurses are active in meeting requests for assistance related to intimate care, in particular a request to use a toilet is responded to within 5 minutes. (Guidance from the Standard Nursing and Midwifery Advisory Committee, 2001)[1]

The nurses there weren't unkind to him, but they were overworked. We often felt that if we asked them if they would clean him up…it would be hours before they came back to clean him up, and in that time he was just lying in a dirty bed with dirty nightwear on, and he didn't want me to go in the room, even. He would say: don't come near me, don't come near me, I smell; and he was a very fastidious man and he really was left lying in his own excrement. (Mid Staffordshire NHS Foundation Trust: evidence to the Independent Inquiry, 2010)[2]

Enabling people to go to the toilet and managing their continence is fundamental. People get very distressed if they are unable, and are not helped, to manage bowel and bladder in a dignified manner.

The word incontinence is of course a dread one. Many people remain too embarrassed to utter or even think it. Dame Josephine Barnes put it in a nutshell over 30 years ago, describing incontinence as:

…a distressing and crippling condition which affects individuals of all ages but is of particular significance in the old. It may make normal life impossible, may cause embarrassment to friends and relatives however well meaning who tend to regard it with disgust. Indeed this attitude goes back to the nursery and to

---

1   Standing Nursing and Midwifery Advisory Committee (2001) *Caring for older people, a nursing priority, practice guidance: Principles, standards and indicators, a resource tool.* London: Department of Health, p.3.

2   Quoted in: Francis, R. (Chair) (2010) *Independent Inquiry into care provided by Mid Staffordshire NHS Foundation Trust January 2005–March 2009.* London: The Stationery Office, p.55.

all our childhoods when our infantile failures were a source of
shame and often of punishment.[3]

True incontinence is generally the result of impairment in the functioning
of the bladder or bowel or both. Poorly assessed and badly managed, there
may be unnecessary use of catheters or pads. Unmanaged, disagreeable,
pungent and even mortifying accidents ensue.

Far worse than this, some hospital patients are suffering these
unpleasant consequences even if their bladder and bowel are in more or
less perfect working order. This is because, lacking the physical ability
on a hospital ward to get to the toilet or commode unaided, they are not
being assisted to do so. The result? Being told by nurses, on a regular
basis, to void bowel and bladder in bed, and then to lie in their own urine
and faeces until staff make time to clean them up, possibly hours later.

Would that such practices were rare. But this does not seem to be
the case and the problem is longstanding. Back in 2001, the Standing
Nursing and Midwifery Committee plainly knew what was going on.
It realised that general exhortation, to get people to the toilet, would
be insufficient. It gave instead specific instruction; requests for the toilet
should be responded to within five minutes.[4] This was accompanied in
2001 by the Department of Health guidance *Essence of Care*, subsequently
revised in 2003 and then again in 2010. It now refers to the importance
of information, screening and assessment, care planning, and an
environment suitable to meet people's needs and preferences.[5] Either way
though, precise or vague, such guidance has singularly failed to have the
desired effect.

By 2006, AGE Concern England and the British Geriatrics Society were
stating that 'people, whatever their age and physical ability, should be able
to choose to use the toilet in private in all care settings'. Accompanying
this statement was a 'decision aid' and a number of standards relating to
access, timeliness, equipment, safety, choice, privacy, cleanliness, hygiene,
respectful language and the environment.[6]

---

3 'Foreword.' In D. Mandelstam (1980) *Incontinence and its management.* 2nd ed. Beckenham: Croom Helm, p.7.

4 Standing Nursing and Midwifery Advisory Committee (2001) *Caring for older people: A nursing priority integrating knowledge, practice and values: A report.* London: Department of Health, p.3.

5 DH (Department of Health) (2010) *Essence of Care: Benchmarks for continence and bladder and bowel care.* London: DH, p.8.

6 British Geriatrics Society, Age Concern England, Department of Geriatric Medicine (Cardiff University), Carers UK, Continence Foundation, Help the Aged, InContact and Royal College of Nursing (2006) *Behind closed doors: Using the toilet in private.* London: British Geriatrics Society.

And, in respect of true incontinence, good practice guidance on the management of continence had already been published by the Department of Health in 2000. It had emphasised the importance of assessment and a proper management and treatment plan for continence.[7] In addition, considerable efforts have been made over the last 30 years to bring incontinence literally out of the closet and to raise awareness of how it can be assessed, treated, cured and managed. For example, continence advisers have emerged as a specialist type of health professional, as have organisations such as the Association for Continence Advice and InContact, providing information and advice to both professionals and the public.

In this light, it is all the more perverse and unfortunate that some hospitals, in the name of health care, should have done so much for so many people – in terms of utterly humiliating them.

AND TOTAL HUMILIATION there has been.

In Mid Cheshire, the Healthcare Commission reported how patients complained about call bells being out of reach or not being answered. This often prevented them from getting to the toilet, commode or bedpan in time – affecting their dignity, morale and health.[8]

Even when a hospital is riddled with infection, it may make no difference. With *Clostridium difficile* on the loose at Maidstone and Tunbridge Wells National Health Service (NHS) Trust, the Healthcare Commission noted in 2007 the accounts given to it of nurses not answering call bells, not assisting people to get to the toilet or commode, and telling them 'to go' in the bed. Some patients would then be left for hours in soiled sheets.[9] In similar circumstances, Stoke Mandeville Hospital oversaw a system of patients not being helped to get to the toilet, and of then having to wait to have their sheets changed.[10]

At Stafford Hospital, the Commission reported that a patient with *Clostridium difficile* could be left for four hours in a soiled bed before the sheets were changed.[11] But, above all, it was the subsequent Independent Inquiry at that hospital which took off the lid, because unlike the

7   DH (Department of Health) (2000) *Good practice in continence services.* London: DH, pp.12–13.
8   Healthcare Commission (2006) *Investigation into Mid Cheshire Hospitals NHS Trust, January 2006.* London: Healthcare Commission, p.34.
9   Healthcare Commission (2007) *Investigation into outbreaks of* Clostridium difficile *at Maidstone and Tunbridge Wells NHS Trust, October 2007.* London: Healthcare Commission, pp.4, 39.
10   Healthcare Commission. *Investigation into outbreaks of* Clostridium difficile *at Stoke Mandeville Hospital, Buckinghamshire Hospitals NHS Trust, July 2006.* London: HC, 2006, p.47.
11   Healthcare Commission (2009) *Investigation into Mid Staffordshire NHS Foundation Trust, March 2009.* London: Healthcare Commission, p.31.

Healthcare Commission, it relayed in detail the experience of patients and their relatives.

THERE IS NO reason to suppose that the physical and mental ordeal of lying helplessly in one's own faeces and urine, regularly and for a substantial duration of time, was any worse in Mid Staffordshire than in other hospitals where it occurs. So a few examples from that hospital serve a wider purpose and justify detailed attention here.

The Inquiry heard that requests for assistance to use a bedpan or the toilet were not responded to. When patients were helped, they were then abandoned on commodes or toilets for far too long. They were often left in sheets soiled with urine and faeces for considerable periods of time. This was especially distressing when the incontinence was caused by *Clostridium difficile*. Some families ended up taking bedding out of the hospital to wash it themselves at home. The Inquiry referred to the 'unimaginable' impact of all this on patients, some in their dying days, and on their families. It described:

> ...patients struggling to care for themselves; this led to injury and a loss of dignity, often in the final days of their lives. The impact of this on them and their families is almost unimaginable. Taken individually, many of the accounts I received indicated a standard of care which was totally unacceptable. Together, they demonstrate a systematic failure of the provision of good care.[12]

Evidence was taken of patients calling for the help of nurses and being ignored. Then, too late, they would be put on the commode and left there before trying to get back to bed themselves and falling 'smack' on the floor. Or of patients waiting an hour for help, soiling the bed and then begging visitors not to make a fuss on their behalf, because the patients feared reprisals from staff.[13]

One relative referred to the staff on one ward as bullies; patients would call out for the toilet, the staff would simply pass by.[14] Buzzers would sound and be unanswered for 20 minutes. Then patients would start shouting for a nurse, and the shouting would go on and on. More than one would be calling at the same time. The shouting would subside

---

12 Francis, R. (Chair) (2010) *Independent Inquiry into care provided by Mid Staffordshire NHS Foundation Trust January 2005–March 2009.* London: The Stationery Office, p.11.

13 Francis, R. (Chair) (2010) *Independent Inquiry into care provided by Mid Staffordshire NHS Foundation Trust January 2005–March 2009.* London: The Stationery Office, pp.53–4.

14 Francis, R. (Chair) (2010) *Independent Inquiry into care provided by Mid Staffordshire NHS Foundation Trust January 2005–March 2009.* London: The Stationery Office, p.45.

into crying and sobbing as the patients wet their beds; they would then shout again before quiet would come.[15]

A relative explained how a nurse warned her to be careful when moving the bedclothes on her mother. This was because the latter's legs were red raw from sitting in faeces and urine-soaked sheets for so long. Yet her mother was such:

> ...a proud, clean lady that she would never have wanted to do that, and she would not have wanted to make extra work for somebody else. That is not my Mum's nature, she would not have done that. But she was left so often in a soaked bed or a urine and faeces – and incredibly, if she ever did get support, if she ever got support onto a bedpan, she had – because the nurses told me it was not in their remit to cut patients' nails, she would have faeces under her nails, and I would say: please get me some soap and water, I will bring the scissors in, I will cut my Mum's nails, but please, she's just been onto a bedpan...at one point they had a basket at the end of the bed that they would put sheets into, and we would go in and they were covered in urine, and they were covered in faeces and the smell. And we would constantly drag this out...[16]

Relatives struggled to provide the care not being provided by the hospital:

> Her daughter told me how her mother experienced severe diarrhoea, and on one occasion when she visited she could not find a nurse to help clean her mother. "...There was not a nurse around, there was not a doctor around. I looked for so long, it was a good half an hour, and there was nobody anywhere. So in the end, I got some rubber gloves and I started to clean my Mum myself. At that point one of the nurses said: your Mum is highly contagious and you should not be cleaning her. I said: where are you; I need some help here, I can't leave my Mum sitting in her own faeces in a ward with visitors and everybody watching her."[17]

In yet another instance, a patient was told to wet the bed, since her immobility prevented her using the toilet facilities unaided. Not only was this embarrassing, but when she did so, a night nurse told her off severely,

15 Francis, R. (Chair) (2010) *Independent Inquiry into care provided by Mid Staffordshire NHS Foundation Trust January 2005–March 2009*. London: The Stationery Office, p.53.
16 Francis, R. (Chair) (2010) *Independent Inquiry into care provided by Mid Staffordshire NHS Foundation Trust January 2005–March 2009*. London: The Stationery Office, p.61.
17 Francis, R. (Chair) (2010) *Independent Inquiry into care provided by Mid Staffordshire NHS Foundation Trust January 2005–March 2009*. London: The Stationery Office, p.349.

which reduced her to tears.[18] In one last example, a woman recalled how she found her husband lying in faeces on numerous occasions, sometimes dried and caked on him:

> She recalled that call bells were rarely answered and in any case were frequently placed out of the reach of patients. She documented that her husband "soiled his bed time and time again because no-one had answered the call-buttons. On numerous occasions when I arrived on the ward, he was lying in faeces and several times he had been lying in it for so long that it dried and caked onto him. Time and time again I had to fetch the necessary equipment from the sluice and attend to him myself because there was no staff in evidence on the ward."[19]

THE MID STAFFORDSHIRE Independent Inquiry, revelatory as it is, does not of course hold anything like a monopoly on the evidence. There are many, perhaps countless, reported incidents of patients being left in utterly demeaning states. Some of these are included elsewhere in this book, part of accounts of other degrading treatment. A few more examples are recounted here.

The Patients' Association reported in 2009 the following experience – in Barnet General Hospital and Edgware Community Hospital – of Mrs Ann McNeill, herself a former nurse who had trained with Claire Rayner. It was recalled by her husband:

> When I visited Ann at both [London hospitals] sometimes I found her lying in her own faeces. She would plead with them to change her, but the answer was always firm: "We will get to you when we have time." She didn't like disturbing the nursing staff, but she was totally compos mentis and she hated the indignity of it. One time the smell of urine from a neighbouring bed on the ward became almost overwhelming. I asked to clean it for Ann's sake.[20]

In 2010, Michael Parkinson, National Dignity Ambassador, detailed his dismay at the accounts sent to him. He had:

> ...received some letters that, quite frankly, appalled me. One lady told me of going to visit her mother after she was admitted to

---

18 Patients' Association (2009) *Patients not numbers, people not statistics.* London: Patients' Association, p.18.

19 Francis, R. (Chair) (2010) *Independent Inquiry into care provided by Mid Staffordshire NHS Foundation Trust January 2005–March 2009.* London: The Stationery Office, p.392.

20 Patients' Association (2009) *Patients not numbers, people not statistics.* London: Patients' Association, p.32.

hospital and finding her in a side room, with the door open, in full view of anyone passing, with no clothes on, covered in her own urine, having obviously been there for ages.[21]

Writing in 2010, the journalist Annabel Wynne recounted how her father had, in 2007, received 'attentive, thorough, caring and respectful' care in the intensive care unit of a hospital for two periods of a fortnight. In between, he had been on the general wards. There, not only was there a general lack of cleanliness, but instead of providing bedpans for patients, the nurses instructed patients to soil themselves in bed. It was not unusual for patients then to lie in their own faeces for an hour or more.[22]

And, at Walsgrave Hospital, a woman related how her mother had been left alone in a waiting room, despite ringing the bell for two-and-a-half hours, in her own faeces and incontinent – having undergone cancer treatment. The staffing shortage was so bad that the daughter was making beds on the ward, giving food to patients and even buying food for patients who had not been given a meal. The hospital apologised for shortcomings in its cleaning and catering services.[23]

Distressed and lying in bodily waste: in March 2010, Mr Donald O'Sullivan's wife recounted how her 75-year-old husband, suffering from dementia, had been cared for during a five-week stay at Chase Farm Hospital; he had originally been admitted for a procedure to clear fluid from his lungs, estimated to require six days only. Continent when admitted, he was immediately put in incontinence pads. On three occasions his family found him greatly distressed and covered in faeces and urine; he often was not given sufficient food and drink. The director of nursing apologised; regular rounds would in future take place to ensure that people's toileting needs were met and that they had access to food and drink.[24] As if anything else should ever have been in contemplation.

According to her family in 2010, Mrs Nancy Bull, in Frimley Park Hospital with inoperable stomach cancer, received very good care until she was moved from one ward to a second, surgical ward; then things began to deteriorate. They found her wearing a nightgown drenched in her own sick, urine and faeces, in which she had been left for some time. The sick had dried onto the clothing. They were forced to change her clothes themselves. They also maintained that her food intake and

21 Parkinson, M. (2010) *My year as National Dignity Ambassador*. London: Department of Health, p.28.
22 Wynne, A. (2006) 'Shortcuts to poor health care.' *The Guardian*, 13 January.
23 'Hospital has third world conditions.' *Rugby Advertiser*, 7 September 2006.
24 Lowe, R. (2010) 'Dementia patient neglected by nurses at Chase Farm, says wife.' *Enfield Independent News*, 31 March.

vomiting were not being monitored. A hospital spokesman, in response to the family's protests, referred to its collaborative working with patients and their relatives.[25]

A puddle of soil and no care: also in 2010, at Darent Valley Hospital, a relative related how:

> My mother has been in Spruce and Beech Wards for the past three weeks after being admitted following a fall which resulted in a mild stroke. One the whole [sic] I have found her to be in a distressed state at visiting times, mainly because she is left for long periods in a chair without access to a buzzer to call staff. One day she was so relieved to see me as she had been left in a thin nightie close to an open window. The buzzer was nowhere to be seen and she had been sitting in a puddle of her own soil. The next day she had a urinary tract infection. The nursing staff appeared to be unconcerned. I expect the Wards are understaffed but its no excuse for neglecting an old lady who is not senile and feels that no-body cares. I am so angry and unimpressed with your hospital.[26]

The lack of proper management of people's bowel, bladder and continence needs can lead organisations and their staff on to still worse practices. At North Lakeland NHS Trust, not only were patients left for long periods of time on commodes and given their meals while so sitting, they were sometimes tied to the commodes. The Commission for Health Improvement (CHI) referred to degradation and cruelty.[27] At least the staff saved themselves the trouble of cleaning up bodies and bedding.

UNDERPINNING MORE OBVIOUS and immediate failure to help people to get to the toilet are other more general deficiencies that may sow the seeds of the poor care and neglect described above. Where there is a genuine bowel or bladder problem, inadequate assessment and care plans will make management of continence more difficult and lead to unnecessary indignities.

A 2006 study by the Royal College of Physicians concluded that only 51 per cent of hospital patients with urinary incontinence had a history

---

25 'Hospital's care of terminally ill pensioner criticised.' *Get Hampshire*, 23 July 2008. Accessed on 20 October 2010 at: www.gethampshire.co.uk/news/s/2032602_hospitals_care_of_terminally_ill_pensioner_criticised.

26 NHS Choices. Accessed on 18 October 2010 at: www.nhs.uk/Services/Hospitals/PatientFeedback/DefaultView.aspx?id=1893&pid=RN707&pageNo=3&sort=1&recordPP=0.

27 CHI (Commission for Health Improvement) (2000) *Investigation into the North Lakeland NHS Trust, November.* London: CHI, p.5.

taken and only 55 per cent a specialist assessment. In only a third of cases was a diagnosis documented. Half the patients had no documented evidence of a specific treatment plan, 58 per cent were given pads and 30 per cent were catheterised. However, lack of accurate diagnosis leads to either unnecessary treatment or inappropriate reliance on containment – including expensive and potentially undignified use of pads.[28]

A further report published in 2010 by the Royal College noted that in acute hospitals staff with the requisite skills to assess continence were not always available; structured training about continence care was taking place in only 49 per cent of such hospitals.[29]

Wider than taking people to the toilet is the more general, but just as vital, matter of managing people's continence appropriately. So, at Gosport War Memorial Hospital, the CHI reported patients' relatives as claiming that patients were more or less automatically catheterised – and that this was done not so much for clinical reasons but so as to save the nurses' time. Relatives referred also to long periods of time elapsing before people were helped to the toilet or commode.[30]

IN SUMMARY, IN some hospitals, in some wards, patients are abandoned to degradation. The case of Mrs Clara Stokes has been described in some detail in Chapter 6. One of the aspects of the lack of care provided was being left in her own bodily waste. As her daughter put it:

> I think dogs are treated better than my mother was. She was left in a pond of her own filth. Worse than an animal.[31]

---

28 Wagg, A., Peel, P., Lowe, D. and Potter, J. (2006) *National audit of continence of care.* London: Royal College of Physicians, pp.6–7.

29 RCP (Royal College of Physicians) (2010) *National audit of continence care: Combined organisational and clinical report, September 2010.* London: RCP, p.8.

30 CHI (Commission for Healthcare Improvement) (2002) *Investigation into the Portsmouth Healthcare NHS Trust: Gosport War Memorial Hospital, July 2002.* London: CHI, p.22.

31 Wilkes, D. (2010) 'How could this happen? Former Land Girl honoured by Brown dies after she is left to "wallow in her own filth" on NHS ward.' *Daily Mail*, 28 April.

8

Keeping the Environment Clean and Managing Infection

> The NHS also commits: to ensure that services are provided in a clean and safe environment that is fit for purpose, based on national best practice. (*The NHS Constitution*, 2010)[1]

> It was difficult to isolate patients because there were few side rooms, and some of these were not available for the isolation of patients with infections because of the reconfiguration of wards and ring-fencing of beds, thought necessary to ensure shorter waiting times for non-emergency patients undergoing surgery. The trust's determination to meet the Government's target for a maximum waiting time in A&E of four hours, led to some patients with diarrhoea being kept in or put on open wards rather than in isolation facilities. (Healthcare Commission: Stoke Mandeville Hospital, 2006)[2]

> Toilets were not cleaned properly with faeces clearly left from several previous uses. My sister often had to clean them herself before she'd let my father use them… We saw dirty and blood stained food trays. We saw soiled and dirty linen left on floors and mixed with fresh supplies. (Patients' Association, 2009)[3]

On the website of the Science Museum is a section devoted to the history of medicine. Within this, is a web page entitled: 'Gateways to death'. It harks back to the 18th century when hospitals were regarded as places in which people died and which positively did harm. In particular, patients would die of infections which they contracted in hospitals. By the mid-1850s, Florence Nightingale had arrived and stressed the importance of cleanliness and of doing the sick no harm.

---

1   DH (Department of Health) (2010) *The NHS Constitution*. London: DH, s.2a.

2   Healthcare Commission (2006) *Investigation into outbreaks of* Clostridium difficile *at Stoke Mandeville Hospital, Buckinghamshire Hospitals NHS Trust, July 2006*. London: Healthcare Commission, p.5.

3   Patients' Association (2009) *Patients not numbers, people not statistics*. London: Patients' Association, p.10.

The site notes, however, that even before then, not all hospitals were uniformly bad. In this country for example, voluntary hospital patients fared better than workhouse infirmaries 'which were large and often overcrowded'.[4] The best known and most notorious description from the 18th century was, in fact, of a French hospital, the Hôtel Dieu in Paris. It was a hotbed of disease.[5] The text concludes with the observation that modern patients have become fearful of contracting lethal infection, and that once again hospitals are being described by some as 'gateways to death'.[6]

The Science Museum's web page is instructive. On the one hand, we must not leap to conclusions when comparing different times and contexts. On the other hand, it is a timely reminder that we should not inadvertently subscribe to what has become known as the Whig interpretation of history.[7] This refers generally to the idea that the history of medicine (or indeed of anything else) is the march of uninterrupted, inevitable and enlightened progress.

We are nowhere near the Hôtel Dieu's large halls containing up to 800 patients crowded in on pallets or heaps of straw, overrun with vermin and filth, unventilated and so foul smelling that attendants would only enter with sponges dipped in vinegar held to their faces.[8] But there is no room either for complacency. Overcrowded hospitals in 21st-century England, with patients nursed in corridors or in poorly staffed and fitted 'escalation' areas, bed heads only 12 inches apart, infected patients nursed on open wards, filthy toilets, and patients left to lie in their own faeces for hours – all of these are nothing to boast about.

Furthermore, the characterisation of hospitals as unsafe places is not confined to disgruntled patients or relatives. This emerged at an inquest in Birmingham. A 44-year-old woman had died with blood clots on her lungs; prior to her death she had been admitted three times within a short space of time to Heartlands Hospital, but discharged home twice. In denying negligence and also the hospital's failure to diagnose a pulmonary embolism, a senior consultant and professor pointed out that, absent a clear diagnosis, it was not a good idea to have kept her in

---

4   Science Museum (2010) *Gateways to death*. Accessed on 24 September 2010 at: www.sciencemuseum.org.uk/broughttolife/techniques/gatewaystodeath.aspx.

5   Garrison, F.H. (1929) *History of medicine*. 4th ed. London: W.B. Saunders, p.400.

6   Science Museum (2010) *Gateways to death*. Accessed on 24 September 2010 at: www.sciencemuseum.org.uk/broughttolife/techniques/gatewaystodeath.aspx.

7   A notion introduced by the historian, Herbert Butterfield in *The Whig interpretation of history*. New York: W.W. Norton, 1965. (Originally published in 1931.)

8   Garrison, F.H. (1929) *History of medicine*. 4th ed. London: W.B. Saunders, p.400.

hospital longer. This was because, given the risk of infection, the city hospital was 'not a terribly safe place to be'.[9]

IN THIS CHAPTER are descriptions of rampant hospital infection, and of systematic lapses in the most basic preventative and containment measures. This is to such an extent that it is understandable if, as the Science Museum notes, there is murmuring about some hospitals once again being 'gateways to death'. And whilst the horrors of some 18th-century hospitals simply cannot be compared with our hospitals today, nonetheless there is also much less excuse now for the absence of reasonable attempts at prevention and management. Our knowledge of the causes of infection, our technology, our cleaning agents and our drugs are a world apart.

This is not to say that all infection can be prevented, particularly with the evolution of so-called 'super bugs', increasingly resistant to antibiotics. But it certainly is to point the finger at those health service policymakers, managers and staff who have, in the last decade and more, effectively, if unwittingly, abandoned at least 150 years of scientific and medical advance and knowledge – as well as common sense.

It should also be noted that in 2009, the National Audit Office reported a decline in the rates of MRSA and *Clostridium difficile*, a discernible trend since 2006. However, a number of riders attach to this. First, such statistics rely on accurate reporting, which cannot be taken for granted; and, even allowing for such a decline, this does not mean that at least some of the deaths which still occur are unavoidable. For instance, although overall rates appear to have fallen, nevertheless 12 per cent of hospitals have seen an increase in MRSA infection and 19 per cent in *Clostridium difficile*.

Second, there are other hospital-based infections that may be increasing. Furthermore, there is no national surveillance system for these, such as urinary tract infections, skin infections and pneumonia. Twenty per cent of National Health Service (NHS) trusts do not carry out surveillance on other infections, whilst most in any case do not provide information to their board about such other infections.[10]

Third, even supposing a corner has been turned and infection control is significantly improving, the events of the last decade seem important to outline, if only to serve as a warning of how politicians and senior

9   'Hospital patient "safer at home".' BBC News, 17 August 2005. Accessed on 20 September 2010 at: http://news.bbc.co.uk/1/hi/england/west_midlands/4160336.stm.

10   NAO (National Audit Office) (2009) *Reducing healthcare associated infections in hospitals in England.* London: NAO, pp.5–10.

management in hospitals came, in effect, to regard infection and patient deaths as collateral damage in the pursuit of higher, political aims. And last, because in any case, it is by no means clear that the war on cleanliness and hygiene – in association with attentive care – has been won. A patient at Southampton General Hospital recorded in early 2009:

> After my operation, I asked to use the toilet. The nurse was annoyed that I had disturbed her and she left me on the commode for over an hour! I was so humiliated as I have significant mobility problems and could not have got off of the commode on my own (the nursing staff were made fully aware of my mobility problems when I arrived at the hospital). Also I was in the hospital for 5 nights and not once was the room I was in (with 3 others) cleaned. A towel covered with blood was left on the floor for 3 days until discovered by a very annoyed senior nurse. The ward was extremely dirty and I understand that several other complaints were received whilst I stayed at the hospital – all regarding the level of cleanliness.[11]

KEEPING HOSPITALS AND patients clean is an obvious thing to do. Filthy toilets, wash basins, wards and furniture do not help. Sick and infectious patients, packed into hospitals in close proximity, not isolated when necessary and moved around in games of musical beds in order to adhere to political objectives – this is not a good idea. In particular it is an even worse notion when super bugs are on the loose. The two on which most attention has been focused are *methicillin-resistant staphylococcus aureus* (MRSA) and *Clostridium difficile* ('C. diff.').

Clostridium difficile is a bacterium, naturally in the gut of some people, which does no harm when it is balanced by other bacteria. However, use of some, broad spectrum, antibiotics can strip the gut of other bacteria, so as to allow the *Clostridium* bacterium to multiply, causing serious problems including mild to severe diarrhoea, blood-stained stools, fever and cramps in the abdomen. These symptoms flow from inflammation of the bowel; the infection can also lead to peritonitis, septicaemia and perforation of the colon.

MRSA can cause skin infection, including boils, styes, carbuncles, cellulitis and impetigo. Pressure ulcers can become infected. MRSA in the bloodstream causes more serious infection, which can spread through the body causing septicaemia, septic shock, osteomyelitis (bone marrow

---

11 NHS Choices. Accessed on 20 October 2010 at: www.nhs.uk/Services/Hospitals/PatientFeedback/DefaultView.aspx?id=1311&pid=RHM01&pageNo=0&sort=4&recordPP=0.

infection), internal abscesses, meningitis, pneumonia and endocarditis (infection of the lining of the heart).[12]

If you are a vulnerable patient you do not want to contract these infections and certainly don't want to be exposed to them unnecessarily. And whilst there are no guarantees, there is no shortage of guidance and policy statements about the need for a clean environment and infection control, in order to improve your chances. The *Code of conduct for NHS managers*, in place since 2002 and thus preceding the major reported scandals, states:

> I will observe the following principles: make the care and safety
> of patients my first concern and act to protect them from risk.[13]

The NHS Plan had already stated in 2000 that it would enable 'the NHS to get the basics right'. Like cleanliness; patients had perceived a 'major deterioration', but they expected 'wards to be clean, furnishings to be tidy. The new resources will allow for a renewed emphasis on clean hospitals.'[14] Notwithstanding this, the deterioration in hospital cleanliness may even have become worse in the years that followed publication of *The NHS Plan*.

It was about 'patient choice', effectively promoting a version of consumerism and market principles. This might explain why it was so enthusiastic about bedside televisions and telephones in hospitals, which were referred to in the same paragraph as basic care and clean wards.[15] Hindsight illuminates, but whilst the government spoke of consumer trappings, lethal infection was running through its hospitals. It really was a case of Nero fiddling while Rome burnt.

By 2006, it was clear that cleanliness and infection control remained an objective rather than actually being attained, as infection held many hospitals in its grip. Department of Health guidance on *Standards for better health* stated that health care organisations should:

> ...keep patients, staff and visitors safe by having systems to
> ensure that...the risk of health care acquired infection to patients
> is reduced, with particular emphasis on high standards of hygiene
> and cleanliness.[16]

---

12 *NHS Choices: Your health, your choices.* Available at: www.nhs.uk/Conditions/Pages/hub.aspx, accessed on 12 July 2010.

13 DH (Department of Health) (2002) *Code of conduct for NHS managers.* London: DH, p.3.

14 Secretary of State for Health (2000) *The NHS Plan: A plan for investment, a plan for reform.* Cm 4818-I. London: The Stationery Office, p.46.

15 Secretary of State for Health (2000) *The NHS Plan: A plan for investment, a plan for reform.* Cm 4818-I. London: The Stationery office, para. 1.17.

16 DH (Department of Health) (2006) *Standards for better health.* London: DH, p.10.

Guidance from the Care Quality Commission (CQC) now demands that health and social care providers comply with legal requirements in respect of the *Code of Practice for health and adult social care on the prevention and control of infections and related guidance.*[17] It states that breach of the *Code* may indicate breach of the relevant regulations; this in turn could lead to the Commission exercising its powers of enforcement. The *Code* itself sets out the following criteria (abbreviated and paraphrased) against which compliance is judged:

- systems to manage and monitor the prevention and control of infection

- provide and maintain a clean and appropriate environment

- provide suitable accurate information on infections to service users and their visitors

- provide suitable accurate information on infections to anybody concerned with providing further support or nursing/medical care

- ensure that people who have or develop an infection are identified promptly and receive the appropriate treatment and care to reduce the risk of passing on the infection to other people

- ensure that all staff and those employed to provide care in all settings are fully involved in the process of preventing and controlling infection

- provide or secure adequate isolation facilities

- secure adequate access to laboratory support

- have and adhere to policies that will help to prevent and control infections

- ensure, so far as is reasonably practicable, that care workers are free of and are protected from exposure to infections that can be caught at work and that all staff are suitably educated in the prevention and control of infection associated with the provision of health and social care.[18]

---

17 CQC (Care Quality Commission) (2009) *Guidance about compliance: Summary of regulations, outcomes and judgement framework.* London: CQC, p.19.

18 DH (Department of Health) (2010) *The Health and Social Care Act 2008 Code of Practice for health and adult social care on the prevention and control of infections and related guidance.* London: DH, p.13.

This is a sizeable list but entailing no more than fairly basic requirements. Yet it comprises more or less a roll call of measures that have precisely not been taken in some hospitals, leading to catastrophic breakdown in infection control.

REPORTS OF INFECTION control going badly astray in the last few years are disturbing. This is, first, because the failure to put in place reasonable measures, aimed at preventing and managing infection, have been associated with the preoccupation with performance and finance-related goals imposed by central government. And second, because the conflict between such goals and patient safety, the former jeopardising the latter, has been known about for a decade.

That is to say, we do not find evidence of diligence, of every reasonably practicable measure having been taken and of policymakers and senior executives having put patient safety first. This makes for an altogether darker scene. It means the scandals that emerged at Stoke Mandeville and in Kent, for example, were not only effectively anticipated and foreseen but, in addition, central government policy was implicated in advance. This is quite plain if one looks back.

In 2004, the National Audit Office published a report on infection in hospitals.[19] A picture of Florence Nightingale adorns the cover; she is giving a wounded soldier in a hospital bed something to drink. A quote from the Florence Nightingale Museum follows, referring to mortality, statistics, infection, death and to her 1863 book, *Notes on hospitals*. The implication is clear; the Office was talking about basic infection control, which is not an alien concept but one spelt out 141 years earlier.

The Office pointed out that already in 2000, in a previous report,[20] it had found that at any one time, 9 per cent of hospital patients were suffering from hospital-acquired infection – resulting in extended stays, disability and, in 5000 cases per year, death. It had also noted in 2000 that good practice was thin on the ground, and that the House of Commons Public Accounts Committee had, in that same year, called for a root and branch shift toward better control of infection.[21]

So in 2004, it was with foreboding that the National Audit Office acknowledged that some progress had been made but that government

---

19 NAO (National Audit Office) (2004) *Improving patient care by reducing the risk of hospital acquired infection: A progress report.* London: NAO.

20 NAO (National Audit Office) (2000) *The management and control of hospital acquired infection in NHS acute trusts in England.* HC 230. London: The Stationery Office.

21 Public Accounts Committee, House of Commons (2000) *The management and control of hospital acquired infection in acute NHS trusts in England.* HC 306. London: The Stationery Office.

policy was not always consistent with good infection control and bed management practice:

> Preventing infections continues to be adversely affected by other NHS trust-wide policies and priorities as identified in our original report. The increased throughput of patients to meet performance targets has resulted in considerable pressure towards higher bed occupancy, which is not always consistent with good infection control and bed management practices. Seventy-one per cent of trusts are still operating with bed occupancy levels higher than the 82 per cent target that the Department told the Committee it hoped to achieve by 2003–04 after this issue was highlighted in our 2000 report. The lack of suitable isolation facilities also remains a concern for trusts, as does the increase in frequency of moving patients and a lack of sufficient beds to separate elective and trauma patients.[22]

It highlighted the conflict between safety and the centrally imposed policy of performance targets – and the resulting high bed occupancy rates, lack of isolation facilities and excessive movement of patients within the hospital. As it turned out, the Office was spot on.

AT PETERBOROUGH DISTRICT Hospital, a patient's daughter offered the following observations about the care of her mother in 2005, suggesting the most basic lapses in the control of infection:

> My mother...had to go into Peterborough District hospital and have a blood transfusion. The day she was due to come home she caught c difficile... She got diarrhoea and had to stay in hospital. Four people on the ward developed c difficile and they all were put in the same 4 bedded ward...some of the people with diarrhoea were soiling the bed so there was a big bin to put things in with a fully functioning foot pedal...the nurses were actually using their hands to open the lid of the soiled bin. Really basic things – one of the patients was receiving injections so the nurses would come in with the injection tray all set up and they would put the tray on the lid of the soil bin...sometimes the nurses would just leave soiled bedding on the floor... They didn't know for example that the alcohol hand wipe isn't any good for c difficile. One would say put on gloves while another would say you don't need to. It was just bad. I spoke to the Matron for the

---

22 NAO (National Audit Office) (2004) *Improving patient care by reducing the risk of hospital acquired infection: A progress report.* London: NAO, p.3.

> ward and she herself had to look on the internet to see what it
> said about infection control about c difficile.[23]

In 2006, the crisis in infection control – about which publicity had been
moderately well suppressed – now made the headlines with a vengeance
in a Healthcare Commission report. True, it took a leak of information to
the national Press for this to happen; when it did, the Commission was
left with no option but to investigate two major outbreaks of *Clostridium
difficile* at Stoke Mandeville Hospital.

The first, between October 2003 and June 2004, was associated with
174 new cases of *Clostridium* and the death of 19 patients, 16 of whom
had acquired the infection in hospital. The infection control team made
various recommendations to control the outbreak, but senior management
and the Trust Board disregarded the advice.

The second ran from October 2004 to June 2005. It was linked to
160 new cases and the deaths of a further 19 patients, 17 of whom
had contracted the infection in hospital. Even after the second outbreak,
senior managers and the Board still failed to follow the advice of the
infection control team and to isolate patients. It was only when matters
were leaked to the Department of Health and to the national Press, that
the Trust took the necessary containment measures.

The Commission concluded, overall, that the first outbreak followed
from a poor environment for caring for patients, poor infection control,
lack of isolation facilities and insufficient priority being given to the
control of infection by senior managers. Some changes were made but
none that risked compromising strategic objectives.

When the second outbreak occurred, it was not controlled because
the Trust was too focused on reconfiguration of services and meeting the
government's targets. The system of clinical governance was dysfunctional,
the Board was not put fully in the picture, and there were serious failings
at the highest level. The Trust had taken the advice of neither its own
infection control team nor the Health Protection Agency.[24]

Contributory factors included an obsession with targets, shortage
of staff, rushed staff not following hygiene procedures, concealment of
the outbreaks from the public and failure to listen to staff concerned

---

23 Patient Opinion. Accessed on 20 September 2010 at: www.patientopinion.org.uk/
opinions/18274.

24 Healthcare Commission (2006) *Investigation into outbreaks of* Clostridium difficile *at Stoke
Mandeville Hospital, Buckinghamshire Hospitals NHS Trust, July 2006.* London: Healthcare
Commission, pp.4–5.

about patient safety.[25] In addition were a lack of hand washing facilities, antiquated bedpan washers and utility rooms (with wash basins) cluttered with uncollected linen and waste bags.[26]

Professor Sir Ian Kennedy, then chair of the Healthcare Commission, averred, in the Foreword to the Commission's report, that the deaths were avoidable:

> I said in the immediate aftermath of the Bristol report [death of a number of babies] that it was not possible to say with confidence that events such as those which took place in Bristol would not happen again. What happened at Stoke Mandeville demonstrates that they are still happening. Patients died when their deaths could have been avoided. It is a matter of the greatest regret that the lessons of Bristol have not been learned and incorporated into every corner of the NHS.[27]

The then Health Minister, Andy Burnham, was quick to offer reassurance that NHS hospitals were tackling matters and reducing levels of infection.[28] What he didn't want was another scandal of the same ilk, reported only a year later, again by the Healthcare Commission. This time it was a severe outbreak in Kent of *Clostridium difficile* at Maidstone and Tunbridge Wells NHS Trust. The events in Kent were arguably more serious than in Buckinghamshire and the political fall-out greater. This was not least because, three years later in 2010, the chief executive of the Trust at the time of the outbreak was still hitting the headlines, in her ultimately successful pursuit of a large financial compensation package. If Stoke Mandeville breached the dam of secrecy and the cover-up of hospital-acquired infection, then the Kent outbreak revealed to the public the spreading floodwaters.

Two HOSPITALS WITHIN Maidstone and Tunbridge Wells NHS Trust were mainly involved, Maidstone Hospital and the Kent and Sussex Hospital. In summary, the infection was 'probably or definitely' the main cause of death for about 90 patients between April 2004 and September 2006 –

25 Healthcare Commission (2006) *Investigation into outbreaks of* Clostridium difficile *at Stoke Mandeville Hospital, Buckinghamshire Hospitals NHS Trust, July 2006.* London: Healthcare Commission, pp.5–8.

26 Healthcare Commission (2006) *Investigation into outbreaks of* Clostridium difficile *at Stoke Mandeville Hospital, Buckinghamshire Hospitals NHS Trust, July 2006.* London: Healthcare Commission, pp.6, 9.

27 Healthcare Commission (2006) *Investigation into outbreaks of* Clostridium difficile *at Stoke Mandeville Hospital, Buckinghamshire Hospitals NHS Trust, July 2006.* London: Healthcare Commission, p.2.

28 Batty, D. (2006) 'Hospital bosses blamed for superbug deaths.' *The Guardian*, 24 July.

and to have probably or definitely contributed to the deaths of 270 patients in that same period. That is not to say that, even of the 90 patients, some would not have died anyway even had they received a reasonable standard of care.[29]

What elicited fierce criticism from the Healthcare Commission were not simply the deaths associated with the infection outbreak. If the Trust had provided good levels of care and taken all reasonable measures, but been up against an unstoppable infection, the Commission would no doubt have been more understanding. What shocked were not only the dreadful standards of care and poor infection control practices, but also that these were causally linked to an all consuming focus by the Trust Board on performance and financial targets, rather than patient care and welfare. The apparent concealment by the Trust of what was occurring merely added fuel to the flames of the Commission's condemnation. The nature of the failure therefore warrants spelling out in some detail.

In response to the initial outbreak of infection, the local infection control team had wanted to isolate patients, but an isolation ward was not made available by the Trust for four months. During this time patients were nursed on open wards, with the result that the infection spread. Part of the reason for this delay was the Trust's preoccupation with using beds and wards consistent with meeting government targets.[30]

The outbreak and poor handling of the infection was associated with poor prescribing of antibiotics, inadequate monitoring of patients for *Clostridium difficile* and for its associated complications such as dehydration, shortage of nursing staff, extremely poor basic nursing care, serious failures in hygiene and cleaning practices, proximity of beds (some bed heads were no more than 12 inches apart) and over-occupancy of beds.

Nurses, other clinical staff, patients and families revealed that nurses were too rushed to wash their hands, to empty and clean commodes, to clean mattresses and equipment properly, and to wear aprons and gloves appropriately and consistently. The high bed occupancy meant that the bed changeover period – between occupation by one patient and occupation by another – was so short that thorough cleaning was compromised.

The pressure on beds meant also that *ad hoc* 'escalation' areas were opened up for patients with inadequate bathroom facilities, laundry and

---

29   Healthcare Commission (2007) *Investigation into outbreaks of* Clostridium difficile *at Maidstone and Tunbridge Wells NHS Trust, October 2007*. London: Healthcare Commission, p.38.

30   Healthcare Commission (2007) *Investigation into outbreaks of* Clostridium difficile *at Maidstone and Tunbridge Wells NHS Trust, October 2007*. London: Healthcare Commission, p.3.

cleaning services. Furthermore, these areas tended to be staffed by agency workers, which adversely affected continuity of care. These factors increased the risk of transmission of infection.[31]

The hospital had a history of broken and worn equipment, furniture, fittings, dishwashers, showers, chair covers and curtains. The Commission found eight bedpan macerators to be dirty, rusty and leaking. Bedpan washers were not working, so bedpans that had been washed were still visibly contaminated with faeces. There were shortages of equipment such as commodes and of supplies including hand wipes, linen and bandages. Nearly half the Trust's commodes needed to be replaced; but months later the condemned commodes were still in use.

Cleaning arrangements were inadequate; at Maidstone Hospital it took place only between 7.30am and midday. Patients and relatives reported dirty floors, commodes and toilets, as well as buckets full of dirty water, blood stains on trolleys and the sides of beds, unemptied bins – and walking frames being shared between patients without being cleaned. An audit of commodes found 98 per cent to be soiled; staff were using alcohol to clean them, even though alcohol is not effective against *Clostridium*. Utility and treatment rooms were being used to prepare hot drinks and food. Refrigerators for clinical items were used for food. Hygiene practices – such as hand washing – were not observed by staff and not enforced generally.[32]

With Stoke Mandeville and then Kent, the banks had burst as both the infections and the newspapers swarmed all over both the hospitals and the hospital mortality statistics. The public at large became dimly, maybe only fleetingly, conscious of what might be a grim underbelly to the modern and improved NHS they had heard so much about. If pretensions, that the NHS as a matter of course was providing safe and hygienic care to patients, were crumbling, then Mid Staffordshire was the coup de grâce that swept, or should have swept, them away.

AT STAFFORD HOSPITAL, the Healthcare Commission heard many concerns about cleanliness and hygiene. The high mortality rate at the hospital appeared to be associated with a range of deficiencies in care, not just a specific infection. Nonetheless, *Clostridium difficile* had surfaced there as well; it was judged by the Independent Inquiry to be a

31   Healthcare Commission (2007) *Investigation into outbreaks of* Clostridium difficile *at Maidstone and Tunbridge Wells NHS Trust, October 2007*. London: Healthcare Commission, pp.4–6.

32   Healthcare Commission (2007) *Investigation into outbreaks of* Clostridium difficile *at Maidstone and Tunbridge Wells NHS Trust, October 2007*. London: Healthcare Commission, pp.44–58.

significant contributor to deaths at the hospital and to be associated with the appalling care provided.[33]

The Healthcare Commission reported that one patient had a chair by her bedside for the five days of her stay; it was covered in dried blood that was not cleaned during the entire period. Excrement trodden into the floor would remain for several days. Curtains were hanging off their hooks, high surfaces, window bars and curtains were dusty. Floors were basically only wiped. Corners were missed.[34]

Toilets were filthy and covered in blood and urine. Relatives would clean toilets before patients used them. Bins would be overflowing, so there was nowhere to put used incontinence pads. In the patient discharge unit, toilets and rooms were filthy. The accident and emergency (A&E) department had dried blood and rubbish on the floor. A ward had excrement splashed on the bedside, armchair and lockers; it was not cleaned up.[35]

Doors to isolation units were commonly left open; medical and nursing staff might not wash their hands, use alcohol gel or wear gloves when handling patients. Dirty commodes and soiled bed sheets were reported.[36]

Balls of dust occupied the corners of rooms, hallways and stairs. Blood was in the lifts and trails of it in the corridors. Rubbish would be stacked in the corridors, including both normal and surgical waste. A cleaner was observed with a pink cloth. She used it to wipe faeces off a bed frame. Using the same cloth she then cleaned the table, the sink, the patient's drip stand and the cupboard next to the table. An audit of commodes found that 35 needed to be replaced, but that up to 50 per cent, supposedly ready for use, were soiled with faeces.[37]

The Independent Inquiry, too, noted that the same cloth might be used to clean both toilets and surfaces on the ward, that hand gel containers were often empty, and that rooms vacated by patients with *Clostridium difficile* were not cleaned before admission of the next patient.

---

33 Francis, R. (Chair) (2010) *Independent Inquiry into care provided by Mid Staffordshire NHS Foundation Trust January 2005–March 2009*. London: The Stationery Office, p.446.

34 Healthcare Commission (2009) *Investigation into Mid Staffordshire NHS Foundation Trust, March 2009*. London: Healthcare Commission, p.36.

35 Healthcare Commission (2009) *Investigation into Mid Staffordshire NHS Foundation Trust, March 2009*. London: Healthcare Commission, p.36.

36 Healthcare Commission (2009) *Investigation into Mid Staffordshire NHS Foundation Trust, March 2009*. London: Healthcare Commission, p.56.

37 Healthcare Commission (2009) *Investigation into Mid Staffordshire NHS Foundation Trust, March 2009*. London: Healthcare Commission, p.85.

The evidence suggested that such failures were not isolated.[38] Bins of soiled pads would be left in patients' rooms, creating a terrible smell; bowls of vomit would be left on patients' tables even during meal times. Relatives would take matters into their own hands to try to clean things up themselves.[39]

One relative reported that the only cleaning in weeks preceded an inspection by Monitor, the organisation responsible for oversight of NHS foundation trusts:

> I have never seen my Mum's locker, bed or anything cleaned during those eight weeks, but that Sunday afternoon they were cleaned by a sister and a staff nurse, and that is the only time we saw two trained nurses together. The following day there was an inspection, but now I know it was by Monitor.[40]

Stoke Mandeville, Maidstone and Mid Staffordshire are thus perhaps the three leading players caught in the spotlight, but they have not been without a solid supporting cast.

ONCE, TWICE, THREE times bitten by the regulator, surely then four times shy, the health service hospitals would rapidly have put their houses in order.

In 2007, the Healthcare Commission issued an improvement notice to Barnet and Chase Farm Hospitals NHS Trust concerning infection control – relating to the adequacy of staff training and information, of root cause analysis of patient infection and of hand washing facilities and bacterial rubs.[41]

A 2008 inspection report about the Princess Royal University Hospital in Bromley also found failures in hygiene and infection control. Amongst these were soiled commodes which were nonetheless marked as clean and ready for use, bed frames and wall-mounted suction bottles covered in dust, visibly dirty bed wheels, blood stains on cot side rails and blood-splashed walls.[42]

---

38 Francis, R. (Chair) (2010) *Independent Inquiry into care provided by Mid Staffordshire NHS Foundation Trust January 2005–March 2009*. London: The Stationery Office, p.13.

39 Francis, R. (Chair) (2010) *Independent Inquiry into care provided by Mid Staffordshire NHS Foundation Trust January 2005–March 2009*. London: The Stationery Office, pp.104–5.

40 Francis, R. (Chair) (2010) *Independent Inquiry into care provided by Mid Staffordshire NHS Foundation Trust January 2005–March 2009*. London: The Stationery Office, p.99.

41 Healthcare Commission (2007) *Improvement notice: Barnet and Chase Farm Hospitals NHS Trust, 5th July 2007*. London: Healthcare Commission.

42 Healthcare Commission (2008) *Improvement notice: Bromley Hospitals NHS Trust: Princess Royal University Trust*. London: Healthcare Commission, pp.2–3.

In 2008, a relative deplored the care of her grandmother at Northwick Park Hospital:

> I visited my grandmother who is 86 years old and recovering from a hip replacement on 17/02/08. She is carrying MRSA so is in her own side room which was simply filthy. The camode had not been emptied, the room smelt of urine, her nightdress was heavily soiled and she had clearly had an "accident" and had not been washed or changed. The windows are a disgrace and the whole place needs a deep clean – no wonder infections are on the rise. The care in this hospital is simply despicable.[43]

In the same year, a patient at the Royal Hallamshire Hospital was aghast at the nurses not washing their hands and not wearing gloves:

> I am a carer for a person who was admitted to ward K1 of the Royal Hallamshire for surgery. Though the medical care was of a good standard, many other aspects (including the nursing) were less than acceptable. I saw a nurse leave an open drugs trolley to attend a patient with diarrhoea, put soiled paper towels in the bin and then go back to the drugs trolley without washing her hands or wearing gloves. On another occasion, I saw another nurse leave an open drugs trolley unattended for 20 minutes![44]

'Short-staffing': part of the explanation given for pressure sores, being shunted from ward to ward, wet beds, bruising, infection and death – as recounted by a relative about his father's stay in late 2008. This was at Good Hope Hospital in Sutton Coldfield, part of the Heart of England NHS Foundation Trust. Admitted with a urinary tract infection, he was left for eight-and-a-half hours on a trolley. Within four days of admission he developed a sacral pressure sore, followed three days later by a grade four sore on his heel. The hospital admitted that it had failed in its pressure care and that his skin was intact on admission. He was moved from ward to ward, receiving no more than ten minutes of rehabilitation each day and none at the weekend. He was constantly left in a wet bed because his needs for the toilet were not met. His arms became bruised from the removal and re-siting of cannulas. Short-staffing was one explanation given for his care. He then contracted both MRSA and *Clostridium difficile* in the hospital. After an 18-week stay, he died. The son tried to complain

43 Patient Opinion. Accessed on 20 September 2010 at: www.patientopinion.org.uk/opinions/9726.
44 Patient Opinion. Accessed on 20 September 2010 at: www.patientopinion.org.uk/opinions/7983.

to the hospital and was then told that it had lost some of his father's notes.[45]

In 2011, making efficiency savings that would see a reduction in 1,600 staff, the same Trust's chief executive stated that patient care would not be affected. He claimed that front-line staffing levels were adequate and would be protected.[46]

In late 2009, the CQC carried out an inspection of Basildon and Thurrock University Hospitals Trust. It found serious lapses in infection control, associated with higher than usual death rates.[47] Using standard mortality rate statistics, the excess deaths could have been as many as 71 over the period of a year.[48]

The Commission issued a warning notice to the Essex-based Trust under the *Health and Social Care Act 2008*. Its findings included the following. In the medical admissions unit there was some damage to doors and door frames, seat cushions were damaged making cleaning difficult, and some patient tables were stained. In the A&E department there was dust on high and low surfaces, floors stained with blood and other fluid, spillages – and black dirt in corners. There was exposed plaster on walls, damage to doors and wall corners. Holes were evident in a chair, footstool and mattress. Six out of twelve privacy curtains were soiled, some with blood. Side rails of patient trolleys were marked and sticky; dust and dirt was found in the trolley frames and dust on equipment stored in the frames.[49]

In September 2010, the Commission lifted all but one of the conditions it had imposed on the Trust as a health care provider, following an inspection two months earlier.[50] Yet, in the same month, a relative of an elderly patient had put it succinctly:

> Cleanliness is a serious issue. Ward was dirty, sheets and floors stained with god knows what. Whilst visisting [sic] soiled items had been left on floor in ward and only after we complained about the smell were they removed. How is the hospital allowed

45 Patient Opinion. Accessed on 20 September 2010 at: www.patientopinion.org.uk/opinions/32499.
46 'Up to 1,600 West Midlands health trust jobs set to go.' *BBC News*, 21 January 2011. Accessed on 21 January 2011 at: www.bbc.co.uk/news/uk-england-12246849.
47 Bowcott, O. (2009) 'Hygiene inquiry into deaths at Essex NHS trust.' *The Guardian*, 26 November.
48 Rose, D. (2009) 'Hospital trust's failings may have led to 71 deaths.' *The Times*, 27 November.
49 CQC (Care Quality Commission) (2009) *Inspection report: The prevention and control of infections, Basildon and Thurrock University Hospitals NHS Foundation Trust*. London: CQC, p.6.
50 CQC (Care Quality Commission) (2010) 'Conditions lifted at Basildon following improvements but more action needed, says CQC.' *News Stories*, 24 September, London: CQC.

to cut corners on cleanliness????? who is checking up to see standards are kept!!!!!![51]

A month earlier, a relative observed, also at the same hospital:

> Staff actually taking patients to the toilet would have been good! Visiting my grandad and my Dad had to help another patient because he was calling for the nurses to help him out of bed and into his wheelchair and they were ignoring him. Not even saying that they will be with him once they have dealt with so and so… just ignoring him. Changing his sheets would have been good considering he was in there for nearly 2 weeks and they were filthy.[52]

East Surrey Hospital, within the Surrey and Sussex NHS Healthcare Trust, came under scrutiny in March 2010. The CQC raised serious concerns about 3 out of 16 infection control measures that were inspected. The problems included dust and debris on furniture, holes exposing inner foam on furniture for patient use, dust on high and low surfaces, dirt accumulated in corners, privacy curtains soiled with blood, clinical equipment trolleys with blood-stained racks, badly soiled cushions on patients' chairs, soiled commodes ready for patient use, a trolley prepared for patient use exuding a foul odour (and badly soiled with wet inner foam) and other trolley mattresses blood stained (and with dirt and even a needle beneath the mattress).[53] Three months later, the Commission issued a follow-up report, stating that its concerns had now been alleviated.[54]

AND SO IT goes on. The Commission tends to report in a dispassionate and detached manner in its attempt to convey objectivity and professionalism. However, its reports mask too opaquely the experiences of patients on the front line, victims of shocking and harrowing care.

At the end of 2009, the coroner returned a narrative verdict on the death of an 82-year-old woman, Mrs Ivie Clarke, in Western Community Hospital in Southampton. He stated that poor levels of care and cleanliness could have caused the infection, *Clostridium difficile*, that resulted in her death. Her daughter had complained that her mother had been bathed

---

51 Patient Opinion. Accessed on 20 September 2010 at: www.patientopinion.org.uk/opinions/39422.

52 NHS Choices. Accessed on 17 October 2010 at: www.nhs.uk/services/hospitals/patientfeedback/defaultview.aspx?id=744&pid=rddh0&sort=4&pageno=14.

53 CQC (Care Quality Commission) (2010) *Inspection report: The prevention and control of infections, Surrey and Sussex Healthcare NHS Trust, March 2010.* London: CQC, pp.4–5.

54 CQC (Care Quality Commission) (2010) *Follow-up report: The prevention and control of infections, Surrey and Sussex Healthcare NHS Trust, June 2010.* London: CQC.

just twice in three weeks and had to wait 30 minutes to be taken to the toilet. Also that her call bell was out of reach, the bedding and equipment were dirty, nurses were rough with her and that she was given insufficient fluids. The coroner noted that the responses by the hospital to these complaints effectively admitted failings. He pointed out that although infection could be picked up in spotless surroundings, poor standards of cleanliness make it more likely. The hospital apologised; at the time it had been rated excellent. Mrs Clarke had been a campaigner for the rights of elderly people.[55]

(All of which is a sharp reminder that even the most prominent campaigners are not spared the very indignities of which they have written and against which they have fought. In late 2010, Claire Rayner, then President of the Patients' Association, died. Alongside the compassionate care she received, things also went awry. Her son reported that at times agency staff knew little or nothing about her and did not try to find out; her calls for assistance were not responded to, and she felt that she was treated by doctors as a set of conditions and readings but not as a person. Her distress was mingled with anger.)[56]

Despairing of clean wards, bathrooms and toilets, relatives sometimes take it on themselves to do the cleaning. And not only relatives. In 2009, a patient ended up doing it herself. Whilst in Colchester General Hospital she stated that only once had a cleaner briefly visited and had not touched the dusty curtains, dirty bed frames and messy floor. She reported that the nurses just let her get on with it. The hospital's reaction was that it had, between 2007 and 2008, scored top marks for cleanliness and patient safety and had been praised for low infection levels.[57] And in autumn 2009, the CQC awarded the hospital 14 out of 14 for safety and cleanliness. Clearly a case of a disgruntled, ungrateful patient?

Maybe not. In November 2009, the chair of Colchester Hospital University NHS Foundation Trust, responsible for the hospital, was sacked by Monitor, on various grounds including, it seemed, the breaching of infection (MRSA) targets, unusually high death rates at the hospital and lack of patient safety.[58] However, apart from 'patient safety indicators', there were also waiting time breaches for A&E admissions, treatment

---

55 Reeve, J. (2009) 'Hospital criticised over care of Ivie Clarke.' *Southern Daily Echo*, 22 December.

56 Patients' Association (2010) *Listen to patients, speak up for change.* London: Patients' Association, p.1.

57 'Colchester General patient had to clean her filthy ward.' *Daily Gazette*, 4 July 2009.

58 Martin, D. (2009) 'Three thousand needless deaths every year in hospital as watchdog fails to spot poor standards.' *Daily Mail*, 28 November.

admissions and cancer treatments.[59] There was a suspicion that it was on these grounds that the chair lost his job, not patient safety grounds and dirty wards.[60]

BY THE END of 2010, so one might have thought, infection control measures would be routinely in hand, well established and, all importantly, sacrosanct and above the ebb and flow of political target, priority and posturing. Not so. Bed occupancy rates in hospitals remain high, at an average of 86.6 per cent for the year 2009–10.[61] Although there is some argument about the correlation between bed occupancy rates and infection, it is generally accepted that above 82 to 85 per cent a tipping point is reached which then makes outbreaks of infection more likely. And, never mind the infection, this militates against patients being on the right ward for their medical condition and thus receiving appropriate treatment.

The Royal College of Surgeons has expressed its agreement with the National Audit Office that the rate should not be above 82 per cent because of infection risks.[62] And, even where the statistics point to an average rate of 86 or 87 per cent, this does not mean that some hospitals may not be running at 95 or even 100 per cent bed occupancy rates.[63]

Responding to a survey, NHS foundation trusts, the elite of NHS trusts, warned in October 2010 that they foresaw difficulties in keeping infection under control, in anticipation of the spending cuts to come.[64] Accurate or not, such a statement can only suggest that infection and safety continue to be regarded as second fiddle to bigger financial and political objectives.

59 'Monitor issues intervention notice to Colchester Hospital University NHS Foundation Trust.' *Monitor News*, 26 November 2009. Accessed on 20 October 2010 at: www.monitor-nhsft.gov.uk/home/news-and-events/media-centre/latest-press-releases/monitor-issues-intervention-notice-colcheste.

60 Bowcott, O. (2009) 'Deadly hospital gave itself top marks.' *The Guardian*, 27 November.

61 DH (Department of Health) (2010) 'Bed availability and occupancy – year ending 31 March 2010.' Statistical Press notice, 29 June 2010. London: DH.

62 RCS (Royal College of Surgeons) (2010) 'High NHS hospital bed occupancy remains a big infection risk, says RCS.' *News*, 30 June. London: RCS.

63 West, D. (2010) 'Hospital bed transfers put thousands of patients at risk of infection.' *Nursing Times*, 5 October.

64 Lister, S. (2010) 'Hospitals fear downturn will hit cancer targets.' *The Times*, 11 August.

9

Helping People Eat and Drink

> Do not let your patients starve and when you offer them nutrition support, do so by the safest, simplest, effective route. (National Institute for Clinical Excellence, 2006)[1]

> I've been sent letters about older people being left without enough to eat and drink, food being taken away before they have had a chance to eat it, food being left at the end of the bed on a tray where they cannot reach it, food they cannot swallow or the reverse, a sloppy, unappetising blob on a plate. Now this is where the time and money argument really falls down for me. It defies all logic to spend vast sums of money to keep people in hospital or a care home, to give them expensive drugs and then to forget to ensure they get the most basic of human needs – enough to eat and drink. Absolutely barmy and cruel beyond belief. (Sir Michael Parkinson: National Dignity Ambassador, 2010)[2]

In 2009, the Health Service Ombudsman published a report of an investigation into the case of a 43-year-old man, Mr Martin Ryan, who had severe learning disabilities, Down's syndrome and epilepsy, and who lived in a care home. In November 2005, he suffered a stroke and was admitted to a hospital ward at Kingston Hospital on which he was, in theory, under the care of a multi-disciplinary team.[3]

For 26 days he received no nutrition; the death certificate recorded that he died of pneumonia and a stroke. He could not swallow; speech and language therapists assessed that he would need feeding through a tube inserted through either his nose or abdominal wall. However, the medical team dithered and did not take a decision about what to do

---

1   NICE (National Institute for Clinical Excellence) (2006) *Nutrition support for adults: Oral nutrition support, enteral tube feeding and parenteral nutrition.* London: NICE, p.3.

2   Parkinson, M. (2010) *My year as National Dignity Ambassador.* London: Department of Health, p.28.

3   Health Service Ombudsman and Local Government Ombudsman (2009) *Six lives: The provision of public services to people with learning disabilities: Part one, overview and summary investigation reports.* HC 203-I. London: The Stationery Office, p.56. See also: Carvel, J. (2009) 'Man with Down's syndrome dies after starving for 26 days in hospital.' *The Guardian,* 24 March.

for 18 days, by which time he was too ill for a tube to be inserted. The Ombudsman recorded the total failure in nursing:

> The Health Service Ombudsman found that the Ward Sister did not take the lead, as she should have done, in monitoring and managing Mr Ryan's condition. She did not put in place arrangements to guide or support members of her nursing team in caring for Mr Ryan's needs. It was clear she was not aware of failings in her team: for example, assessments were poor, care plans were inadequate and the delivery and evaluation of nursing care was below a reasonable standard in the circumstances. There was no evidence of nursing actions aimed at meeting Mr Ryan's nutritional needs.[4]

However, even in such extreme circumstances, the Ombudsman's language remained measured, suggesting a reluctance to spell out the obvious effect of depriving a person of nutrition for nearly four weeks. With studied under-statement, she conceded that people do need food to live. She said that 'although it was impossible to prove that malnutrition and starvation contributed to or caused Mr Ryan's death, it was likely that the failure to feed him for a prolonged period was one of a number of failings that led to his death'.[5]

The Ombudsman did at least find maladministration. But Mr Ryan's mother put it altogether more compellingly: she had thought her son would be 'in good hands' in the hospital; instead he had 'starved to death'.[6]

MAN PLAINLY DOES not live by bread alone, he needs water also. Yet in some of our hospitals it seems that sick patients are nonetheless expected to survive with neither. Or, perhaps they are simply not expected to survive. If they are resourceful and able to do so, they will drink from flower vases on the hospital ward, as some patients were observed doing on a number of occasions by Julie Bailey when visiting her mother at

---

4   Health Service Ombudsman and Local Government Ombudsman (2009) *Six lives: The provision of public services to people with learning disabilities: Part one, overview and summary investigation reports.* HC 203-I. London: The Stationery Office, p.58.

5   Health Service Ombudsman and Local Government Ombudsman (2009) *Six lives: The provision of public services to people with learning disabilities: Part one, overview and summary investigation reports.* HC 203-I. London: The Stationery Office, p.59.

6   Health Service Ombudsman and Local Government Ombudsman (2009) *Six lives: The provision of public services to people with learning disabilities: Part one, overview and summary investigation reports.* HC 203-I. London: The Stationery Office, p.56.

Stafford Hospital.[7] Within her hundreds of pages of evidence to the public inquiry, she characterised the chaotic scenes at the hospital as akin to Bedlam.[8]

The Hackney Society has produced a succinct work sheet for children, outlining the history of health care in Hackney. It notes that Victorian workhouse infirmaries could often offer little to patients suffering from, for example, cholera, smallpox and fever. But it does make the observation that the availability of food, water and a bed might marginally improve the chances of recovery.[9] And Florence Nightingale had pointed out in her *Notes on nursing,* published in 1860:

> Every careful observer of the sick will agree in this that thousands of patients are annually starved in the midst of plenty, from want of attention to the ways which alone make it possible for them to take food. This want of attention is as remarkable in those who urge upon the sick to do what is quite impossible to them...[10]

This is surely a straightforward reminder that there is nothing more basic and important than ensuring that sick people are given food and drink. It is more fundamental even than helping people to the toilet. Without food and drink there would be little or nothing to excrete. Admitting people to hospital for care and treatment for illness, disease or accident, and then denying them the very basics of life, is grotesque.

Even more so when one considers that denial of hydration and nutrition is taking place at the hands of health care professionals and their managers, on whom patients are entirely dependent. Where such denial occurs, it indicates inescapably a sheer recklessness, on the part of organisations or individuals or both, as to the welfare of their patients or even whether they live or die.

Moving forward from Victorian times to the present, we can now perform cures on people that might previously have been regarded as virtually miraculous. But patients do still need to eat and drink. Making just this point, in 2009, the Nutrition Action Plan Delivery Board, a body set up by the government, published its final report. It referred to continued widespread reports of malnutrition, both in hospital and the community, at the hands of professional carers. In particular it noted

---

7   '"Huge concerns" exist still at Stafford Hospital, inquiry told.' *Birmingham Post,* 24 November 2010.

8   'Cure the NHS campaigner tells of Mid Staffs bedlam (The Press Association).' *Nursing Times,* 23 November 2010.

9   Hackney Society (2010) *The story of health care in Hackney.* London: Hackney Society, p.1.

10 Nightingale, F. (1860) *Notes on nursing: What it is, and what it is not.* New York: Appleton (1st American ed.), p.69.

that 239 patients were reported to have died from malnutrition in English hospitals during 2007. However, this figure represented only 0.5 per cent of the number of people in hospital who die in a malnourished state. Given that malnutrition predisposes to disease, delays recovery and increases mortality, it followed that the effect on mortality rates was far greater than the number of people formally reported to have died directly from it.[11]

The Board thus drew attention to the caution and hesitance attached to implicating malnutrition directly as cause of death, particularly when those dying are sick, anyway, from other conditions. It was not exaggerating this point; even in the case of Mr Martin Ryan, denied nutrition for 26 days, official cause of death still glossed over the contribution of the malnutrition.

Objective signs of malnutrition aside, the whole matter goes wider. Outside of hospital, we put huge store by what we eat and drink and when. Physically and psychologically, even in the course of a single period of 24 hours, intake of nutrition and fluid is essential, simply in order to grapple, reasonably, with everyday life. Yet somehow hospital patients, arguably in extra need of such sustenance to aid recovery, are denied it.

Just where, then, has all the food and drink gone?

FAILURE TO HELP hospital patients eat and drink was raised in the original Dignity on the Ward campaign in 1997,[12] and then subsequently in the Health Advisory Service (HAS) report of 2000, *Not because they are old*.[13]

The NHS Plan of 2000 then stepped in. It stated that people would have decent food to meet their needs and that they would be helped to eat it:

> ...half of all hospitals will have new "ward housekeepers" in place by 2004 to ensure that the quality, presentation and quantity of meals meets patient needs; that patients, particularly elderly people, are able to eat the meals on offer; and that the service patients receive is genuinely available round-the-clock.[14]

11 Lishman, G. (Chair) (2009) *Nutrition Action Plan Delivery Board end of year progress report.* London: Department of Health, p.3.

12 Durham, M. and Bright, M. (1997) 'Join our campaign for the old.' *The Observer*, 5 October. Also: Bright, M. (1997) 'Charity calls for abuse inquiry.' *The Observer*, 26 October.

13 HAS (Health Advisory Service) (2000) *Not because they are old: An independent inquiry into the care of older people on acute wards in general hospitals.* London: HAS, p.11.

14 Secretary of State for Health (2000) *The NHS Plan: A plan for investment, a plan for reform.* Cm 4818-I. London: The Stationery Office, p.47.

The *National Service Framework for Older People* arrived soon after, duly including the need for people to be helped to eat and drink, as well as be given appropriate nutrition.[15] This was reinforced by further Department of Health good practice guidance about the nursing of older people, also issued in 2001. It referred to dietary care plans and assistance to implement them:

> If risk is identified, a dietary care plan is devised with appropriate members of the multi-disciplinary team to ensure that older people receive adequate nutrition and hydration. This includes physical assistance with eating and drinking. Nursing staff will ensure that this is provided.[16]

The guidance was swelled even further in 2001 by the *Essence of Care*, now in a revised 2010 edition. It states that patients should be enabled to consume food and drink to meet their needs and preferences.[17]

Notwithstanding this quantity of direction at the beginning of the decade, on the ground it was a different story to that told, or at least advocated, in the guidance. Patients were being condemned to picking up not only a few crumbs of comfort but also of food.

For instance, in 2002, Walsall Manor Hospital admitted that they had allowed an 86-year-old man, Mr Frederick Thomas, to die after they failed to give him sufficient food and drink for nearly a fortnight. He had undergone a successful hip operation but became severely dehydrated after nurses failed to put on him a drip, as ordered by the doctors. By the time this was realised, it was too late and he died on his 60th wedding anniversary. His daughter commented:

> I thought it was just a broken hip, not a death sentence. Even my dog gets a bowl of water every day. They treated him like he didn't exist. I have got them to hold their hands up and admit responsibility.

The hospital did indeed concede the failure to record adequately his food and fluid intake, to institute a drip to improve fluid intake and to ask the dietician to write up a care plan for his food needs.[18]

---

15 DH (Department of Health) (2001) *National Service Framework for Older People.* London: DH, p.55.

16 Standing Nursing and Midwifery Advisory Committee (2001) *Caring for older people, a nursing priority, practice guidance: Principles, standards and indicators, a resource tool.* London: Department of Health, p.14.

17 DH (Department of Health) (2010) *Essence of Care: Benchmarks for food and drink.* London: DH, p.1.

18 Britten, N. (2002) 'Hospital admits man, 86, died from lack of food.' *Daily Telegraph*, 8 August.

In 2005, a coroner expressed incredulity at the treatment of a hospital patient in Manchester, complaining that it was 'totally unsatisfactory in a major city in a Western democracy that families have to take food into a hospital because their loved ones are not being fed properly by staff'.[19]

The case had involved a 91-year-old woman, Mrs Sarah Ingham, who died in pain weighing five stone. During her three-month stay in Tameside General Hospital in 2004 she lost three-and-a-half stone after staff apparently failed to give her the prescribed soft diet. She had originally been admitted after a fall which had led to a dislocated hip and broken knee. But both injuries were missed and her pain was attributed instead to pressure sores. She was sent home. Readmitted, the injuries were diagnosed and part of her artificial hip removed; however, the operation wound became infected and a chest infection followed.

Her family had become so concerned about her deterioration that they took in their own food to give her. She was then sent home even though she was dying, the hospital telling the family she was ready for discharge. She died two weeks later. The coroner recorded accidental death but criticised the care Mrs Ingham had received.[20]

By 2006, AGE Concern England, aware that government guidance was not doing the trick, produced *Hungry to be heard*. This report referred to the importance of the following to avoid malnutrition in hospital patients: listening to patients and relatives, ward staff being 'food aware', staff following their professional codes and guidance, assessment for signs and risk of malnutrition, protected meal times, a red tray system (indicating help required by patient) and use of volunteers.[21] The report also contained a number of examples of patients effectively being deprived of sustenance (summarised and paraphrased):

- a depressed post-surgical patient who had stopped eating and is given no encouragement to do so
- a meal arriving with the cover on and is taken away in the same state, the food untouched

19 Fresco, A. (2005) 'Woman, 91, dies weighing 5st as hospital "fails to feed her".' *The Times*, 4 October.
20 Fresco, A. (2005) 'Woman, 91, dies weighing 5st as hospital "fails to feed her".' *The Times*, 4 October.
21 Age Concern England (2006) *Hungry to be heard: The scandal of malnourished older people in hospital.* London: Age Concern England, pp.20–6.

- a patient with Parkinson's disease being given no encouragement to eat and fortifying drinks being left out of reach resulting in dehydration

- a patient with Coeliac disease (inability to digest gluten) continually given inappropriate food despite his wife persistently telling staff about his dietary needs

- meals being left out of reach of patients – including an 88-year-old woman recovering from a severe infection – to such an extent that relatives set up a rota of visits to ensure that the patients actually get their food

- a patient suffering weight loss because she could not eat her food unassisted – the hospital had a notice encouraging relatives to come in to help at meal times, but not all relatives of course have the time to do this

- an elderly woman with dementia, requiring pureed food because of swallowing problems, being given lumpy food

- the family of a 92-year-old woman (confused and barely conscious because of medication and so often leaving her food untouched) being told that the nurses did not have time to help her eat or drink. The ward sister suggested the family come in and help her eat.[22]

Although they were not holding up its hands publicly, at least some in the Department of Health must have been uneasily aware that all was not well. In that same year of 2006, guidance on standards for better health care stated that:

> ...health care organisations should ensure that patients are provided with a choice and that it is prepared safely and provides a balanced diet...and patients' individual nutritional, personal and clinical dietary requirements are met, including any necessary help with feeding and access to food 24 hours a day.[23]

Still in that same year the National Institute for Clinical Excellence (NICE) published detailed guidance about nutritional support for adults in both hospital and the community. It dealt not just with assistance but also causes of malnutrition, screening of patients, clinically appropriate

---

22 Age Concern England (2006) *Hungry to be heard: The scandal of malnourished older people in hospital.* London: Age Concern England, pp.14–19.

23 DH (Department of Health) (2006) *Standards for better health.* London: DH, p.14.

diet, methods of assistance, etc. The guidance, though detailed, has a simple overall rationale and aim. It points out that the consequences of malnutrition include vulnerability to infection, delayed wound healing, impaired recovery, precipitation of other medical conditions, longer hospital stays and threat to life.[24] Overall, its gist, including its startling opening statement, quoted at the beginning of this chapter, is to the effect that patients should not be left to starve.[25]

The problem was that as the guidance piled up, so too did the bad news. In 2006, the Healthcare Commission reported, at Mid Cheshire Hospitals National Health Service (NHS) Trust, a significant lack of assistance for patients with eating, not to mention medication. Indeed, the Trust's own survey had found that necessary assistance was given only about 50 per cent of the time with eating and drinking.[26] In the same year, the commission had observed that at Stoke Mandeville Hospital, the shortage of nurses meant that patients had not been receiving their food supplements.[27]

In 2007, the coroner condemned as unacceptable the care given to an 86-year-old woman, Mrs Minnie White, at Louth Hospital. He characterised the failure to provide nourishment and basic medical attention as neglect, though not as the cause of death. She was admitted following a scooter accident, discharged the same day, but immediately readmitted after collapsing at home. She then contracted *Clostridium difficile* at the hospital, and suffered with diarrhoea and ulcerative colitis until she died. The doctor concerned admitted her condition worsened because of inappropriate medication and of a failure to consider putting her on a drip when she became malnourished and dehydrated. It had also been an error to transfer her to a non-acute intermediate care facility in another hospital. Her bedside table was left dirty, and her daughter had to wash her mother's soiled nightwear. Nurses and junior doctors failed to keep monitoring charts of the patient's condition. The coroner condemned these failures as 'inexcusable'.[28]

24 NICE (National Institute for Clinical Excellence) (2006) *Nutrition support for adults: Oral nutrition support, enteral tube feeding and parenteral nutrition.* London: NICE, p.2.
25 NICE (National Institute for Clinical Excellence) (2006) *Nutrition support for adults: Oral nutrition support, enteral tube feeding and parenteral nutrition.* London: NICE, p.3.
26 Healthcare Commission (2006) *Investigation into Mid Cheshire Hospitals NHS Trust, January 2006.* London: Healthcare Commission, p.34.
27 Healthcare Commission (2006) *Investigation into outbreaks of* Clostridium difficile *at Stoke Mandeville Hospital, Buckinghamshire Hospitals NHS Trust, July 2006.* London: Healthcare Commission, p.47.
28 Ladbroke, C. (2007) 'Louth hospital neglected patient says coroner.' *Louth Leader*, 30 August.

Even when the need to maintain adequate nutrition and hydration is acutely obvious, appropriate care may still not be forthcoming. In the case of patients who had become infected with *Clostridium difficile* at Maidstone and Tunbridge Wells NHS Trust, there was no evidence of assessment and management of fluid and electrolyte losses – notwithstanding the degree of such loss owing to diarrhoea. Likewise, nutritional management seemed to be absent, despite evidence of the declining nutritional status of patients.[29]

Belatedly in 2007, former Health Minister, Ivan Lewis, would admit to older people not being given food and drink in hospitals and care homes:

> ...some older people are still being served their dinners with plastic cutlery, even though they have suffered a paralysing stroke which makes it pretty impossible for them to eat properly. Some have a tray placed on the end of the bed, tantalising with hot food. It may be just an inch out of reach but it might as well be a mile. To a bed-ridden pensioner, it must seem like torture. We wouldn't put up with this happening to our children, so why should we find it acceptable for our older people?[30]

These were shades of the concern expressed ten years earlier by a predecessor Health Minister, Frank Dobson. As the reports and criticism piled up, so the government was forced back to the table, much as it had been at the end of the 1990s. There followed an action plan for improving nutritional care, as it quietly conceded that:

> ...the very people who are being cared for by health and social care services are at times not getting the right nutritional care to support them to eat and drink.[31]

It referred to five key issues: awareness of the link between nutrition and good health, accessible guidance, nutritional screening in health and social care, training for front-line staff and managers about the importance of nutrition for good health – and the strengthening of inspection and regulation.[32] Also, the Nutrition Action Plan Delivery Board was set up to facilitate improvement.

29 Healthcare Commission (2007) *Investigation into outbreaks of* Clostridium difficile *at Maidstone and Tunbridge Wells NHS Trust, October 2007*. London: Healthcare Commission, p.34.

30 Womack, S. (2007) 'Starving on a spoonful of mash a day.' *Daily Telegraph*, 26 January.

31 DH (Department of Health) (2007) *Improving nutritional care: A joint action plan from the Department of Health and Nutrition Summit stakeholders*. London: DH, p.3.

32 DH (Department of Health) (2007) *Improving nutritional care: A joint action plan from the Department of Health and Nutrition Summit stakeholders*. London: DH, p.3.

AN AGE CONCERN England survey in 2008 indicated that almost 50 per cent of NHS trusts had not introduced a system of 'protected meal times' for nurses to help people eat and drink, and about a third had not introduced the 'red tray' system to indicate that a particular patient needed help with eating.[33] A flavour of this was given by a patient of Royal Doncaster Infirmary in 2007:

> It would have been better if there were more cleaners on the ward and if the nurses would answer the patients buzzers when they go off. I was opposite a patient who could not feed herself, did she get help? NO. It was myself who fed and watered her, it was only when we had almost finished feeding her that a nurse came to take over and the food trolley was coming to collect the trays.[34]

By 2010, the Mid Staffordshire Independent Inquiry reported what had been happening at Stafford Hospital from 2005 to 2009. The nutritional failures at this NHS trust were far from minimal:

- lack of menus

- provision of inappropriate food for patients' conditions

- failure to provide a meal

- meals placed out of reach and taken away without being touched

- patients not helped to unwrap the meal or cutlery

- patients not encouraged to eat

- relatives and others denied access at meal times

- visitors having to assist other patients with their meals

- visitors prevented from helping feeding

- water not available at the bedside

- water intake not encouraged or monitored

- drip feeds not monitored adequately

- monitoring and appropriate records of fluid balance not maintained.

The Inquiry also heard the following sort of evidence about how patients were deprived of food:

---

33   Salter, J. (2008) 'Age Concern charity warns that old people going hungry in hospital.' *Daily Telegraph*, 24 August.

34   Patient Opinion. Accessed on 20 October 2010 at: www.patientopinion.org.uk/opinions/1812.

Without saying anything, the healthcare assistant placed a tray of food on the table in front of the other patient, who was immobile and unable to reach the tray, and left again. She returned approximately 15 minutes later and collected the tray of untouched food.[35]

It summed up by referring to a systemic failure to ensure that one of the basic responsibilities of a hospital was fulfilled:

...the provision of food and water is one of the most basic responsibilities of a hospital and its staff. Patients are often unable to provide for themselves. Each patient requires individual consideration. The deficiencies observed in the evidence were not confined to one ward or period. Frequently the explanation appears to have been a lack of staff, but sometimes staff were present but lacked a sufficiently caring attitude. There was evidence of unacceptable standards of care as a result of systemic failings. What has been shown is more than can be explained by the personal failings of a few members of staff.[36]

A drink may be forthcoming in hospital but only at a cost in emotional distress to the patient, as recorded in 2009 by the husband of Mrs Ann McNeill about her care in Barnet General Hospital:

...there were a number of times I was shocked at the lack of dignity and compassion shown to her. She told me of one time that she had awoken in the night, dreadfully thirsty and unable to reach her drink. She pressed her buzzer for assistance. When the nurse arrived he said "What do you mean by waking me at this time of night? What do you want?"[37]

The Patients' Association also recorded the following occurrence of dehydration, when a doctor expressed incredulity at how Mrs Oenone Hewlett had become so dehydrated in St Mark's Hospital:

Sometimes several days went by without any records at all – this is especially so regarding food and drink intake, elimination and measures of her blood pressure and weight. This meant that as [her] condition deteriorated there was no recognition of her decline, and when her weight loss became critical, no action was taken...the doctor thought she must have been at home

---

35 Francis, R. (Chair) (2010) *Independent Inquiry into care provided by Mid Staffordshire NHS Foundation Trust January 2005–March 2009*. London: The Stationery Office, p.43.

36 Francis, R. (Chair) (2010) *Independent Inquiry into care provided by Mid Staffordshire NHS Foundation Trust January 2005–March 2009*. London: The Stationery Office, p.12.

37 Patients' Association (2009) *Patients not numbers, people not statistics*. London: Patients' Association, p.32.

alone and neglecting herself. We had to explain she had been in hospital. He couldn't understand how she could've become so dehydrated.[38]

The Association's 2009 report, detailing what happened to 16 patients in hospital, made the news for a few days. It was heartening that it caused a stir, but perhaps surprising because it was really saying nothing new. It had collated and publicised but a few of the accounts, which were being reported regularly, albeit more piecemeal, in the Press.

MRS JEAN ARTHUR, an 89-year-old woman, died from heart and kidney failure at Wansbeck General Hospital in 2008. At the inquest, her son related how family members would frequently find her food untouched, and that hospital staff did not make sufficient effort to ensure she was eating well. He also said that sedation was used against the family's wishes, and that a catheter and wound dressings were not changed frequently enough. The coroner returned a narrative verdict, doubting that the problems with food had significantly contributed to her death. But he noted that Northumbria Healthcare Trust had acknowledged shortcomings, and that he would write to the Trust asking it to consider actively how to improve the regime for helping patients eat and drink.[39]

A doctor and his wife, both health care professionals themselves, commented on the care in 2008 of the doctor's 89-year-old mother at St Martin's Hospital, Canterbury, and on the deprivation of nutrition and hydration, together with the development of pressure sores:

> [She was] suffering from severe depression with features of psychosis... Despite our best efforts, on admission...she was very frail, malnourished and very depressed. We made this very clear to the nursing staff and we expected basic nursing assessments to be performed (Waterlow, MUST etc.). As far as we know they were not. Indeed, she was not even weighed on admission. Medication was not helpful, the nursing care she received was terrible and within days she had developed bleeding sacral sores... These sores were not noticed by the nursing staff, but found by me on one of my daily visits, when I noticed blood on her chair. At around the same time we noticed she had developed a foot drop, but despite pointing it out nothing was done about it. She continued to eat and drink poorly and lose weight. The staff appeared to put little or no effort into encouraging her to

38 Patients' Association (2009) *Patients not numbers, people not statistics.* London: Patients' Association, p.21.

39 'Elsdon man criticises care.' *The Journal Rothbury,* 12 September 2009.

eat or drink, and their lack of care was reported to us by other patients. Food and drink would be put in front of her and taken away when it hadn't been consumed. The bulk of the care of patients was devolved to nursing assistants, whilst the trained staff spent the majority of their time in the office. It was only on my suggestion that she was given Resource drinks to supplement her poor food intake.[40]

In 2009, the Healthcare Commission upheld a complaint against Airedale General Hospital, made by a woman about the care in 2006 of her 84-year-old father, Mr John Farrow, a war veteran. He had been unable to feed himself and had also been given the wrong food. Staff said they were too busy to help. He then developed ulcers and blisters in his mouth which made it difficult for him to drink. For nearly two weeks after his admission, she had been unable to speak to a specialist; he died aged 84 from heart failure and renal problems.[41]

Even patients with obvious sensory impairment may fare no better. In 2009, a 92-year-old woman, Mrs Irene Hudson, partially deaf and blind in one eye, was admitted to Lewisham Hospital with severe leg pain. She also had dementia and needed help with eating and taking medication. In less than two weeks she lost half a stone. She could not remove the lid and cling film on her food; medication was left in little cups that she sometimes missed. It took a week for nurses to put a notice on the bed alerting staff to her blindness. The hospital apologised and vowed to avoid a repeat performance.[42]

A cavalier and reckless attitude to people's nutritional needs can even work the other way and just as lethally. A coroner gave a narrative verdict when stating that a 76-year-old man, Mr Bernard Bennett, had in 2008 died of fluid overload at Kettering General Hospital. He had been given intravenous fluids because of a belief that he was dehydrated, following an operation on his bowel. The hospital apologised for deficiencies in his care. This was linked to a lack of note taking and recording by staff.[43]

And fatal outcomes may be achieved not just cumulatively over time but instantaneously. Another coroner expressed strong criticism following the death of a patient in 2009 at the Royal Sussex County Hospital; he

40   Patient Opinion. Accessed on 20 October 2010 at: www.patientopinion.org.uk/opinions/8670.
41   Waites, M. (2009) 'NHS complaints system attacked.' *Yorkshire Post*, 10 February.
42   Goodchild, S. (2010) 'Woman, 92, left "to starve in hospital".' *Evening Standard*, 5 January.
43   'Kettering General Hospital apologises for man's death.' *Evening Telegraph* (Northamptonshire), 3 April 2010.

had choked on his own dentures as he ate alone, even though he was meant to be receiving assistance. This precipitated a fatal heart attack.[44]

WITH SUCH OCCURRENCES still being regularly reported, the Care Quality Commission's (CQC) guidance of 2009 had plenty to say about nutrition. It states that people should be encouraged and supported to have adequate nutrition and hydration, and be given a choice of nutritionally balanced food and drink.[45]

A second set of guidance from the Commission went into some detail, perhaps an indication of the mountain to climb. Staff should identify, and continue to review, those people at risk of poor nutrition or dehydration. Action should be taken where such risk is identified, and this should be set out in a care plan. Referral should be made to appropriate services. People should be supported with their eating and drinking needs with sensitivity and respect for their dignity and ability – and enabled to eat and drink as independently as possible.

The guidance then gets back to the obvious, affirming that all assistance necessary should be provided to ensure people eat and drink. This includes provision of appropriate equipment and people being helped into an appropriate position to allow them to eat and drink safely. Meal times should not be interrupted except in case of emergency. Special diets or dietary supplements should be arranged as needed with appropriate advice.[46]

BY 2009, THE government showed signs of wanting to move on and also silence the Nutrition Action Plan Delivery Board it had set up three years before. Taking a final published bow in 2009, the Board reiterated ten key characteristics of good nutritional care. In summary, these included safe delivery of a food service and nutritional care, an environment conducive to enjoyment of a meal, a multi-disciplinary approach to nutritional care, specific guidance from the care provider for staff, screening of people for malnourishment, flexible facilities and services, care plans, appropriate skills and training for staff and volunteers – and a care provider policy on food service and nutritional care.[47]

---

44 'Major nursing overhaul at Royal Sussex after patient deaths.' *The Argus*, 12 March 2010.

45 CQC (Care Quality Commission) (2009) *Guidance about compliance: Summary of regulations, outcomes and judgement framework.* London: CQC, p.14.

46 CQC (Care Quality Commission) (2009) *Guidance about compliance: Essential standards of quality and safety.* London: CQC, pp.77–9.

47 Lishman, G. (Chair) (2009) *Nutrition Action Plan Delivery Board end of year progress report.* London: Department of Health, p.8.

Winding up the Board, the Minister, Phil Hope, referred to programmes underway to improve matters.[48] The Board was unconvinced:

> ...a significant and continuing problem with malnutrition and help with eating... The Board feels that the attention of Ministers and others should be drawn to the direct human cost of malnutrition and failures to help with eating in hospital and care settings.[49]

Its final report exhibits barely suppressed frustration and anger with central government. One observation stands out, which characterises more generally the attempts to deal with neglectful care within the health service. It lamented that it had in effect been preaching to the converted, whereas the people who mattered – that is, those in charge – remained outside the circle and would remain so, until they were held accountable:

> ...we are concerned that our work has simply not connected with many of the people who need to hear the core messages: managers, service providers and Board members. We have talked with, and have succeeded in extending, the circle of people who understand and respond to the nutritional needs of the people with whom they work. However, it is essential that the management and regulatory structures of health and care providers accept a wider responsibility which ensures that all professional staff, at all levels of the services, see issues around nutrition and help with eating and drinking as a core part of their responsibilities, for which they will be held to account.[50]

This clash reflects the fact that central government is captivated too easily by task forces, working groups, initiatives, indicators and gathering of associated statistics. For instance, protected meal times are one such. The assumption would be that if they were reported to the Department of Health or to the CQC as being in place, then all would be well.

The truth in fact may be the exact opposite and the protected meal times, perversely and in some circumstances, exacerbate the very evil they were designed to eradicate. In other words, the corrosive effect of insufficient or uncaring staff is capable of souring and undermining the best of intentions. Evidence given to a parliamentary committee in 2009 included the following instance, involving just such protection leading not to improved nutritional status but to slow starvation:

---

48 Hope, P. (2010) (Minister of State of Department of Health) *Hansard.* House of Commons Written Statements, 25 February, col. 75WS.

49 Lishman, G. (Chair) (2009) *Nutrition Action Plan Delivery Board end of year progress report.* London: Department of Health, pp.3, 6.

50 Lishman, G. (Chair) (2009) *Nutrition Action Plan Delivery Board end of year progress report.* London: Department of Health, p.4.

She grew very thin and it was obvious to visitors that, although she has always had an excellent appetite, she found great physical difficulty in feeding herself and using a cup. Visitors would have been only too willing to help her but they were discouraged from staying during meal times. She appeared to be slowly starving to death.[51]

The Mid Staffordshire Inquiry records that whilst patients needed help from relatives to eat and drink, nonetheless it tells also of visitors being prevented from doing so on grounds of health and safety. A 90-year-old patient, formerly a nurse herself, had plenty to say about this:

After her experience, she met with the Chief Executive to discuss her complaint. She was so concerned with other patients that she volunteered to visit the wards to help feed them. She was told, however, that this was not possible because health and safety regulations would not permit it. She concluded her written evidence to me with the following stark summary: "malnutrition and starvation…was one of the hazards of being in a geriatric ward at Stafford".[52]

The sheer perversity of pleading both health and safety and protected meal times – when the consequence of doing so is to put the health and very life of patients at risk – is clearly lost on some health care managers and staff. An account given to the organisation, Age UK, sums it up:

My dad had to undergo surgery to remove half a lung. As we had no faith in the NHS in caring for Dad, my brother booked into a hotel nearby and stayed with Dad at the hospital. Although my brother was available to ensure that Dad got food and drinks every mealtime, he was ordered off the ward as they had "protected mealtimes". Every time my brother came back, Dad's tray of food was untouched – it was left out of my dad's reach. My brother tried to get my dad to eat, but by this time his food had gone cold. Dad was told by a nurse to drink a glass of water every hour. Given that my dad could not get out of bed and no water was given to him, I still wonder how they thought he was going to manage this.[53]

---

51 House of Lords and House of Commons Joint Committee on Human Rights (2007) *The human rights of older people in healthcare: Eighteenth report of Session 2006–07.* HL 156-I, HC 378-I. London: The Stationery Office, p.12.

52 Francis, R. (Chair) *Independent Inquiry into care provided by Mid Staffordshire NHS Foundation Trust January 2005–March 2009.* London: The Stationery Office, p.293.

53 Quoted in: Age UK (2010) *Still hungry to be heard: The scandal of people in later life becoming malnourished in hospital.* London: Age UK, p.13.

IN ANY CASE, the evidence continued to suggest that the weight of argument lay with the Nutrition Action Plan Delivery Board and not with the Minister. Figures were released, indicating that in 2008–09, 185,446 people were discharged from English hospitals with a diagnosis of malnourishment, compared with 175,003 who were admitted malnourished.[54] The following year, the number of patients recorded leaving hospital malnourished, compared to those entering it in such a state, had risen to over 13,000.[55]

Of course not all malnourishment that develops in hospital can be laid at the door of the institution. Malnutrition is generally down to insufficient or poorly-balanced diet; alternatively it might be associated with faulty digestive processes. Thus, people may have eating or swallowing difficulties or lose appetite in depression. Gallstones or stomach ulcers may make eating painful and cause diarrhoea or vomiting, by which means nutrients are lost. Severe illness or surgery may lead to lack of nutrition. And intestinal disorders can hinder absorption of food.[56] It may be a natural consequence of a disease such as cancer or dementia. For example, some years ago, allegations were made by staff that 11 hospital patients were deliberately starved at Kingsway Hospital in Derby, in order to hasten their deaths.[57] The inquest concluded that they died of natural causes, although the coroner did raise issues about practices on the ward concerned.[58] Even making these allowances, a serious concern remains.

Age UK published in 2010 *Still hungry to be heard*, a follow-up to Age Concern England's 2007 report. It maintained that a serious problem still remained. Some hospitals had made progress, others had not, and whether you were helped at meal times could even vary across wards in the same hospital.[59]

On the ground, unsettling accounts had not dried up unlike, in some cases, the food and drink. February 2010 saw 22-year-old Mr Kane

54 Smith, R. (2010) 'Thousands of patients leave hospital malnourished.' *Daily Telegraph*, 22 January.
55 Borland, S. (2010) '13,500 patients "left to starve" on NHS wards: Elderly suffering most as malnutrition cases hit new high.' *Daily Mail*, 6 December.
56 Personal communication: NHS Information Centre, December 2010.
57 Rogers, L. (2004) 'Coroner seeks inquiry into "mass euthanasia" at hospital.' *The Times*, 8 February.
58 'Elderly patients died of natural causes at Derby Hospital.' Alexander Harris, Solicitors, 21 March 2005. Accessed on 7 September 2010 at: www.alexanderharris.co.uk/News/ClinicalDentalNegligence/Pages/ElderlypatientsdiedofnaturalcausesatDerbyHospital.aspx.
59 Quoted in: Age UK (2010) *Still hungry to be heard: The scandal of people in later life becoming malnourished in hospital.* London: Age UK, p.5.

Gorny die of dehydration at St George's Hospital in Tooting, South London. The coroner referred the death to the police for investigation by homicide and serious crime detectives. Before he died, the patient had rung the police and asked for help, claiming that he was being denied drinks on the hospital ward. The hospital stated that it had now introduced new procedures to prevent a reoccurrence.[60]

In May 2010, Southampton General Hospital apologised for failings with food. Private caterers, with whom the hospital had a contract, had failed in a number of ways to ensure that Mrs Florence Smith, a 96-year-old woman with pressure sores, received the food she needed. On admission, she was underweight and needed building up. But catering staff ignored her side ward on several occasions, sometimes they did not give her the next day's menu, didn't understand her needs and brought the wrong food. On one occasion, she requested soup but received a diabetic patient's food; on another, a glass of milk but none of the requested food. She correctly missed food prior to an operation, but because she was unable to fill out the menu on that day, no food came the next.[61]

Also in 2010, the CQC reported on the health care provided for older patients with organic mental health disease at Totnes Hospital in Devon. It found that, in many instances, the rationale for decisions about care were not being documented; in addition, basic nursing elements such as weight, fluid and nutrition measurement were not being recorded. Underweight patients were usually without care plans for nutrition or dietary supplements, with any advice from dieticians going unrecorded.[62]

OVER 30 YEARS ago, the most famous punk band of all, the Sex Pistols, shocked respectable society with a succession of songs that were deemed to be rather crude and aggressive. They sang in one song, released as a single in July 1977, how they were 'pretty vacant', followed up by the observation that 'we don't care'. Inspirational to some, for others their music conveyed, and conveys, mindlessness and anarchy.

What on earth has this band, and more particularly these sentiments, got to do with food and drink in hospitals? In one sense, nothing; presumably the band did not have in mind the starvation and dehydration of older people in health care institutions. Yet perhaps their (at the time)

60 Jamieson, A. (2010) 'Police probe of hospital patient who begged for water.' *Daily Mail*, 6 March.

61 'Claims that underweight patient "not fed properly" at Southampton General Hospital.' *Southern Daily Echo*, 14 May 2010.

62 CQC (Care Quality Commission) (2010) *Investigation into the mental health care for older people provided by Devon Partnership NHS Trust, June 2010*. London: CQC, pp.10, 12.

shockingly raw sentiments about society were more prescient than they may have suspected. The mental vacuity and nihilism expressed have, unexpectedly, become accurate, dispiriting, descriptors. Not for punk rockers and their successors but, instead, for hospitals run by the State. Hospitals which, quite matter-of-factly and with chilly detachment, deprive their most vulnerable patients of the very stuff of life. With barely the bat of an eyelid.

10

Pressure Sores and Falls

Agreed person-focused outcome: people experience care that maintains or improves the condition of their skin and underlying tissues. (Department of Health: *Essence of Care*, 2010)[1]

I was also invited to meet the group known as *Cure the NHS*, and I spent a Friday afternoon with them at the café and I saw photographs of pressure sores there which frankly were truly shocking. I have never seen anything like it. Really gruesome and a very sad indictment of what was going on. I don't know if those were people that had the pressure sores and were admitted and they got worse, or whether or not they came in without the pressure sores and developed them, but either way, it was as bad as it gets. (General Secretary of the Royal College of Nursing: evidence to the Mid Staffordshire Independent Inquiry, 2009)[2]

A theme of this book is the lack of care and attention sometimes provided in hospital, particularly for older people. Two particular consequences of this come in the form of pressure sores and falls.

Not all, but many of these, are avoidable. The problem is well known. Still they persist. At best, allowing them to flourish is a terrible waste of money; where is the rationale of having people in hospital, receiving expensive treatment and taking up expensive bed space – only to undermine all this with life-threatening (and agonising) sores and falls, the consequences of which entail still further expense?

At worst, it is sheer cruelty on the part of those hospitals that oversee, routinely, their excessive incidence. Government guidance urges, in civilised tones, that they must be avoided where possible or at least reasonably managed. But about the underlying neglectful care, there is nothing civilised.

THE DAUGHTER OF an 86-year-old war veteran of the 1944 D-Day landings, Mr Kenneth Ballinger, recounted how she remained haunted

---

1   DH (Department of Health) (2010) *Essence of Care: Benchmarks for prevention and management of pressure ulcers*. London: DH, p.7.

2   Francis, R. (Chair) (2010) *Independent Inquiry into care provided by Mid Staffordshire NHS Foundation Trust January 2005–March 2009*. London: The Stationery Office, p.96 (evidence from the General Secretary of the Royal College of Nursing).

by her father's screams of agony in Leeds General Infirmary. He had been admitted in 2006 after a fall. He died, however, not from this, but instead from multiple bedsores, including one the size of a fist; his hip bone was exposed and he had no skin left on his heels. The Leeds Teaching Hospitals NHS Trust conceded mistakes had been made and reached an out of court settlement with the family of £20,000. The mistakes included not carrying out a pressure sore prevention plan within 24 hours of admission, leaving him in soiled bedding and leaving him to feed himself despite being aware he was unable to do this.[3]

Pressure sores and ulcers develop when skin and underlying tissue become damaged. In more serious cases they expose muscle, tendon and bone. Great pain, suffering, septicaemia and sometimes death follow.

They are reported to cost the National Heath Service (NHS) a great deal of money to treat. Worse than this, they are often caused or made worse by the lack of, or inappropriate, care and treatment in hospital. This might typically involve a dearth of assessment, of basic nursing care (including regular, physical turning of the patient) and monitoring, of appropriate equipment and of communication between wards or different organisations when a patient is being moved.

It is not realistic to say that a patient should never have pressure sores in hospital; a sore may have developed elsewhere prior to admission. And, on occasion, a person may be so vulnerable to tissue breakdown that prevention of some sore areas is very difficult. However, there is a view that the development of new pressure sores in hospital should, in principle, be an infrequent event. It is commonly claimed that old fashioned nursing alone, without the benefit of special pressure-relieving beds and other aids, would in days gone by have prevented most pressure sores. As one relative in 2010, a nurse herself, saw things at the Royal Chesterfield Hospital when her mother's untended skin led to agony:

> She could not move around the bed and was on a ripple mattress. I asked if she could be moved more to prevent a pressure sore. I was told by an HCA that "we don't need to be that any more, because of the special mattresses". I was horrified. Any Spinal Injuries Nurse (who do this...so called "basic" care so superbly) would have recoiled at that remark... And, so do i, as a Nurse for the past 25 years!... Anyway...you know what's coming next... she got a sore sacrum. The Nurse came to see her and said it was very superficial and clean and it was so painful because it was superficial (which i understand). Mum deteriorated and could not

---

3   'Payout over veteran neglect death', BBC News, 17 November 2009. Accessed on 16 August 2010 at: http://news.bbc.co.uk/1/mobile/england/west_yorkshire/8365237.stm.

get out of bed any more. She needed very good skin care and pressure care. The day that she died (Monday 26th April)…she was turned and repositioned for comfort…low and behold a huge sore on her Sacrum, about the size of the palm of your hand, and with now much fuller thickness. She asked to be moved as her bottom was "agony"…her word. I was appalled and extremely angry that she was going to die like that.[4]

If the development of most pressure sores is avoidable, then the government-run NHS Choices information page makes disturbing reading. Up to October 2010, it stated that pressure ulcers are widespread, and 'that between four and 10% of all patients admitted to hospital will develop at least one pressure ulcer. For elderly people with mobility problems, the figure can be as high as 70%.'[5] The statement is disarming, deadpan, damning and silent about the fact that this should not be happening.

This is not the way the General Secretary of the Royal College of Nursing saw it when giving evidence to the Mid Staffordshire Independent Inquiry. Using words such as 'truly shocking' and 'gruesome' in commenting on patients' pressure sores at the hospital, she went on to say:

> …with…people that are seriously ill, sometimes it is very difficult to avoid pressure sores, but they should be at an absolute minimum. You will hear from people – from different eras – that would pride themselves that you would never see a pressure sore within a ward. I still go to lots and lots of hospitals where they can demonstrate that they don't have pressure sores, but to say never, it would be very, very difficult, but they should be at an absolute minimum. Where you have a high incidence of pressure sores, that is definitely an indicator that something is fundamentally wrong.[6]

An experienced nurse, also giving evidence to the Inquiry, was asked if patients used to get pressure sores, and answered:

> Very rarely, and you were on the mat for it if you did. This is a very, very important thing. It was a matter of shame if you got a pressure sore… We had to twice a day go round with a tray, whatever your rank, you went around every patient, you rubbed

---

4   Patient Opinion. Accessed on 20 October 2010 at: www.patientopinion.org.uk/opinions/32062.

5   NHS Choices. 'Pressure ulcers.' Accessed on 20 September 2010 at: www.nhs.uk/conditions/Pressure-ulcers/Pages/Introduction.aspx.

6   Francis, R. (Chair) (2010) *Independent Inquiry into care provided by Mid Staffordshire NHS Foundation Trust January 2005–March 2009*. London: The Stationery Office, p.96.

their elbows, their heels and their back with – first you did it with soap and water and then you wiped that off and then you rubbed it with spirit and then you rubbed it with – powdered it with talc. That was a twice-daily routine. That is why we didn't have bed sores. We very rarely got an abscess, very rarely.[7]

Accordingly, Department of Health practice guidance for nurses states that pressure 'damage prevention and management forms an important part of nursing assessment and care'. Nursing assessments should be carried out to determine risk and, working in partnership with other staff, nurses should work to prevent pressure damage and manage it.[8] Further guidance, called the *Essence of Care*, states that: 'People [should] experience care that maintains or improves the condition of their skin and underlying tissues.' It talks about screening and assessment, information, care planning, preventative equipment and preventative care regimes such as regular repositioning of the patient.[9]

Despite this guidance, significant failure continues to be reported in practice. As already noted, it is thought that between 4 and 10 per cent of patients admitted to NHS acute hospitals develop new pressure sores.[10] Taking the lower figure of 4 per cent, this would mean that 320,000 people developed pressure sores in hospital in the United Kingdom in 2000.[11]

The expense to the NHS of treating and managing pressure sores is well documented and accepted. For example, some data suggest that the cost of treating sores varies from £1064 for a grade one ulcer to £10,551 for a grade four. Total annual costs in the United Kingdom have been estimated in the past at between £1.4–£2.1 billion, some 4 per cent of total NHS expenditure.[12]

---

7 Francis, R. (Chair) (2010) *Independent Inquiry into care provided by Mid Staffordshire NHS Foundation Trust January 2005–March 2009.* London: The Stationery Office, p.95.

8 Standing Nursing and Midwifery Advisory Committee (2001) *Caring for older people, a nursing priority, practice guidance: Principles, standards and indicators, a resource tool.* London: Department of Health, p.18.

9 DH (Department of Health) (2010) *Essence of Care: Benchmarks for prevention and management of pressure ulcers.* London: DH, pp.7–8.

10 RCN (Royal College of Nursing) and NICE (National Institute for Clinical Excellence) (2005) *The management of pressure ulcers in primary and secondary care: A clinical practice guideline.* London: RCN, p.25.

11 Bennett, G., Dealey, C. and Posnett, J. (2004) 'The cost of pressure ulcers in the UK.' *Age and Ageing 33*, 230–35.

12 RCN (Royal College of Nursing) and NICE (National Institute for Clinical Excellence) (2005) *The management of pressure ulcers in primary and secondary care: A clinical practice guideline.* London: RCN, pp.25–6.

The suffering and cost is illustrated in the following account of what happened to a man's wife in 2007 at the Royal Bolton Hospital, where she had developed an undetected and untreated pressure sore:

> My wife kept falling without warning and went into Royal Bolton, on ward 4. She came out with a bedsore on her bottom and had not been treated for this or notified that it was there.
>
> It was only when my wife came home that the West Houghton District nurses found my wife had a bedsore on her bottom. It hadn't been treated and consequently she has been in an orthopaedic bed for 13 months. She is still in bed and treated daily by West Houghton District nurses (once a day). We have care people 3 times per day.
>
> The Bolton hospital nurses never mentioned this sore, it was only when she came out of this hospital that the nurses from West Houghton Clinic found it. This is unacceptable. I am so angry that they let this happen to my wife. The nurses were run off their feet, but they still should have found it!
>
> My wife and I are both in our eighties. I have to look after the house and care for my wife. We are too old for this business![13]

If these figures are correct for the incidence of pressure sores developing in hospital, then the following examples are but a minute sample.

THE INDEPENDENT INQUIRY at Stafford Hospital found evidence of people having bad experiences with pressure sores including avoidable skin breakdown. This suggested lack of care – resulting from too few staff, inconsistent use of assessment techniques and too little multi-disciplinary working.[14] One relative gave evidence to the Inquiry about the lack of dressings and cream:

> Her husband developed large pressure sores on both of his heels. She recalled that "time and time again his dressing had come off and his wounds were exposed to the air... This was at the time when MRSA was rife in the hospital". She had to dress the wounds herself but the hospital did not even have the necessary creams and dressings for her to use. She recalled that "his wounds smelled dreadfully and needed to be cared for properly".[15]

---

13 Patient Opinion. Accessed on 20 October 2010 at: www.patientopinion.org.uk/opinions/2576.
14 Francis, R. (Chair) (2010) *Independent Inquiry into care provided by Mid Staffordshire NHS Foundation Trust January 2005–March 2009.* London: The Stationery Office, p.13.
15 Francis, R. (Chair) (2010) *Independent Inquiry into care provided by Mid Staffordshire NHS Foundation Trust January 2005–March 2009.* London: The Stationery Office, p.393.

And it was not just a case of people being admitted with pressure sores but of the development of sores through poor hospital care:

> Another witness told me how a pressure sore her mother had incurred before her admission to Stafford had been resolved while she was being cared for by her family at home with the assistance of a pressure-relieving air bed. After her admission, the patient's sore returned. Her daughter told me: "The pressure sore came back. By the time we got her back from the hospital, the pressure sore came back and she was only in there Monday afternoon to Thursday, and we fetched her by 5 o'clock on the Friday and the pressure sore had come back again. I do not think we ever got are rid of it after that."[16]

Figures put forward by the Healthcare Commission were that, of a sample of 38 patients at Stafford Hospital, 55 per cent had pressure damage, but only four of these patients had pressure damage before admission to hospital.[17]

At Maidstone and Tunbridge Wells NHS Trust, where patients were dying from an uncontrolled outbreak of *Clostridium difficile*, the Healthcare Commission expressed concern about the speed with which new pressure sores developed – not all of which could be directly associated with loose stools in the form of diarrhoea. For instance, some were on an unconnected body part, people's heels. Existing sores deteriorated quickly, and even the local primary care trust (PCT) had complained to the Trust.[18]

In May 2010, the Care Quality Commission (CQC) issued a warning to the Weston General Hospital in Weston-Super-Mare, that the hospital had too high an incidence of pressure sores. This followed a complaint made about the care received by Mr Robert Collins prior to his death. The complaint, to the Commission, was made by the nursing home to which he was discharged from the hospital. His son-in-law had also complained, to the hospital, discovering that a chart to assess pressure sores was not properly kept and that Mr Collins' diabetes (a risk factor for pressure sores) was not taken into account. Mr Collins developed grade four pressure sores, where muscle, tendon or bone is exposed.[19]

---

16 Francis, R. (Chair) (2010) *Independent Inquiry into care provided by Mid Staffordshire NHS Foundation Trust January 2005–March 2009.* London: The Stationery Office, p.96.

17 Healthcare Commission (2009) *Investigation into Mid Staffordshire NHS Foundation Trust, March 2009.* London: Healthcare Commission, pp.64–5.

18 Healthcare Commission (2007) *Investigation into outbreaks of* Clostridium difficile *at Maidstone and Tunbridge Wells NHS Trust, October 2007.* London: Healthcare Commission, pp.35, 66.

19 'Town given warning over bedsores.' *Weston-super-Mare-People,* 27 May 2010. Accessed on 20 September 2010 at: www.westonsupermarepeople.co.uk/news/Town-hospital-given-warning-bedsores/story-4565438-detail/story.html.

ASIDE FROM FORMAL reports by regulatory commissions, there are many accounts published in the Press and also on the websites of some legal firms.

Avoidable pain and death may certainly follow from pressure sores, as revealed in the following account provided by the family. When they visited their grandmother, Mrs Pamela Goddard, suffering from cancer in East Surrey Hospital, they often found her lying in faeces and urine – and had to prompt staff to come and wash and change her. She had pressure sores. She had been referred to a tissue viability nurse who never came – the nurse was on annual leave for ten days but no explanation of this was given.[20]

When admitted for radiation treatment, two months before her death, an incipient sore was noted; however, during Mrs Goddard's stay this became 'raging', which left her groaning in pain. The family had regularly turned her when she had still been at home, in order to manage the sore area; they claimed that in hospital this was not done. The explanation apparently given by hospital staff was that either there was only one nurse available (but that two were required) or that the equipment was broken. The family stated that they had tried to get the nurses to do something but that there seemed to be institutional inertia – and Mrs Goddard 'was basically in torture over a four-week period. Then she was drugged up and left to die. It's unconscionable, very sad.' The cause of death was given as septicaemia from the pressure sore.[21]

'Joan's gone now. She passed away in agony just don't let it happen to other people.' These were the words of the son-in-law of Mrs Joan Street, an 87-year-old woman admitted in 2009 to William Harvey Hospital in Ashford, for a routine hip operation, but who developed bedsores in her lower back. Cause of death was recorded as acute tracheo-bronchitis and a sacral pressure sore. The inquest established that she had been assessed by the hospital as being at high risk of pressure sores, but recording of both the ulcers and pain management was not complete. The chronology was that broken skin was recorded a week after her operation and a pressure-relieving mattress not provided for a further five days. She died eight weeks later. East Kent University Hospitals NHS Trust admitted failures and offered the family £7500 in compensation.[22]

20 'Hospital care: Pamela Goddard's bed sores were inadequately treated.' *Daily Telegraph*, 27 August 2009.

21 Johnston, I. (2009) 'Patient lived with cancer for 50 years before dying of bedsore.' *Daily Telegraph*, 5 July.

22 'Kent hospital admits failures over 87-year-old's death.' *BBC News*, 20 August 2010. Accessed on 20 September 2010 at: www.bbc.co.uk/news/uk-england-kent-11043750.

In March 2010, the Belfast Health and Social Care Trust admitted liability and made a £40,000 out of court settlement in relation to the death of Mrs Lily Convill. Her family had claimed she was not treated properly and died from septicaemia as a result. She was admitted to Royal Victoria Hospital with a suspected broken hip. For about two weeks, staff were undecided about whether it was broken; in the meantime she was allowed to develop a pressure sore on her heel, which deteriorated until the whole heel turned black and gangrenous.[23]

Mrs Joan Hollis, a 74-year-old woman, was admitted to Derbyshire Royal Infirmary suffering from lung disease. Before she died, she developed pressure sores which resulted in her dying in avoidable pain and discomfort. The doctor responsible for the post mortem examination identified that she had died with infected sores, one centimetre long on her leg, and four centimetres long and deeply penetrating at the base of her back. He stated to the inquest, held in January 2009, that, without the sores, she would probably have died in less pain and discomfort. The Derby Hospitals Trust apologised to the family for the failings in care. The family had not wanted to apportion blame, but had been appalled as they watched their mother suffer so.[24]

The suffering and neglected patient need not be elderly, though often seems to be. In 1999, a 37-year-old man with multiple sclerosis was admitted to the Royal United Bath Hospital NHS Trust with pneumonia. Transferred to a neurological ward, visitors regularly found him lying in his own faeces and urine, unwashed and with food and medication out of reach. The family had raised concerns about his vulnerability to pressure sores, but a special mattress was only located on the day he was discharged, ten days after admission.

By then he had developed a pressure sore on his buttock, as large as a man's fist; his general practitioner (GP) was so disturbed that he wrote a letter of complaint to the hospital. He was then nursed by his family and by district nurses; the pressure sore needed 18 months' treatment, but it was believed that the sore had accelerated his multiple sclerosis. He no longer talked, no longer enjoyed television or music. He barely moved and, because of the pressure sore, lay on his side a lot. An expert stated that the energy required to recover from such a sore would have provoked deterioration in his condition of multiple sclerosis. He lost a lot

---

23 'Belfast Trust pays damages over pensioner's death.' BBC News, 1 March 2010. Accessed on 1 September 2010 at: http://news.bbc.co.uk/1/hi/northern_ireland/8544259.stm.

24 Walsh, A. (2009) 'Hospital trust sorry as pensioner spends last days suffering.' *Derby Telegraph*, 27 January.

of weight. A legal settlement with the Trust was reached by solicitors for about £90,000; he then died less than a year later.[25]

ASSUMING THAT THERE is not a collective loss of memory of many older nurses, or too many rose-tinted spectacles focused on the past, it seems extraordinary that pressure sores should be so prevalent in hospitals despite the existence of many sophisticated pressure-relieving aids, including beds, mattresses and cushions.

It is therefore impossible to escape the conclusion – whether through lack of competence, training, staffing numbers or appropriate management-led policies – that patients are being left to develop penetrating pressure ulcers in hospitals. There is an irony in that a veteran soldier, perhaps a hero, who escaped being killed in a world war, should finally succumb to grisly wounds caused by a hospital's neglect.

PRESSURE SORES ARE one consequence of not attending to patients, particularly the elderly; falls another.

Falls in older people have been identified by the Department of Health as a major issue. In particular, it notes that they are at particular risk of falling in hospital, and that efforts should be made to record such incidents, learn from them and minimise them.[26]

At Stafford Hospital there was 'striking evidence' of the incidence of falls – and of these repeatedly being unobserved, unreported or reported inaccurately and belatedly by staff, who were either too few in number or insufficiently qualified to cope.[27] For example, a 90-year-old woman suffered three falls within five days after which she died, despite being known to be at risk of falling (the very reason she was admitted); there was no evidence of preventative measures taken or of effective planning.[28] The sound of patients going smack on the floor was part of the routine:

> In Mum's bay the woman in the next bed, she would sound the buzzer and it would just go off and off and off and then the same – it was the same thing, she would just call out for the nurse. When the nurse did come, she would be put on to the commode

25 *PGM v Royal United Hospital Bath NHS Trust*. Withy King Solicitors. Accessed on 20 September 2010 at: www.withyking.co.uk/site/individuals/srvclinicalneg/failure10.html.

26 DH (Department of Health) (2001) *National Service Framework for Older People*. London: DH, p.80.

27 Francis, R. (Chair) (2010) *Independent Inquiry into care provided by Mid Staffordshire NHS Foundation Trust January 2005–March 2009*. London: The Stationery Office, p.11.

28 Francis, R. (Chair) (2010) *Independent Inquiry into care provided by Mid Staffordshire NHS Foundation Trust January 2005–March 2009*. London: The Stationery Office, p.66.

and it was obviously too late. The nurse would put her back into the bed, you could hear her – she would wait on the commode for half an hour and very often she would just try to make it herself and just go smack on to the floor. So you would have to go searching – if you couldn't do it yourself, you would have to go searching, and I mean searching, for the staff. Very often you would just give up. I would just have to give up.[29]

The Patients' Association likewise reported in 2009 repeated omissions to keep a patient safe and the thumps as he hit the floor on several occasions:

I went to the hospital the next morning and I was told my husband had fallen out of bed and as a result cut his head badly while trying to get himself to the toilet. There was still blood on the pillowcase and blood on the floor. When I spoke to the nursing staff asking why my husband had fallen out of bed, the comment was "we heard the terrible thump on the floor" and when I asked the nursing staff why the guard rails were not up on the bed, they said that they had "forgotten…" My husband fell out of bed again (!) while trying to go to the toilet and when I went back in to see him, there was blood again on the pillowcase and again his head was badly cut and there was also blood on the floor. I asked why again the guard rails were not up on the bed and the answer was again that they had forgotten. Not surprisingly, my husband wanted to go home.[30]

The Association related also how a woman's mother had suffered at least seven falls since being in hospital over a short period, leading to a subdural haemorrhage. The daughter observed of another patient:

There was an elderly lady in a bed next to Mum, I don't know what her diagnosis was but it was clear she didn't know where she was or what she was doing. The first day I met her she was in a hospital gown, no underwear and walking around with dried blood down the gown and her foot. I was horrified to see not only had she not been washed and changed but also that she was sitting on my Mum's bed and even tried putting her foot in my hand bag. I also witnessed her standing by the door urinating, as she went to walk, she almost slipped over, at which point my husband went to grab her to stop her fall whilst calling out for one of the nurses who were standing only two feet away

29   Francis, R. (Chair) (2010) *Independent Inquiry into care provided by Mid Staffordshire NHS Foundation Trust January 2005–March 2009*. London: The Stationery Office, p.53.

30   Patients' Association (2009) *Patients not numbers, people not statistics*. London: Patients' Association, p.44.

chatting. On another occasion the same lady fell in the toilet next to my Mum's bed, we heard a loud crash, she had fallen into the shower screen and smashed it. She had wet the floor so the nurses covered it with paper towels and put her back in bed. The shower screen was cleared up but when I took my Mum to the toilet the following night the floor was exactly how the nurses had left it the previous night, urine all over the floor.[31]

ABSENCE OF RISK assessment seems to be a common theme. Mrs Iris Dodd was an 83-year-old woman living at home. She fell on 24 August 2009 and was admitted to the Gloucestershire Royal Hospital. Three days later she fell on the ward, whilst going to the toilet. On 2 September she fell again; this precipitated a major bleed on the brain, a subdural haematoma, from which she probably died. Despite the fact that she was admitted because of a fall, the staff caring for her did not know this and no risk assessment was carried out. In any case, staff were unaware of procedures and protocols for patients at risk of falling. The coroner criticised the failure to implement a falls prevention policy and to assess the risk.[32]

Similarly, an absence of risk assessment was the downfall of Mrs Olive Unwin, who had been admitted to the Royal Berkshire Hospital in 2008 with a chest infection. Within 90 minutes of admission, she had climbed out of bed, fallen and hit her head; death followed a few days later. Her daughter stated that had the nurses read her mother's patient notes straight away, they would have known she suffered from confusion and so was at risk.[33]

So, the risk assessment may simply come too late. Mrs Ivy Bunn, 90 years old, was admitted to Stafford Hospital in October 2008. Within seven days, she suffered three falls, the last of which killed her. It was only after the first two that a risk assessment was carried out; in addition, her liquids were not monitored and regular neurological observations were not carried out as they should have been. Her family pointed out that she had been a capable and independent woman and that they were

31 Patients' Association (2009) *Patients not numbers, people not statistics*. London: Patients' Association, pp.65–72.

32 'Hospital staff criticised after pensioner's death.' *This is Gloucestershire*, 29 March 2010. Accessed on 20 October 2010 at: www.thisisgloucestershire.co.uk/news/Hospital-staff-criticised-pensioner-s-death/article-1950227-detail/article.html.

33 'Elderly woman died after fall at hospital.' *Getreading*, 6 November 2008. Accessed on 16 August 2010 at: www.getreading.co.uk/news/s/2038831_elderly_woman_died_after_fall_at_hospital.

appalled by the lack of care she received. The hospital stated that lessons had been learnt.[34]

A patient may fall and die even when there *has* been an assessment of risk. For instance, a coroner expressed strong criticism of the death of a 72-year-old man, Mr Brian Waller, at the Royal Sussex County Hospital in 2009. He had fallen out of bed, even though he was wearing a wrist band with 'risk of falls' written on it, to alert staff. He landed on his head, broke his neck and died six days later.[35] The hospital in question was the very same which had been exposed in 2005 by a Panorama programme and the 'whistleblowing' nurse, Margaret Haywood.

In February 2009, a 77-year-old man, Mr John Hooper, fell at the Royal Oldham Hospital on his way to the toilet, having passed the nursing station. He had difficulty walking but no help was offered. The coroner considered that as a matter of course, and out of respect for his dignity, he should have been assisted. He died from the consequent brain haemorrhage. The coroner criticised the risk assessment procedures for vulnerable patients and requested that the hospital send him updated procedures. However, in the coroner's view, this failing did not amount to neglect on the part of the nursing staff.[36]

Of course, if nurses don't answer call bells, risk assessments and care plans may anyway be redundant. A patient noted, in 2010, of Airedale Hospital:

> ...patient care is dreadful – elderly patients left crying out for help and the nurses failed to answer the buzzer even after 40 minutes, two patients in their eighties were allowed to have falls on the ward and both broke their hip, no understanding of how to nurse patients on general wards with dementia, almost total lack of communication with relatives...utterly dreadful.[37]

Sometimes hospitals fail to deal with the consequences of falls after they have occurred. Mrs Mary Churchman, 95 years old, was admitted to the Royal Bolton Hospital with a badly broken thigh bone and a shattered knee cap. Only her hip was X-rayed, so both fractures were missed. She

34 'Hospital issue apology over fall pensioner.' *This is Staffordshire*, 4 September 2010. Accessed on 24 January 2011 at: www.thisisstaffordshire.co.uk/news/Hospital-issue-apology-fall-pensioner/article-2609263-detail/article.html.

35 'Major nursing overhaul at Royal Sussex after patient deaths.' *The Argus (Brighton)*, 12 March 2010.

36 Ayala, B. (2010) 'Coroner attacks falls risk policy for vulnerable.' *Oldham Evening Chronicle*, 10 February.

37 NHS Choices. Accessed on 18 October 2010 at: www.nhs.uk/Services/Hospitals/PatientFeedback/DefaultView.aspx?id=805&pid=RCF22&pageNo=2&sort=1&recordPP=0.

was sent to an intermediate care home, where she spent four days in agony until a physiotherapist intervened and had her sent back to hospital. She then contracted both MRSA and *Clostridium difficile* in the hospital, both of which she survived; she returned home two months later after her readmission. The hospital apologised, stating, with no hint of irony, that it had reminded staff that they should examine the 'whole leg'.[38]

Similarly, a coroner raised concerns with the Heart of England NHS Foundation Trust following the death of Mr Arthur Burley. Ninety-five years old, he had suffered a fall at the nursing home in which he lived and hit his head. He was taken to Heartlands Hospital but then returned to the nursing home a few hours later. He deteriorated and was then admitted later the same day to Solihull Hospital. The coroner found that he should have been given a computed tomography (CT) scan, kept under observation and had his blood thinning medication, warfarin, stopped immediately. The bleed was belatedly identified but even then the plasma he needed was not made available for 23 hours. The notes from his admission to the first hospital were not available to the second hospital, even though both were part of the same foundation trust. The advice of a neuro-surgeon was sought but not received for 12 hours. The coroner stated that there was no doubt that these failures made his survival much less likely, but stopped short of labelling them as the cause of death.[39]

In 2001, as already noted, the *National Service Framework for Older People* drew attention to falls, the threat they to pose to elderly people and to the need to set up local falls prevention services.[40] Six years later, in June 2007, a 64-year-old man, Mr Anthony Horobin, fell and fractured his skull in the Princess Royal Hospital in Telford. He died. Criticised by the coroner, the Trust promised to set up a falls prevention service. It got only as far as a 'falls task force', without actually setting up a team to do anything about the problem.

In November of that same year, another patient died at the hospital, this time 89-year-old Mr Francis Steele, who had fallen out of bed. The inquest jury pinpointed failures by both Trust and nurses in relation to his death; the verdict was accidental death which was caused – or contributed to – by individual failure, itself flowing from systematic failure. The latter,

38 Lavender, J. (2010) 'OAP sent home from hospital with broken leg.' *This is Lancashire*, 11 February 2008. Accessed on 30 July 2010 at: www.thisislancashire.co.uk/news/2033694. oap_sent_home_from_hospital_with_broken_leg.
39 'Falls pensioner died after Heartlands Hospital blunders.' *Birmingham Post*, 25 August 2009.
40 DH (Department of Health) (2001) *National Service Framework for Older People.* London: DH, p.77.

in turn, was due to chronic staff shortages and a lack of training. By 2010, the time of the second inquest, the falls prevention service still had not been set up. The hospital spokesman gave an assurance, that despite this delay and the two deaths, the Trust took falls 'very seriously'.[41]

IT SEEMS FAIR to say that both pressure sores and falls have become an accepted fact of life in at least some, maybe many, hospitals. Whilst nobody claims they could all be prevented, it appears that many could.

The risks are familiar, the consequences serious, painful and potentially fatal. It is difficult to account for this continuing phenomenon other than by the sheer indifference of politicians, hospital managers and staff. This leads, when considered in the cold light of day, sometimes to what is in effect punishment being inflicted on patients, largely the elderly, for being sick and vulnerable. If one didn't know better, a notion of sadism might even come into mind.

---

41 'OAP's death happened despite hospital safety pledge.' *Shropshire Star*, 24 May 2010.

11

Hospital Beds, Admissions, Stays and Discharges

Needs-based models where patients are allocated on admission either to specialist wards for older people or to general wards, based on locally agreed criteria. Decisions on the most appropriate ward are based on perceived clinical need. (Department of Health: *National Service Framework for Older People*, 2001)[1]

Staff on general wards and relatives of patients told us that many patients had to move from one ward to another, some several times. We note that this is not uncommon in acute hospitals. Ward managers, junior doctors and senior nurses also told us about patients having multiple moves and said this was not uncommon. There were reports of patients, including some with *C. difficile*, being moved up to six times in one stay... Many of the ward moves took place at night. For the period February to April 2006, at Maidstone Hospital 21% (514) ward moves happened between 9pm and 6am. (Healthcare Commission, 2007)[2]

And so to beds. Ever present, snaking in and out of poor and neglectful care, is the issue of how people get admitted to hospital beds, how their stays progress and how they are discharged. Unwaveringly, what emerges is a tale of insufficient numbers of hospital beds, chaotic admission processes, harmful movement of patients from ward to ward during their stay – and premature, undignified and inappropriate discharges.

A REDUCTION IN hospital beds has long been part of overall government policy (albeit unspoken) to shift a proportion of secondary (hospital) care to primary (community) care. However, closures of beds and associated reductions in staff attending them have outstripped the development of alternative community services. There has in addition almost certainly been a misjudgement as to how much complex need, involving

---

1   DH (Department of Health) (2001) *National Service Framework for Older People*. London: DH, p.59.

2   Healthcare Commission (2007) *Investigation into outbreaks of* Clostridium difficile *at Maidstone and Tunbridge Wells NHS Trust, October 2007*. London: Healthcare Commission, p.71.

medical instability, can be dealt with outside of hospital. Together with government emphasis on the throughput of patients, this state of affairs has put immense pressure on the occupation of those hospital beds remaining. The policy has gone astray.

It all started with a National Beds Inquiry commissioned in 1998 by the Secretary of State for Health. The results indicated a system under pressure, with capacity sorely tested.[3] Following the Inquiry, it was announced that implementation of *The NHS Plan* meant that there would be 7000 new beds in total. Of these, some 2000 were to be in general and acute wards. There would in addition be 5000 extra intermediate care beds, some in community or cottage hospitals, some in specially designated wards in acute hospitals, some in purpose-built new facilities – and some in redesigned nursing homes and residential homes.[4] Intermediate care was, and is, a somewhat vague term. It is associated generally with the provision of simpler and quicker forms of rehabilitation, outside of an acute hospital setting. It is not associated with more complex rehabilitation.[5]

In 2000, the Audit Commission expressed the view, in its perceptive report called *The way to go home*, that simpler rehabilitation and reablement outside of acute hospitals – called intermediate care – was indeed a promising development. It warned, however, that it should not come at the expense of older people with more complex needs, who were not medically stable and required intensive inpatient rehabilitation.[6] The warning has gone unheeded.

BY THE MID-2000s, there were increasing pressures to save money by reducing the number of hospital beds and of attendant staff. Elderly care and rehabilitation beds in acute hospitals seemed to be at particular risk, as well as community hospital beds. When, following the 2005 General Election, the Health Secretary, Patricia Hewitt, called for massive savings, National Health Service (NHS) trusts were falling over themselves to shed both beds and staff, by the score and sometimes by the hundred. For instance, in 2006 the *Southern Daily Echo* reported the upcoming loss of 564 jobs and 140 beds in Southampton – following 600 posts and

---

3   DH (Department of Health) (2000) *Shaping the future NHS: Long term planning for hospitals and related services. Consultation document on the findings of the National Beds Inquiry.* London: DH.

4   DH (Department of Health) (2001) 'Implementing *The NHS Plan*: developing services following the National Beds Inquiry.' Health Service Circular 2001/03. London: DH, para. 7.

5   DH (Department of Health) (2009) *Intermediate care: Halfway home.* London: DH.

6   Audit Commission (2000) *The way to go home: Rehabilitation and remedial services for older people.* London: Audit Commission, p.21.

109 beds lost the previous year.[7] This was not such an atypical newspaper headline for the period.

The NHS budget was over-spent, by a relatively small amount, but the demands emanating from the Secretary of State at the time verged on the hysterical. Local NHS chief executives were told to come within budget at all costs, whatever it took.[8] Patricia Hewitt's avowal that she would take personal responsibility for the savings was bad news for everybody; it caused even more stress than usual for all those chief executives and the harassed tiers of management beneath – and more importantly loss of services for patients, particularly the more vulnerable. In time honoured political fashion, this was happening just after the 2005 General Election, when promises could be broken for a year or two and then hopefully forgotten about by the time of the next vote.

In addition, the threat to community hospitals and their beds was widespread and arguably unprecedented. In 2006, a hastily formed body called CHANT, Community Hospitals Acting Nationally Together, pulled together a petition of 300,000 signatures to protest at the threat across England.[9] The scale was not surprising; across the country there was a remarkable number of protest marches and petitions at the time.[10]

In Cumbria alone, where nine community hospitals were threatened, a weekend of action was accompanied by a petition of almost 70,000 signatures. In all, at one time, some 100 community hospitals were under threat; a nurse consultant, Linda Nazarko, encapsulated what all this could mean to vulnerable older people and to why the closure of such non-acute beds would be so harmful:

> It is cold and dark. We are expecting very cold weather. There is a shortage of flu vaccine and an epidemic is predicted. People are falling ill and the hospitals are crammed to capacity... Acute hospitals are closing beds, freezing posts, cutting back on agency staff and even making staff redundant in order to save money. Yet many people considered medically fit may not be well enough to go home. Community hospitals can help ease these pressures... They offer sub-acute care so that acute hospitals can discharge quicker, and provide ongoing rehabilitation following illness or

---

7   Makin, J. (2006) 'Job cuts will lead to a better service.' *Southern Daily Echo*, 28 June.

8   See: 'NHS must make surplus next year.' BBC News, 11 December 2006. Accessed on 20 September 2010 at: http://news.bbc.co.uk/1/hi/6161535.stm.

9   Stuart, G. (Chair of CHANT) (2006) 'One thousand campaigners from across the country attended a rally in Westminster yesterday to protest against closures and cutbacks to community hospitals.' News release, 29 March. London: CHANT.

10 Mandelstam, M. (2006) *Betraying the NHS: Health abandoned.* London: Jessica Kingsley Publishers, pp.112–16.

> injury and high-quality palliative care… However, now it seems
> that PCTs may close up to 100 community hospitals to save
> money.[11]

Although some community hospitals and their beds were saved, nonetheless the gist of the newspaper headlines was not misleading. By 2008, it had become clear that instead of an increase in NHS beds, as promised in 2000, there had in fact been a huge decrease. The statistics revealed a loss of 32,000 NHS hospital beds, one in six, in the ten-year period between 1997 and 2007. In 2007 alone, 8400 beds were lost. In 1997 there were nearly 190,000 NHS beds in England; by 2007, this figure had dropped to 160,000.[12]

WITHIN THIS OVERALL picture, the British Geriatrics Society has drawn attention to the loss of many inpatient rehabilitation beds, without obvious replacement – at least in terms of complex, slower stream rehabilitation services.[13] At the time of writing, closures of rehabilitation and elderly care beds are continuing.[14] And a new coalition government is now working out how to apply a severe brake on public spending. It is almost certain, therefore, that despite all the problems for older people associated with such closures – including neglectful care – more beds will be lost, without genuine alternatives available either in principle or practice.

Central government has by no means denied this colossal bed loss, despite the promises made in 2000 of more beds. The explanation given generally is that people have shorter hospital stays, more day surgery and that some people's chronic needs can be met in their own homes by well resourced community teams. All of which is true, but only up to a point. In the ongoing struggle to save money, such arguments have been taken too far.

An illustration of the fanciful thinking that has taken hold came in East Anglia. The Suffolk West Primary Care Trust (PCT) was overseeing the closure of significant numbers of acute beds in the West Suffolk Hospitals NHS Trust at Bury St Edmunds. It also proposed to shut large numbers of community hospital beds as well. Its director of clinical services stated

---

11 Nazarko, L. (2006) 'It is the worst possible time for cuts in the NHS.' *Nursing Times*, 3 January, p.13.

12 Donnelly, L. (2008) 'NHS hospitals lose 32,000 beds in a decade.' *Daily Telegraph*, 24 May.

13 British Geriatrics Society (2007) *Rehabilitation beds report on the second England council survey.* London: British Geriatrics Society.

14 Bowcott, O. (2010) 'Fears that community hospitals face the threat of being shut down.' *The Guardian*, 27 January.

in 2006 that there was no problem: 'There are thousands of beds in West Suffolk: in people's own homes.'[15]

In 2010, in an annual report containing more pictures than text, NHS Suffolk (the enlarged PCT) expressed great disappointment with the performance of the acute hospitals, from which the PCT itself had overseen the removal of so many beds. Why the disappointment? Against a target of stroke patients spending 90 per cent of their stay on the right ward, namely a stroke unit, only 35 per cent had been achieved.[16] This was highly predictable, given the cull of beds that had taken place in Suffolk.

The difficulty is that not everybody's medical, nursing and rehabilitation needs can be met in the community; acute and non-acute hospital beds are still obviously required in sufficient numbers. Second, even when care and rehabilitation is possible in principle in the community, nonetheless well-resourced, adequately skilled community teams do not come cheap, and this can mean a corresponding reluctance to fund them sufficiently.

For instance, at Maidstone and Tunbridge Wells NHS Trust, excessive bed occupancy and resulting infection were partly, in the NHS Trust's view, the result of the local PCT's failure to treat more patients in the community, despite its promises to do so.[17] A view shared by many hospitals, frustrated at effectively being ordered from above to close beds, at the lack of alternative community solutions, at the continuing demand for beds – and at the perpetual anxiety thereby engendered.

The anxiety and frustration are inevitable; the hospitals are trying to balance an equation that cannot, by definition, be balanced – because of the awkward and contradictory variables placed within it by central government.

IMPERSONAL MOVEMENT OF patients from ward to ward might seem akin to the progress of manufacturing a product in a factory. Governments talk of productivity in the health service; perhaps this is what they mean. But even this unsettling analogy is inapt. Products are moved down the production line to the right part of the factory to enable efficient assembly; if they go to the wrong place, they will not be finished or will be flawed. If they are missing a part, not checked or inspected and yet still sent out, the products are likely to fail or to be recalled.

---

15 'Thousands of beds at home.' *Suffolk Free Press*, 13 April 2006.

16 NHS Suffolk (2010) *Annual report 2009–10*. Bramford: NHS Suffolk, pp.3, 26.

17 Healthcare Commission (2007) *Investigation into outbreaks of* Clostridium difficile *at Maidstone and Tunbridge Wells NHS Trust, October 2007*. London: Healthcare Commission, p.102.

This is precisely what happens too often in acute hospitals; patients, particularly the elderly, may not only be moved frequently and randomly but are placed on inappropriate wards before being discharged prematurely. Evidence points to the clinical needs of patients too often held to be secondary to finance and other priorities, with resulting detriment and sometimes death occurring.

A surgical patient might end up on a medical ward or vice versa, in which case he or she may not see the appropriate consultant or nursing staff. Patients in the wrong place are sometimes referred to as 'outliers'. This status can lead not only to inadequate treatment and care, but also to distress and anxiety for patients, who are unable to obtain adequate information about what is going on. Avoiding all this grief, the patient may instead simply be sent home too early, medically unstable, to die or to be readmitted almost immediately.

The ascendancy of bureaucracy and managerialism over patient care was illustrated simply and devastatingly in the case of the schoolgirl, Clementine Nicholson. Admitted with meningitis to University Hospital Coventry, she was at first treated appropriately with antibiotics and fluids on a resuscitation unit; she then disappeared and was lost for an hour, during which time the doctors were searching for her. This was because a bed manager had her moved to two inappropriate wards without the consent of the relevant clinicians. By the time she was finally transferred to the intensive care unit, where she should have been, she was effectively moribund.

The coroner gave a narrative verdict but identified a number of faults; he could not be certain that they contributed to her death but this could not be ruled out. The 'associate director for clinical performance' at the hospital expressed regret that the girl had in effect 'been moved by an electronic bed management system'.[18]

In short, moving people around in hospital for non-clinical reasons – or indeed discharging them from a hospital inappropriately – is bad for them.

OVERCROWDING EXPLAINS A lot. If there aren't enough beds in a hospital to allow people to be on the right ward for the length of time required, things will clearly and inevitably go awry. And the effects have been known, for some time, to be not just unfavourable but potentially

---

18 'Dying Warwickshire schoolgirl "lost" by Coventry hospital, inquest told.' *Birmingham Post*, 6 October 2010. Also: 'Coventry University Hospital criticised over Clementine Nicholson.' *Coventry Telegraph*, 7 October 2010.

disastrous. This was even before the Healthcare Commission hit the headlines, with its condemnation of events at Stoke Mandeville in 2006 and Maidstone and Tunbridge Wells in 2007.

Already in 2002, the Commission for Health Improvement (CHI) had reported on the chaos in East Kent Hospitals NHS Trust, which comprised the Queen Elizabeth the Queen Mother Hospital in Margate, the William Harvey Hospital in Ashford and the Kent and Canterbury Hospital, as well as two community hospitals.

The Commission had found that overcrowding in the hospital's accident and emergency (A&E) department put patients at clinical risk and staff under excessive pressure. People were simply admitted to any bed, which meant staff were caring for patients without the appropriate skills, and doctors were seeking their patients throughout the hospital. This caused delays in arranging treatment and obtaining drugs; one patient had to wait *14 hours* for a cannula to be changed because of the difficulty in finding the responsible doctor.

Associated with this state of affairs came other failings. Trays were regularly delivered to the ward with dirty cutlery; food was often cold. Toilets and washing facilities were insufficient for the number of patients, who sometimes had to be physically examined in open areas. Patients might be left in corridors for days rather than hours.[19]

At Maidstone and Tunbridge Wells NHS Trust, which was riddled with infection, the high bed occupancy and frequent bed moves were reported to be distressing for patients. Astonishingly, some were moved up to six times during their stay, moves often made during the night. Doctors complained as well as relatives – sometimes they did not get to see their patients for days.[20] Spread of infection was thus facilitated:

> At the private part of the board meeting in July 2005, it was reported that patients were moved frequently between wards, increasing the risk of cross-infection. Senior nurses raised concerns at their monthly meetings about the movement of patients.[21]

And at Stoke Mandeville Hospital, clinical staff had repeatedly expressed concern about moving patients to different wards because of the likely spread of infection. But no effective action was taken to stop this.

---

19 CHI (Commission for Health Improvement) (2002) *Clinical performance review: East Kent Hospitals NHS Trust.* London: CHI, pp.5–10.

20 Healthcare Commission (2007) *Investigation into outbreaks of* Clostridium difficile *at Maidstone and Tunbridge Wells NHS Trust, October 2007.* London: Healthcare Commission, p.71.

21 Healthcare Commission (2007) *Investigation into outbreaks of* Clostridium difficile *at Maidstone and Tunbridge Wells NHS Trust, October 2007.* London: Healthcare Commission, p.71.

Between 38 to 50 per cent of moves were not for clinical reasons, but caused by bed capacity issues.[22] At the hospital, patients were exposed to potentially lethal infection because of priorities and targets which overrode the need to isolate infected patients. Instead they were left occupying beds in open wards instead of side rooms.[23]

The Healthcare Commission reported in 2006 also, at Mid Cheshire NHS Hospitals Trust, that excessive bed occupancy had meant that every day between 15 and 40 patients who should have been on medical wards were instead on surgical wards. Consequently, patients would not get to see their consultant for days or even at all. Bed managers, rather than clinicians, determined where patients should be treated. Continuity of care was lost as patients were moved; and criteria for controlling movement of patients were often not adhered to because of pressure to meet the A&E four-hour waiting target.[24]

Nurses felt they were under pressure to move patients who were not fit to be moved. Significant numbers of moves occurred right through the night from 6pm onwards and after midnight. Some patients were moved several times; families reported the distress this caused. In addition, the frequent moves led to the spread of infection. The pressure on beds also meant the wrong mix of patients on some wards – with frail, older and vulnerable patients being placed with patients who were aggressive because of alcohol or dementia.[25]

Similarly, at Stafford Hospital, the clinical inappropriateness of switching patients around was abundantly plain. For instance, an emergency assessment unit – used to transfer patients from A&E to avoid a breach of the four-hour waiting time target – was under-staffed. Those staff on it did not have the skills to look after surgical patients or other traumatic injuries. People with surgical or trauma-related needs would also be sent to medical wards because of the shortage of appropriate beds. This meant that patients might be cared for by nurses who lacked the necessary skills and equipment – for example, for lower limb traction. Sometimes patients ended up in a no man's land between two wards;

---

22 Healthcare Commission (2006) *Investigation into outbreaks of* Clostridium difficile *at Stoke Mandeville Hospital, Buckinghamshire Hospitals NHS Trust, July 2006.* London: Healthcare Commission, p.5.

23 Healthcare Commission (2006) *Investigation into outbreaks of* Clostridium difficile *at Stoke Mandeville Hospital, Buckinghamshire Hospitals NHS Trust, July 2006.* London: Healthcare Commission, pp.5, 45.

24 Healthcare Commission (2006) *Investigation into Mid Cheshire Hospitals NHS Trust, January 2006.* London: Healthcare Commission, pp.35–7.

25 Healthcare Commission (2006) *Investigation into Mid Cheshire Hospitals NHS Trust, January 2006.* London: Healthcare Commission, pp.35–7.

there was no reception area, no nurses' station, no telephone and no access to a computer. In addition, some beds could not be observed by staff.[26]

WITH SUCH GOINGS on within a hospital, discharge from it is inevitably a fraught and contentious matter. The pressure to get patients out of acute hospitals tends to be, well, acute. There is of course a rational way of looking at this. Hospital stays cost the NHS a lot of money; furthermore, unnecessarily long hospital stays can be bad for the patient. Dependency, lack of stimulus and sometimes risk of infection are factors.

But rather less attention has been paid to premature discharge. It is, however, particularly relevant in the context of older, vulnerable patients who are regarded, pejoratively, as 'bed blockers'. In the numbers game of bed occupancy in hospitals, they are too often seen as clogging up the works, even if they have reversible medical conditions which just need a bit of time and effort to sort out. They are awkward statistics threatening the hospital's throughput of patients.

Just like, perhaps, 77-year-old Mrs Jean Garside, into whose death an inquest was held in April 2010. She had been transferred in the middle of the night from an acute ward in the Royal Oldham Hospital to a discharge lounge, because of bed shortages. Later the next day she was discharged to a nursing home but readmitted within 24 hours; she died three weeks later. She had acute kidney failure and was in a diabetic coma; at the inquest, her family questioned the decision to move her to the discharge lounge, given the round-the-clock care she required.

A hospital consultant admitted at the inquest that the hospital had problems finding beds for acutely ill patients; this sometimes meant nocturnal patient transfers. Mrs Garside died of *Clostridium difficile* precipitated by antibiotics used to treat another infection, and exacerbated by end-stage dementia. The coroner did not believe the transfer to the lounge had a bearing on her death, but that if it had, he would have pursued that issue.[27]

With such occurrences in mind, the latest Department of Health guidance, published in 2010, says all the right things. It stresses the importance of appropriate discharge from hospital. It notes that pressure to discharge or transfer patients and release beds means that there is

---

26 Healthcare Commission (2009) *Investigation into Mid Staffordshire NHS Foundation Trust, March 2009.* London: Healthcare Commission, p.128.

27 Berry, M. (2010) 'Family attacks transfer after death of frail patient.' *Oldham Evening Chronicle,* 22 April.

less time for assessment and discharge or transfer. It points out that the consequences of getting it wrong cut both ways, leading to either premature or delayed discharge. The former means that people may be discharged with unmet needs, poorly prepared for home, likely to be readmitted and having to use inappropriate or more costly services. Alternatively, delayed discharge risks infection, depression or low mood, boredom, frustration, loss of independence and confidence and inappropriate use of NHS resources.[28]

The guidance emphasises that expected dates of discharge need to be given, and agreement reached with patients and carers about how to make discharge safe. It reminds staff to communicate properly and to show compassion for patients in order to gain their trust. It observes that staff may be so busy and efficient that they become accustomed to their own environment and 'immune to distractions'.[29] Distractions like patients?

The trouble is that guidance from the Department of Health has been preaching good practice about hospital discharges since at least 1989;[30] the gist of it all has been much the same, as has the frequent departure from it in practice.

IT IS UNSURPRISING that the guidance warns about premature discharge. Figures obtained in 2010 show that in 1998, 359,719 people were discharged but had to be readmitted within 28 days. By 2007–08 this figure had risen to £546,354; of these, 159,134 were aged 75 years or more.[31] This is commonly referred to as a revolving door syndrome.

For example, evidence given in 2007 to the Joint Committee on Human Rights expressed concern about rushed discharges which deprived people of choice, resulted in inappropriate placements (miles away from their families), led to inadequate care or discharge when they were still unwell, gave no chance for people to come to terms with momentous decisions about where and how they would live – and deprived people

28 DH (Department of Health) (2010) *Ready to go? Planning the discharge and the transfer of patients from hospital and intermediate care.* London: DH, p.4.

29 DH (Department of Health) (2010) *Ready to go? Planning the discharge and the transfer of patients from hospital and intermediate care.* London: DH, pp.16, 19, 28.

30 See: DH (Department of Health) (1989) *Discharge of patients from hospital.* London: DH. Also: DH (Department of Health) (1995) *NHS responsibilities for meeting continuing health care needs.* London: DH. Also: DH (Department of Health) (2003) *Discharge from hospital: Pathway, process and practice.* London: DH.

31 Chapman, J. (2010) '500,000 hospital patients sent home too soon every year (and 1,500 a day readmitted for emergency care).' *Daily Mail,* 1 February.

of rehabilitation opportunities.[32] In its evidence to the Committee, the British Geriatrics Society put it bluntly:

> ...what we do as geriatricians is to try and thwart some of the attempts to discharge people prematurely... I do not have the words for how stupid and how wrong such a policy is.[33]

Also giving evidence, the Royal College of Nursing (RCN) echoed this: 'it is clearly harmful to discharge someone who is not ready to be discharged and to discharge them before services have been put in place. That is something that concerns us a lot.'[34]

Elsewhere, a nurse, writing anonymously, described rather more graphically just what these two organisations were trying to get across to the Committee:

> Three hours and that trolley has to go to the assessment unit, whether there are beds there or not. Failure to do so results in purple-faced people ringing each other and firing off emails saying the word nobody must utter: "breach". Hence people not on trolleys in A and E any more, but waiting on trolleys in the assessment unit, who are in turn trying to discharge patients to the wards, who in turn are trying to discharge patients.[35]

At Mid Staffordshire NHS Foundation Trust, staff reported that discharge from hospital was based on a bed being required by somebody else rather than what was right for the patient. Inappropriate discharges to people's own homes, or to another hospital, would take place and result in readmissions within the week.[36] This, of course, is tantamount to an absurd abandonment of clinical principle; it means that an illusory clinical decision is made for one person – with reference not to that patient's needs, but to those of somebody else.

The Independent Inquiry further noted:

---

32 House of Lords and House of Commons Joint Committee on Human Rights (2007) *The human rights of older people in healthcare. Eighteenth Report of Session 2006–07*. HL 156-I, HC 378-I. London: The Stationery Office, pp.17–18.

33 House of Lords and House of Commons Joint Committee on Human Rights (2007) *The human rights of older people in healthcare. Eighteenth Report of Session 2006–07*. HL 156-I, HC 378-I. London: The Stationery Office, p.18.

34 House of Lords and House of Commons Joint Committee on Human Rights (2007) *The human rights of older people in healthcare. Eighteenth Report of Session 2006–07*. HL 156-I, HC 378-I. London: The Stationery Office, pp.17–18.

35 Moffat, Karen (a pseudonym) (2006) 'Nurses can't walk away.' *The Guardian*, 28 April.

36 Healthcare Commission (2009) *Investigation into Mid Staffordshire NHS Foundation Trust, March 2009*. London: Healthcare Commission, p.68.

- discharge from A&E without appropriate diagnosis or management
- premature discharge from wards
- protracted discharge processes
- failure to communicate arrangements to patients and their families
- discharge at an inappropriate time or in an inappropriate condition
- failure to ensure adequate support.

It went on to tackle headlong the issue of how targets affect discharge from hospital. It stated clearly that easing the pressure on A&E should not result in patients on other wards being discharged before they are ready. It averred also that adequate discharge arrangements should be in place and any waiting area for discharged patients should be properly equipped.[37]

One item of evidence related to an elderly woman discharged back home, suffering from *Clostridium difficile*, her family left unable to cope and sobbing:

> The daughter of one elderly patient told me her reaction to her mother being discharged home still very ill, suffering from c. difficile, and with no support:

> "When…we got her home, she just had no energy; she was sleeping all the time, she couldn't get out of bed, she couldn't do nothing and this terrible diarrhoea, it was every hour and a half, day and night, and I have never smelt anything – I can't say it smelt like death because I do not know but I have never smelt nothing like it. It wasn't like normal excretion, it just wasn't. It was horrendous… My Mum couldn't help us. My husband was having to like ease her to it that way and then cuddle her and sort of shuffle to the commode which we had at the side of the bed and I had to like get my Mum onto there and then I would clean my Mum and then it was the shuffle again to get her back on the bed. She couldn't – she just – we didn't know what to do. I mean we were sobbing, we had nobody to talk to."[38]

---

37 Francis, R. (Chair) (2010) *Independent Inquiry into care provided by Mid Staffordshire NHS Foundation Trust January 2005–March 2009.* London: The Stationery Office, p.15.

38 Francis, R. (Chair) (2010) *Independent Inquiry into care provided by Mid Staffordshire NHS Foundation Trust January 2005–March 2009.* London: The Stationery Office, p.140.

Protracted discharge arrangements at Mid Stafford could result in patients arriving home, freezing cold and disorientated:

> The wife of an 80-year-old man who was discharged from Ward 7 in Stafford Hospital in February 2009 recalled the delay her husband experienced on the day of his discharge and the impact this had on his health: "…we were told that the ambulance would bring him home. It was booked for 10 o'clock and he arrived at 3.10, absolutely freezing cold, quite disorientated, hardly able to communicate… He just had his dressing gown and a cotton cellular blanket round him. It was very cold weather. It was 6 February."[39]

And likewise, a woman, discharged at 3.30am in the morning in midwinter:

> Another 73-year-old woman was discharged from A&E at 3.30am in mid-winter: it turned out she still had a cannula in her arm. Her paramedic son told me: "I didn't think it was acceptable. She had been transferred then from the bed in the resuscitation room down to the clinical decisions unit, which I think is either a four- or a six-bedded unit. Mum was the only person in there. It wouldn't have hurt anybody to leave her in there comfortable overnight rather than sending her out in what was, as Dad said, a bitterly cold night in just a nightie and a blanket round her. I could not have physically lifted her in the car myself. Luckily, two of my friends were there, they had just brought another patient in, and they helped me to put her in the front seat of the car."[40]

Mid Staffordshire, as ever, stands out but is only part of a broader picture involving huge pressure on acute hospital beds. This situation has fuelled regular accounts of inappropriate, unsafe and undignified arrangements for hospital discharge.

PREMATURE DISCHARGE MAY not only be clinically bad for people but the rushed mechanism of it adds to the harm. It may involve sending people out of hospital, alone, in the middle of the night, in freezing weather, under-dressed – and without family being informed.

In January 2010, Mrs Hazel Jarvis, an 80-year-old woman, was reported to have been admitted to Broomfield Hospital in Chelmsford on New Year's Eve suffering hernia pain. She received tests and was

---

39 Francis, R. (Chair) (2010) *Independent Inquiry into care provided by Mid Staffordshire NHS Foundation Trust January 2005–March 2009*. London: The Stationery Office, p.142.

40 Francis, R. (Chair) (2010) *Independent Inquiry into care provided by Mid Staffordshire NHS Foundation Trust January 2005–March 2009*. London: The Stationery Office, p.145.

discharged at 10pm in freezing weather; a nurse said there was nothing wrong. She still looked unwell and had slurred speech. Her son and daughter came to collect her; she collapsed in the hospital car park, was immediately readmitted and died the next day. She had in fact suffered a ruptured bowel.[41]

In Leeds, the daughter of a 74-year-old woman, Mrs Elsie Allanson, reported that her mother had suffered a mini-stroke making walking difficult. Seven hours after being admitted to St James' Hospital, she was sent home in a taxi (paid for by the NHS Trust) at 2am in freezing weather in February 2010. It had snowed all day; none of her children were informed about the discharge. She arrived home cold and wet; the taxi driver took her things to the door and almost carried her in.[42]

Another 2am discharge, back in 2003, was condemned by the Southwark coroner. Ninety-five-year-old Mrs Frances Archer had been diagnosed with a broken pubic bone following a fall in a care home. She was seen in the A&E department of King's College Hospital and referred to the orthopaedic team; at that point the documentation became scarce and things got confused. She should have been referred to the medical team; instead she was discharged at 11pm, arriving back at the care home at 1am. By the morning she was unresponsive and breathing with difficulty. She was readmitted to hospital, where the development of a severe systemic infection was diagnosed; she died the next day. The coroner noted the lack of medical referral and of formal discharge, but did not find these causative of death.[43]

Mr Glyn Jones was an 89-year-old man suffering from dementia. He had been a member of the Welsh Guards and taken part in the D-Day landings. Admitted to the Royal Glamorgan Hospital with fluid on the lungs, he was reported as being discharged, in May 2010, alone, in his pyjamas. His family was not informed, and when he arrived at his home by ambulance, he could not get in. Fortunately a passing (paid) carer knew the key code and let him in, staying with him until he was settled and the house warm. His daughter had told the hospital that his carers needed 48 hours' notice of discharge from hospital. When she had

41 'Broomfield Hospital sent elderly woman home to die in freezing home.' *Daily Gazette* (Essex), 27 January 2010.
42 Allanson, E. (2010) 'Elderly woman sent from Leeds hospital in gown and slippers.' *Yorkshire Evening Post*, 19 March.
43 'Woman, 95, dies after 2am hospital discharge.' *Daily Mail*, 27 August 2003.

arrived at the hospital to visit him, there was another patient in his bed; he had been sent home.[44]

A 99-year-old woman with a cut head and two broken ribs was sent home from the Princess Royal Hospital in Telford at 1am in March 2009 – because otherwise she would have had to spend the night on a trolley. Four days later, back in the hospital, Mrs Walker died from bronchial pneumonia and cardiac arrest. The coroner recorded accidental death but said he would not have wanted his grandmother treated in that manner. One of the hospital doctors lamented the loss of community hospital beds as contributing to the pressure on the hospital.[45]

The director of nursing of Tameside Hospital Foundation Trust apologised after a 76-year-old woman was sent home in a taxi. She could not get on the seat, so she sat on the floor of the taxi, with her head between a nurse's legs. The director stated that this was entirely unacceptable.[46]

IN CONTRAST TO these instances of inappropriate discharge, the following report repays some study because of the number of people involved, the reasoning given and the background. On 20 December 2007, at Ipswich Hospital in Suffolk, a number of patients were woken up in the middle of the night and sent home there and then. The explanation from the hospital was that on the medical wards there were 21 patients to admit with only six available beds, and on surgical wards seven patients to be admitted with only one available bed. The hospital spokeswoman stated:

> Some of the patients had to be woken up so they could be discharged, but there were very sick people who needed to come in. Those who went home were all ready and happy to leave and we organised transport for them. It is that time of year when most hospitals are busy, especially this one which is extremely busy with people who need emergency care and trying to bring down waiting times.[47]

The explanation is instructive. First, the idea that the patients 'were all ready and happy to leave' to be discharged, with no notice, in the middle

---

44 Brindley, M. (2010) 'Author's father is sent home from hospital alone in just his pyjamas.' *Western Mail*, 6 May. Accessed on 5 August 2010 at: www.walesonline.co.uk/news/health-news/2010/05/06/author-furious-her-father-with-dementia-was-discharged-from-hospital-alone-in-just-his-pyjamas-91466-26386025.

45 Johnson, P. (2009) 'Injured widow, 99, sent home from hospital.' *Shropshire Star*, 12 August.

46 Dlyak, P. (Director of Nursing) (2010) 'Sent home from hospital on the floor of a taxi.' *Patient Opinion*. Accessed on 20 August 2010 at: www.patientopinion.org.uk/opinions/29378.

47 Bond, A. (2007) 'Hospital hit by bed crisis.' *East Anglian Daily Times*, 22 December.

of the night, is risible. Given the continual pressure the hospital was under – a more or less continual state of black alert for many weeks – they would not have been occupying beds in the first place had they not had a clinical need to do so. In any case, how many of us express happiness when woken in the middle of the night and turfed out of bed – even at the best of times, let alone when sick in hospital?

Second, the incident, as the hospital conceded, was partly to do with hitting the waiting time target. Third, the spokeswoman did not mention that the incident came against a background of the closure of both acute and community hospital beds in East Suffolk. It fell to the Ipswich Hospital Patient and Public Involvement Forum to point this out.[48] In fact, Department of Health statistics obtained at the end of 2007 showed that hospital beds in Suffolk had decreased by 20 per cent in the past ten years, above the national average.[49]

It was not reported how the discharged patients fared.

IN THE FOLLOWING case, reported in 2007, the outcome *was* known; the patient did badly. An 83-year-old pensioner, Mrs Annie Edge, suffering from dementia, died after being sent home from Warrington Hospital in the middle of the night, without any of her family being informed. She was found dead the next day, clutching a bible, at home where she lived alone. She had been admitted at 1am in the morning with pains in her right shoulder. Three hours later she was taken home by ambulance, without her family being informed, even though her notes indicated that she lived alone. The only record of her hospital visit was that she had been given a cup of tea; this was despite the fact that, when found, she had a sling on her arm and orange sticky pads from echocardiogram tests. The hospital issued an unreserved apology for not informing the family of both her admission and discharge.[50]

The Patient's Association commented that such practice was all too common and that in its view: 'This isn't about hospitals being under pressure – it's about basic humanity and providing the most elementary care that vulnerable people need.'[51]

Perhaps the case of Mr John Platt, a dying 101-year-old man, is also what the Association had in mind. In 2006, he was sent home from

48 Bond, A. (2007) 'Hospital hit by bed crisis.' *East Anglian Daily Times*, 22 December.
49 'Suffolk's NHS beds cut by 20 per cent.' *Ipswich Evening Star*, 19 December 2007.
50 Tozer, J. (2007) 'Why was my mum sent home from hospital to die alone?' *Daily Mail*, 9 February.
51 Tozer, J. (2007) 'Why was my mum sent home from hospital to die alone?' *Daily Mail*, 9 February.

Salisbury District Hospital. He was wearing only an incontinence pad and poorly fitting pyjamas. During his stay of five days on a mixed-sex ward, his hearing aid had been stepped on and crushed, his false teeth went missing – and his soiled pyjamas were piled up in the locker by his bed for the duration of his stay. He could not eat unaided, and he was discharged in an incontinent and confused state, clutching a bag with dirty clothes mixed in with the clean. He died a few days later after arriving back at his home. He had been awarded the Distinguished Service Order (DSO) during the Second World War. His family referred to degradation and humiliation; his daughter-in-law said:

> Everybody's got to die. He was obviously going to die and he wanted to die. It wasn't because he was a heavily decorated soldier – but I felt they didn't acknowledge he was an old man of 101 who deserved respect.[52]

Referring to his treatment as disgraceful, she went on to describe the nonchalant way in which staff regarded what had happened, suggesting that such care must be endemic:

> All that he had at the end of his 101 years was his dignity and they took that away from him. You just don't do that to people… I was so furious. I think respect in that situation is the same as compassion. I just can't believe that any hospital would keep excrement-covered clothing in a locker for five days. I got the impression this lack of attention must be endemic because it was so lightly treated.

The hospital apologised for some aspects of the care provided for Mr Platt and also acknowledged the concerns about the patients' personal effects. Solemnly, it stated that it took complaints seriously so that it could learn from such experiences.[53]

THERE IS NO doubt that some patients, typically older, are moved around in hospital to their detriment and for non-clinical reasons. Desperate measures are then taken in order to get them out of hospital. This is because of shortages of beds and of political and financial priorities which

---

52 Dreaper, J. (2008) 'Compassion key to good health care.' BBC News, 30 December. Accessed on 20 August 2010 at: http://news.bbc.co.uk/1/hi/health/7797548.stm. Also: Nelson, S. (2008) 'Hospital sends war hero, 101, home to die wearing a nappy and clutching a bag of soiled clothes.' *Daily Mail*, 31 December.

53 Dreaper, J. (2008) 'Compassion key to good health care.' BBC News, 30 December. Accessed on 20 August 2010 at: http://news.bbc.co.uk/1/hi/health/7797548.stm. Also: Nelson, S. (2008) 'Hospital sends war hero, 101, home to die wearing a nappy and clutching a bag of soiled clothes.' *Daily Mail*, 31 December.

conflict with proper patient care. It is almost as though patients, often helpless and afflicted to greater or lesser extent by illness, are sometimes viewed as wrecks beyond salvage, broken up still further and reduced to mere flotsam and jetsam, cut adrift on the hospital wards. How it is that elderly people have come to be treated in this way is outlined in the next chapter.

The final and fitting word on beds comes in the form of the following piece:

> So Prime Minister, Mr Health Secretary and NHS Management Executive, as you return bleary-eyed from your Christmas break (no doubt well rested and well fed) spare a thought for the poor, sickly old patient lying hurting and exhausted on an NHS trolley…hang on a minute, we can't let patients lie around on trolleys, that would muck up the waiting time statistics. Quick, shove her into any bed you can find. What? We haven't got any beds. Well MAKE SOME. How about shoving those patients from the Elderly Ward into that old shed at the back – the one with the crib and baby in it? Yes I know it's the Obs and Gynae Ward. They'll be fine there, even if they don't get any physiotherapy and the staff there haven't a clue about caring for elderly people. The old gerries won't complaint; half of them are deaf and demented anyway. Tomorrow we can move them somewhere else – the laundry perhaps – with a bit of luck some of them might catch pneumonia there and create a few more beds. Happy New Year by the way. That new patient doesn't look too well, does she? No, poor old sod. Good job she's got the NHS to fall back on.[54]

A joke maybe? Hardly. It was submitted to The Journal newspaper in 2000 by Mr Kay, a highly-qualified ward manager at Wansbeck Hospital. His employer, Northumbria Healthcare NHS Trust, took both a dim view and disciplinary action against him; consequently he went to an employment tribunal in 2001 and won his case. Ten years on, such comments about the care of elderly people in our hospitals resonate still.

---

54 *Kay v Northumbria Healthcare NHS Trust.* Employment Tribunal case no. 6405617/00, 29 November 2001 (Newcastle upon Tyne). From: Bowers, J. *et al.* (2007) *Whistleblowing: Law and Practice.* Oxford: Oxford University Press, pp.575–577.

12

Older People: The Unwanted

> It is a sign of how far we have drifted from the idea of universal health care that the Secretary of State needs to make a public statement that older patients in the NHS should have equal rights. Two-thirds of those using the NHS are over the age of 65. Instructing hospitals to take their needs into account is not far removed from telling those who run Disneyland that it would be good if they catered for the needs of children. (Martin Bright, 2001)[1]

This book is not just about older people. They do, however, feature prominently, for the reasons explained in this chapter. And also because a caricature of how National Health Service (NHS) acute hospitals treat the elderly might read as follows.

The health service really doesn't want older people in hospitals. It tries to avoid admitting them; if they are admitted, they are not properly diagnosed. They are not kept nourished and hydrated, kept clean, taken to the toilet or cared for. They are allowed to develop lethal and agonising pressure sores, exposed unnecessarily to infection and, untended, left to fall, smack, on the floor. They are denied pain relief, or alternatively are over-prescribed drugs that lead to premature death. They are deprived of slower stream, more complex rehabilitation. They may not even be spoken to. Everything is done to make it quite clear that they are not welcome. If still alive, they are then discharged from hospital prematurely. It is hoped that they will take themselves and their complex needs elsewhere, to a nursing home, to rot in their own homes or to the grave. And, at least if they are then neglected or even abused, this will be at the hands of somebody else.

Such a description is of course a total insult to all those hospital wards and units that pride themselves on looking after their patients, of whatever age, properly. However, as the many examples contained in this book reveal, it is at the same time not, and as we might wish, just parody.

For instance, an 86-year-old woman, Mrs Phyllis Foster, was admitted to Whipps Cross Hospital with heart and kidney problems. She stayed a month before being discharged, but during her hospital stay she had

---

1   Bright, M. (2001) 'A blow struck for dignity.' *Society Guardian*, 1 April.

developed pressure sores on her feet and had been given a wrong and dangerous dose of warfarin. She was discharged home without her personal belongings or a commode, even though the latter had been deemed necessary for a safe discharge. The overdose meant she had to be readmitted five days later. After being transferred to another hospital, St Margaret's in Epping, she suffered a number of falls, some of which were not recorded. She was discharged for a second time, again without the walking frame she needed for getting to the toilet and without her personal belongings. Two days later she was readmitted; within three days she died.

Her son complained; the Healthcare Commission criticised the hospitals for the discharges, the bedsores, treatment of her back pain and a 'do not resuscitate' instruction on her notes. This last had been placed there with no consultation with either mother or son. Threatened with legal action for negligence, the hospitals settled the compensation claim out of court.[2]

AND IT IS precisely because the above passage is not quite caricature that it is useful to recall a bit of history. It would be foolish to suggest we have not moved on from 19th-century workhouses, but equally it would be short-sighted to think that we are a race apart and that descriptions from history have no bearing on our current treatment of the sick and the old.

Consider, for instance, the principle that came to be known as 'less eligibility' and which underpinned the *Poor Law Amendment Act 1834*.[3] It was explained in a report of the same year by the Poor Law Commissioners as follows: 'The first and most essential of all conditions, a principle which we find universally admitted, even by those whose practice is at variance with it, is, that his situation on the whole shall not be made really or apparently so eligible as the situation of the independent labourer of the lowest class.'[4] In other words, conditions in the workhouse were to be made so bad that only absolute desperation would drive somebody to it.

This principle was referred to early on in the story of *Oliver Twist*. If we substitute the elderly for the workhouse orphans there are uncomfortable

---

2 'Watchdog finds elderly Theydon Bois woman continually let down by hospitals.' *Attwaters Solicitors News*, 11 November 2009. Accessed on 20 August 2010 at: www.attwaters. co.uk/2009/11/watchdog-finds-elderly-theydon-bois-woman-continually-let-down-by-hospitals.

3 *An Act for the Amendment and Better Administration of the Laws Relating to the Poor in England and Wales [4 & 5 Will. IV cap. 76]*.

4 Commissioners for Inquiring into the Administration and Practical Operation of the Poor Laws (1834) *Report from His Majesty's Commissioners for inquiring into the administration and practical operation of the poor laws*. London: House of Commons, Part 2, Section 1, para. CXV.

resemblances. For instance, in relation to nutrition which, as we have seen, has become a serious matter for some older people in hospital, we read: 'at the very time a child had contrived to exist upon the smallest possible portion of   Food, it did perversely happen in eight-and-a-half cases out of ten, either that it sickened from want and cold, or fell into the fire from neglect…in any one of which cases, the miserable little being was summoned into another world.' The rule was that 'all poor people should have the alternative…of being starved by a gradual process in the house, or by a quick one out it.'[5]

We know also that government and health service policy is directed toward keeping the elderly in particular out of hospital. It really is only a short step then to making conditions so bad that they will not want to come in or, if they do, they will deteriorate rapidly and die. Certainly, some of what is described in this book is not so far off this mark.

In *Oliver Twist*, the poor care and nutrition of the orphans meant that the children were dying (emphasis added):

> It was rather expensive at first, in consequence of the increase in the undertaker's bill, and the necessity of taking in the clothes of all the paupers, which fluttered loosely about their wasted, shrunken forms, after a week or two's gruel. But the number of inmates got thin as well as the paupers; *and the board were in ecstasies.*[6]

In keeping with NHS trust boards now, in terms of the power they wield and the authoritative, apparently well informed statements that they make, the workhouse board comprised 'very sage, deep, philosophical men'.[7] By comparison, we know that trust boards have in recent times made many vainglorious statements and indeed congratulated themselves on adhering to priorities and achieving aims, objectives and targets — even when this has been at the expense of people's welfare. This occurred in Mid Staffordshire, where the self-praise and ecstasy, in the midst of degradation and death (literally), took the form of pay rises for Board members.[8]

To draw parallels and comparisons may seem far-fetched. But less eligibility is to a degree, rearing its head, albeit unspoken. This is the logical outcome of some of the policies and approaches adopted; more

---

5   Dickens, C. (1907) *Oliver Twist*. London: J.M. Dent, pp.5, 11.

6   Dickens, C. (1907) *Oliver Twist*. London: J.M. Dent, p.11.

7   Dickens, C. (1907) *Oliver Twist*. London: J.M, Dent, pp.5, 11.

8   Evans, M. (2010) 'Failed hospital bosses given pay rises while crisis unfolded: senior managers who oversaw one of the worst scandals in the history of the NHS awarded themselves bumper pay increases at the same time as hundreds of patients were needlessly dying, it can be disclosed.' *Daily Telegraph*, 26 February.

needy and complex patients are not wanted. Often, not always, these are the elderly. This is not an over-statement: at times, good clinical and nursing care of such patients has been actively abandoned by hospitals, whose gaze is fixed on other matters and on a different type of health care, namely, for easier and less complicated patients.

The following views reflect this and the idea that people may end up being fearful and reluctant to enter hospital; the principle of less eligibility in action. For instance, in 2009 a patient at the Queen's Medical Centre, Nottingham University Hospitals NHS Trust, put it this way:

> ...it was so dirty I feared getting infection all the time. Nurses at times left people in to soil there beds when they had been calling for help for ages alarms conected to patiant were left ringing for more the half an hour during the night, being unable to get out of bed not given bowels [sic] to wash hands after using a bed pan... I hope I never have to go into this hospital ever again![9]

A relative described in 2010 a feeling of horror about the Royal Liverpool University Hospital:

> The room my mother was in at first, stunk of urine. Took me a lot of dettol to clean it. A staff member was shrieking with laughter outside the room my mother was dying in. Other nurses did not seem to recognise a dying patient.
>
> My first experience with this hospital was 4 years ago, when my mother had a hip replacement, got collinstrum difficile [sic] plus pressure sores and leg ulcers. I took her out after 5 weeks of horror, not knowing she had c.diff till the day I extracted her. Care of an elderly patient with dementia is simply a disgrace. It seems obvious, if you put an elderly person sitting in a chair all day they will get swollen legs, which will take its toll on thin skin surfaces and leave them open to infection. At one stage my mother was sharing a toilet with 2 elderly male patients. I cleaned it myself every day, it was disgusting. I cannot even come within sight of the Royal liverpool hospital now, without feeling sick and starting to shake. I do not believe that nurses today actually care about people, and I do not know why they took up the profession. My experiences with this hospital fill me with horror.[10]

Talking of Warrington Hospital in 2010, a relative (who was herself a nurse) felt that an animal clinic might be a better bet:

---

9   Patient Opinion. Accessed on 20 September 2010 at: www.patientopinion.org.uk/opinions/24332.

10   Patient Opinion. Accessed on 20 October 2010 at: www.patientopinion.org.uk/opinions/31122.

The level of care that my relative received was barely adequate. As a qualified nurse I can truthfully say I was horrified by the poor quality of basic nursing and medical standards. This applies to both Doctors and nusing [sic] staff alike. Very poor record keeping. Case records incomplete and woefully inaccurate. Medication not given on time. Inappropriate Physiotherapy forced on someone already in intense pain which caused further damage. Pain relief inadequate. I could go on and on, the list would make very depressing reading. Frankly, given a choice I would rather attend an Animal Clinic than Warrington General Hospital.[11]

Posting a comment in 2009 about Manchester Royal Infirmary, the following observer believed that a factory floor would be cleaner:

The general condition of the wards left a lot to be desired, the basics of house keeping and cleanliness are not being adhered to. In summary I work in a electronics manufacturing environment and I would sooner recover after an operation on the shop floor at work, as the housekeeping far exceeds the standard observed with the royal Manchester hospital.[12]

Absolutely ideal, according to the principle of less eligibility, is the following comment by a relative in 2010, about dying rather than ending up in Colchester General Hospital. He had observed the care given to his frail, elderly and terminally ill, 86-year-old father (emphasis added):

My father was brought into the hospital as he was unable to look after himself – he has terminal cancer and is 86 years old – he is very frail and confused. No one bothered to check his medication even though I had listed everything on a sheet and enclosed all the medication…the Wivenhoe Ward staff did not bother to contact me or find out what was wrong with him – he was left sitting in a chair – cold and confused and in pain – 2 paracetemol [sic] were given to him in 22 hours – no morphine – no nothing – its absolute disgrace. They tried saying he did not have any medication with him – I showed them the bag it was in next to his bed. The man in the bed opposite him phoned me to say he was very concerned about my dad and I should contact the ward as a matter of urgency. He had been up all night wandering around, packing and then unpacking and shaking. No one helped him… Left in dirty pyjamas all day with no covers – unable to

---

11 Patient Opinion. Accessed on 20 October 2010 at: www.patientopinion.org.uk/opinions/31299.
12 NHS Choices. Accessed on 20 September 2010 at: www.nhs.uk/Services/Hospitals/ PatientFeedback/DefaultView.aspx?id=1559&pid=RW3MR&pageNo=8&sort=1&record PP=0.

> eat – he needs help with a soft diet – utterley confused and lonely
> with no empathy from the staff. Yesterday I arrived to find the
> tumour on his neck weaping [sic] a fluid – I had to ask 3 times
> from 4pm for someone to look at it – eventually a nurse looked
> at it at 5pm – took a swop [sic] but said it was too late in the day
> to get a Dr – they finished at 5pm. *They call it the caring profession
> – what an absolute joke – they could not care less – there is no empathy
> with elderley [sic], frail and sick people, no compassion and certainly no
> caring. I hope to god I die before I end up in a hospital as grim as this – it
> feels like a workhouse!*[13]

At least Oliver Twist was able both to eat some gruel and then to ask for more; some patients are in a worse position. They are unable physically or mentally to take nourishment for themselves, let alone ask for more.

REVERTING TO THE more recent past, the government and the NHS have form in showing a distinct antipathy toward older people in relation to hospital care. Since at least the late 1980s, many long-stay NHS beds have been closed and older people with chronic health needs have gone elsewhere, largely to nursing homes. The theory was that they would still be an NHS responsibility and that their nursing home placements would be fully paid by the health service, and therefore be free of charge – just as hospital stays would be.

It has not worked out like this. Even for people with clearly complex and multiple health needs, the NHS began to say that they had 'social care' rather than 'health care' needs, in which case, if they had the money, they would have to pay nursing home bills themselves. This has meant that whilst the NHS does still fully fund some patients, many others have wrongly been denied NHS 'continuing health care' status. They have had to pay for nursing home care from their savings and the equity of their homes; alternatively local councils have had to pick up the tab of those lacking financial resources of their own.

This was, and is, not an official policy; it has been achieved on the quiet with no transparent, political debate, in or out of Parliament. It is this that has made it so objectionable; financial necessity and transparent, if controversial, policymaking are one thing, disingenuousness and political cowardice quite another. But what was happening did not go totally unnoticed. By 1994, the Health Service Ombudsman had issued a special report, aghast at the abandonment by Leeds Health Authority of patients

---

13 NHS Choices. Accessed on 20 September 2010 at: www.nhs.uk/Services/Hospitals/
PatientFeedback/DefaultView.aspx?id=13&pid=RDEE4&pageNo=5&sort=1&recordPP=0.

with complex medical needs.[14] In 1999, the Court of Appeal intervened in the case of Pamela Coughlan, again catching the NHS red handed in denying responsibility for a person with clear health care needs.[15] Hospitals though, with the bit between their teeth, were undeterred in their determination to turn away the elderly.

A new Health Service Ombudsman, inundated with complaints about continuing health care, published a scathing report in 2003, in which she reserved her ire for the Department of Health; it was overseeing an unfair, illogical and opaque policy.[16] The Department even had to appear to back down, by agreeing to refund a total of many hundreds of thousands of pounds to people who had wrongly been forced to pay for their care. New guidance was issued in 2007 and then reissued in 2009.[17]

Despite this, we have witnessed an inexorable and continuing shift of responsibility for people's health care needs away from the NHS. The unwritten policy and practice are nothing to do with whether a person has health care needs or not, and everything to do with the Department of Health's and local NHS trusts' beliefs that they do not want responsibility for older people with chronic health care needs. In other words, the recategorising of health care as social care has no basis in diagnosis or condition but is almost entirely political.

Even the belated concession by government, that the NHS would at least contribute something financially to people's nursing needs in care homes, was disingenuous. Many of those residents would formerly have had all their needs met and paid for by the NHS; and, in any case, the weekly hundred pounds or so barely makes inroads into the huge weekly fees payable for nursing home care. As Claire Rayner, health campaigner, retorted: they said they would make people's nursing care free in future; they were lying.[18]

And it has not just been a distaste for those with chronic, perhaps irreversible health care needs. This dismissive attitude has spread to those who would benefit from active treatment and rehabilitation. Professors John Grimley Evans and Raymond C. Tallis, eminent geriatricians both,

---

14 Health Service Commissioner (1994) *Failure to provide long term NHS care for brain damaged patient*. London: HMSO.

15 *R v North and East Devon Health Authority, ex p Coughlan* (1999) 2 CCLR 285, Court of Appeal.

16 Health Service Ombudsman (2003) *NHS funding for long term care*. London: The Stationery Office.

17 DH (Department of Health) (2009) *National Framework for NHS continuing health care and NHS-funded nursing care*. London: DH.

18 Rayner, C. (2001) 'Claire Rayner: I'm leaving the Labour Party after 50 faithful years.' *The Independent*, 26 September.

wrote in 2001 about the policy of intermediate care (simpler reablement out of hospital) and the *National Service Framework for Older People*.

They saw these policies as part of a longstanding political and managerial agenda to keep old people out of hospital, in the hope that 'somehow they would disappear from the system'. It was convenient for the caste of management to confuse convalescence out of hospital with a need for rehabilitation within. They also foresaw what has indeed come to pass, the premature discharge of people from hospital direct to intermediate care 'bypassing the skilled diagnostic evaluation that the complexities of disease and disability in old age require'. The trouble was, of course, that specialist rehabilitation was expensive. Nobody was owning up to all this, but, as they noted, 'practice is substance, policy mere spin'.[19]

IN LATE 2010, the National Confidential Enquiry into Patient Outcome and Death published an observational study of 800 elderly patients who had all died within 30 days of surgery. Entitled *An age old problem*, the report made no bones about its 'depressing' findings. These included the fact that underlying problems beyond the surgical were not diagnosed or understood, and competent input by hospital consultants with expertise in care of the elderly was often lacking. This meant that recovery from surgery could be jeopardised, always supposing the surgery was performed in a timely manner, which in nearly 30 per cent of cases it was not.

Compared to a typical younger adult, an older person with a fractured hip was more likely to be already dehydrated, have nutritional problems, have thrombotic (blood coagulation) complications, experience slower healing, and be at risk of tissue breakdown (pressure sores). Some singularly damning findings emerged. Only 36 per cent of patients received 'good care'; and even this did not mean 'exceptionally brilliant' but merely 'appropriate'. This was particularly troubling because the patients considered in the study were of the type that will become more prevalent as the population of people aged over 85 doubles within the next 25 years.

The study did not even find that, whether or not they were receiving appropriate medical diagnosis and intervention, patients received adequate pain relief. This, in the Enquiry's view, indicated 'what must sometimes be an organisational failure to respond to suffering'.

---

19 Grimley Evans, J. and Tallis, R. (2001) 'A new beginning for care for elderly people? Not if the psychopathology of this new national framework gets in the way.' *British Medical Journal*, 7 April, pp.807–8.

It came, strangely enough (or not so strangely) to the same sort of conclusion as Martin Bright, quoted at the head of this chapter, namely a pattern 'of "one size fits all medicine" being applied to a heterogeneous population with varying needs and falling short in ways which are both predictable and preventable'.[20]

So, JOURNALISTIC COMPARISONS with Disneyland aside, there is a respectable and cogent view that the NHS is, generally speaking, not designed for older patients, particularly because, compared to other age groups, they tend to have more complex needs. If this is true, such a state of affairs is an absurdity, as they are the main users of acute hospital beds. But it is of course not just outlandish; unfortunate consequences attach.

If a hospital is not set up – in terms of staffing, expertise and resources – to treat and care for elderly people with complex needs, neglect is at least one foreseeable outcome. This is not as tendentious as it may sound. The Mid Staffordshire Independent Inquiry was in no doubt about the link between inadequate services for older people and neglect:

> It will have become apparent that many of the cases in which patients and their families have reported concerns have involved elderly patients. The multiple needs of such patients in terms of diagnosis, management, communication and nursing care are in many ways distinct from those of younger patients. The latter can more often be safely treated only for the condition for which they have been admitted. Older patients will often present with a complex of medical and care problems requiring a skilled and all-embracing multi-disciplinary team approach.[21]

Beyond Stafford Hospital, it seems incontrovertible that older people are bearing the brunt of the following characteristics of hospital care: bed shortages; high bed occupancy rates in hospitals; being placed on the 'wrong' ward; being subject to moves from ward to ward for non-clinical reasons; shortfalls in the numbers and skills of staff to diagnose, treat and provide care; premature discharge from hospital; the giving way of more intensive, slower stream rehabilitation to shorter, lighter rehabilitation, 'reablement' or intermediate care; and persistent negative attitudes toward elderly patients. Pull these together and it is unsurprising that not just poor care but neglect is the end product.

---

20 Wilkinson, K., Martin, I.C., Gough, M.J. *et al.* (2010) *An age old problem: A review of the care received by elderly patients undergoing surgery.* London: National Confidential Enquiry into Patient Outcome and Death, pp.4–7.

21 Francis, R. (Chair) (2010) *Independent Inquiry into care provided by Mid Staffordshire NHS Foundation Trust January 2005–March 2009.* London: The Stationery Office, p.400.

AND THERE CERTAINLY are a lot of elderly people using the NHS. It is not entirely clear how all the reported statistics dovetail but the gist is plain. The NHS Confederation has claimed that the NHS spends 80 per cent of its time and 80 per cent of its resources on the elderly.[22] The Department of Health put this figure at 43 per cent of resources and 65 per cent of hospital beds – bearing in mind that people over 65 make up about 16 per cent of the population.[23] Then in October 2010, the statistics revealed that hospital admissions and stays for people over 75 had risen 66 per cent over a decade, whilst people over 60 accounted for over 50 per cent of hospital admissions in the year 2009–10.[24]

In 2007, Professor Ian Philp, writing for the Department of Health, acknowledged this numerical argument and also that existing health services are not designed for older patients. His report stated that by 2025:

> ...the number of people in the UK aged over 85 will have increased by two thirds. Why is that important? Because it is older people who are the main users of health and social care services. Older people are three times more likely than younger people to be admitted to hospital following attendance at an emergency department. Once there older people are also more likely to stay and suffer life threatening infections, falls and delirium. Older patients often have multiple health problems, are taking a variety of medication and often present to the health service with non-specific problems like falls and confusion. Our existing services were not designed with older people's needs in mind.[25]

So it is not then merely a question of numbers but also the nature and complexity of need. In 2007 also, the British Geriatrics Society gave evidence to a joint parliamentary committee. It regretted the failure to recognise the increasing complexity, frailty and dependency of older people in hospital and care home settings over the last five to ten years – and to provide staff with appropriate skills and in sufficient numbers

22 In evidence to: House of Lords and House of Commons Joint Committee on Human Rights (2007) *The human rights of older people in healthcare. Eighteenth Report of Session 2006–07.* HL 156-I, HC 378-I. London: The Stationery Office, p.21.

23 Philp, I. (2007) *A recipe for care: Not a single ingredient, clinical case for change.* London: Department of Health, p.1.

24 Lister, S. (2010) 'NHS under pressure as the number of elderly patients rises.' *The Times*, 29 October.

25 Philp, I. (2007) *A recipe for care: Not a single ingredient, clinical case for change.* London: Department of Health, p.1.

to meet these changes.[26] As ever, it had all been said before. In 2001, the Standing Nursing and Midwifery Advisory Committee had explained that:

> Older patients often have complex health care needs. They may have more than one diagnosis, requiring treatment for chronic illness and disability as well as the acute episode that has brought them into hospital. Sensory impairments, dementia or other mental health problems may create barriers to communication.[27]

The Audit Commission had a year earlier warned against prematurely writing off older people who had suffered an acute episode but also had underlying multiple pathology. But it in turn was quoting from a 1994 Royal College of Physicians (RCP) report, delineating how easily this could happen; inadequate diagnosis might indicate a general, irreversible breakdown, when in fact there was an underlying, reversible problem:

> Focal disease may have a global impact in a biologically aged patient such that a common and familiar acute condition may present in atypical fashion. An elderly patient with pneumonia may present with the effects of cerebral hypoxia and toxaemia, confusion, impaired mobility and urinary incontinence. The presentation may seem rather unfavourable, with a reversible underlying problem presenting as an apparently irreversible general breakdown. The presence of other concurrent diseases increases the chance of a particular condition leading to dependency and loss of function: so-called "multiple pathology".[28]

The *National Service Framework for Older People*, too, chimed in. It urged early involvement of consultants in old age medicine or rehabilitation. This would be so that appropriate treatment and management decisions could be made for the elderly with atypical disease presentation or complex needs.[29]

We should not think that because all this was written so long ago, that it has long since been sorted out. In 2010, a geriatrician essentially repeated it:

---

26 House of Lords and House of Commons Joint Committee on Human Rights (2007) *The human rights of older people in healthcare. Eighteenth Report of Session 2006–07.* HL 156-I, HC 378-I. London: The Stationery Office, p.58.

27 Standing Nursing and Midwifery Advisory Committee (2001) *Caring for older people: A nursing priority integrating knowledge, practice and values: A report.* London: Department of Health, p.3.

28 Audit Commission (2000) *The way to go home: Rehabilitation and remedial services for older people.* London: Audit Commission, p.9. Quoting from: RCP (Royal College of Physicians) (1994) *Ensuring equity and quality of care for elderly people.* London: RCP.

29 DH (Department of Health) (2001) *National Service Framework for Older People.* London: DH, p.51.

High quality management of frail older people is challenging because as geriatricians know all too well, they usually present non-specifically which can make the immediate diagnosis obscure. Junior doctors and most non-geriatrician receiving consultants will have minimal training in geriatric medicine and the formulation of the non-specific presentation. Add to that the challenge of multiple co-morbidities – especially cognitive impairment, polypharmacy, functional decline and institutional ageism, and it is of little surprise that frail older people get a raw deal.[30]

THE IMPORTANCE OF what all these were, and are, saying cannot be over stated. Not heeding this message leads inexorably to a paradox; the greater, because the more complex the needs of older people, the less chance of them receiving the health treatment and care they require. This contradiction surfaces because if you are a hospital chief executive and have too few beds (and staff), you do not want them occupied by slow movers. Clearly, you do not want to provide intensive, slower stream inpatient treatment, care and rehabilitation. And, above all, you need to discharge people quickly. But how can you do this if they have medical needs, are not medically stable, require being in a hospital setting and need to receive considerable amounts of treatment, nursing and rehabilitation? It is surprisingly simple.

Don't make the diagnosis, or at least not the searching, thorough one. Ignore what the RCP, the Audit Commission, the *National Service Framework for Older People*, the Standing Nursing and Midwifery Advisory Committee and the British Geriatrics Society have all advised. And if, for want of investment, staff are not available – with sufficient expertise or time or both to diagnose, care and treat – this abandonment of patients can be achieved with remarkable ease. If you deliberately ill-equip your institution for a particular task, you can indeed – in all earnestness – then plead that you are ill-equipped to perform it.

In this vein, the passing over of older people's needs, particularly people with multiple pathology, is achieved sometimes by diagnoses such as 'acopia' (inability to cope) or 'social admission'. As soon as that tag is applied, serious health care intervention is over. However, there is a firm view amongst clinicians and other health care professionals who

30 Conroy, S. (2010) 'Ageism 1, geriatric medicine 0.' *British Geriatrics Society Newsletter*, 7 June.

are specialists in elderly care that such dismissive diagnoses are often wrong.[31]

The suggestion that a hospital might simply ignore a person's medical needs is counter-intuitive. But at Mid Staffordshire NHS Foundation Trust a whole range of omissions were found in the recording of people's needs and condition:

- no clear registration of patients' transfer from one ward to another
- no consistent use of care plans
- incomplete nursing records
- lack of appropriate nutrition and hydration charts
- sparse details of social history, past medical history and other important background information
- authors of records not clearly identifying themselves
- failure to record assessment scores
- inaccurate recording of time of death.

Relatives took to altering and correcting the records themselves.[32] This is suggestive of perhaps exactly the type of therapeutic nihilism that can descend on clinicians and health care professionals.[33]

IT HAPPENED TO 88-year-old Mrs Margaret Shepherd. She had been admitted in 2006 to Leeds General Infirmary, following a car accident which gave her minor fractures. She died eight days later, having suffered a stroke due to a blood clot in an artery. The coroner deemed some aspects of her treatment unacceptable and the note taking woeful. In the two days following her stroke, immediately prior to her collapse and death, she was not attended, examined or diagnosed by a doctor. This constituted a serious omission, despite the fact that diagnosis and treatment would not have prevented her death. The coroner pointed out that if it is not in the notes, then it hasn't happened. Leeds Teaching

31 Oliver, D. (2008) '"Acopia" and "social admission" are not diagnoses: Why older people deserve better.' *Journal of the Royal Society of Medicine 101*, 168–74.

32 Francis, R. (Chair) (2010) *Independent Inquiry into care provided by Mid Staffordshire NHS Foundation Trust January 2005–March 2009.* London: The Stationery Office, p.14.

33 Oliver, D. (2008) '"Acopia" and "social admission" are not diagnoses: Why older people deserve better.' *Journal of the Royal Society of Medicine 101*, 168–74.

Hospitals NHS Trust apologised for what it claimed were individual errors in note keeping, rather than a systematic problem.[34]

In effect, the coroner criticised the hospital for literally ignoring Mrs Shepherd's medical needs, and allowing her to die without an exploration of what could have been done.

At Stafford Hospital, a 66-year-old woman, Mrs Gillian Astbury, died in 2007 because staff did not give her the insulin she needed. She had been admitted after she had fallen at home and broken her pelvis and arm. She died following a 40-hour gap in her insulin injections. The primary cause of death was the resulting ketoacidosis involving excess acid in the bloodstream. Secondarily, she died from a urinary infection and *Clostridium difficile*.

Her death was due to a catalogue of errors. Following a transfer to the orthopaedic ward, there was a breakdown in communication, which included inadequate record keeping and lack of checks. The ward was short-staffed, with two nurses covering 22 patients. Shift handovers were not documented, and patients' records not checked. Those staff who did know about Mrs Astbury's diabetes forgot to tell others about it. Although a blood test revealed she had dangerously high blood sugar levels, no treatment was given. The food she was given was inappropriate, and even when a high blood sugar level became apparent, no action was taken. The senior staff nurse on duty at the time referred to Mrs Astbury's care as 'appalling'.

The inquest jury concluded that Mrs Astbury's death was due to gross failings in care, as well as lack of communication between staff, the failure to consult patient notes, giving of the wrong diet and deficiencies generally across the hospital.[35]

Mr Ivor Hitchman, 77 years old, went into Gloucestershire Royal Hospital for a knee operation. Despite a successful operation, he then died of *Clostridium difficile*. The inquest concluded that staff had failed to follow instructions, keep proper records and to recognise his symptoms. A renal consultant had asked for close monitoring of his fluid intake and output, and for blood tests to be carried out every day. This did not happen because staff did not look at the notes and instructions were not transferred properly between shifts. During the time that this monitoring did not take place, he developed the lethal infection. An independent expert had described the care given to him as 'appalling'.

---

34 Wardrop, M. (2009) 'Coroner criticises "unacceptable" treatment of Mike Tindall's grandmother.' *Daily Telegraph*, 30 April.

35 Grainger, L. (2010) '"Appalling" standards in care led to the death of Hednesford grandmother.' *Cannock Chase Post*, 16 September.

The NHS Trust publicly accepted the coroner's criticism about communication between staff and record keeping; it sought legalistic refuge, however, in the fact that the coroner stopped short of a verdict of neglect — and also that, even if the hospital had provided proper care, it might not have prevented Mr Hitchman's death.[36]

Death from natural causes but condition aggravated by neglect: this was the summing up of the coroner about the death in 2007 of Mr George Angelides at Leicester General Hospital, run by the University Hospitals Leicester NHS Trust. Amongst points made by his family were that a stomach feeding tube was not checked and cleaned, his catheter was left to spill and overflow, inappropriate dressings were used to cover sores — and no record was kept for four months about the management and treatment of those sores.[37]

AT GOSPORT WAR Memorial Hospital, gross laxity in prescribing practices for older people was exposed in 2002 by the Commission for Health Improvement (CHI). The problem came to light following a police investigation into the possibly unlawful killing of several patients in 1998. The Commission found systemic failure, including absence of local prescribing guidelines, of supervision, of appraisal and of multi-disciplinary assessment.

High levels of prescribing went unquestioned. Of particular concern was the inappropriate combined subcutaneous administration of diamorphine, midazolam and haloperidol. This carried a risk of depressing respiratory function in older patients, leading to death. Such was the absence of adequate assessment that prescribing practice used for patients with palliative care needs — that is, for those patients who were dying — were in fact applied to patients who were there for quite the opposite reason, namely, rehabilitation.[38] In other words, the inference was that people's lives were being brought to an end prematurely and indiscriminately.

The same sort of issue surfaced a decade later at Totnes Hospital in Devon. It involved failure to diagnose and monitor people's needs,

---

36 'Gloucestershire Royal Hospital criticised after superbug death of pensioner.' *This is Gloucestershire*, 6 October 2010. Accessed on 20 October 2010 at: www.thisisgloucestershire. co.uk/news/Gloucester-hospital-staff-failed-pensioner/article-2723438-detail/article.html.

37 'Coroner raps Leicester hospital over death of granddad.' *This is Leicestershire*, 2 November 2009. Accessed on 20 December 2010 at: www.thisisleicestershire.co.uk/news/Coroner-raps-Leicester-hospital-death-granddad/article-1472767-detail/article.html.

38 CHI (Commission for Healthcare Improvement) (2002) *Investigation into the Portsmouth Healthcare NHS Trust: Gosport War Memorial Hospital, July 2002*. London: CHI, pp.viii, 12.

coupled with inappropriate prescription of powerful palliative care drugs with the potential to shorten life. The Care Quality Commission (CQC) investigated, following concerns about medication, pain relief and assessment for older people with organic mental health problems such as dementia. The Trust had already conducted its own review, finding a lack of timely, appropriate and simple examinations of people's physical and mental states. Records of ward rounds were often not kept. Most patients did not have a nursing care plan.[39]

The effects of polypharmacy and the side effects were apparently not considered; the importance of monitoring food and fluid intake was not appreciated. Palliative care was not properly understood, and there was a lack of stepped, gradated, care and pain relief. There was a surprisingly swift move to deliver drugs by injection without considering the underlying causes of the person's condition, and a lack of multi-disciplinary response to the distress of patients. Syringe drivers to administer opioids were used unusually frequently. The director had stated:

> ...patients would be unlikely to live long when prescribed these drugs at these doses. They [staff] continued to prescribe high doses and there is no record that they, on any occasion, considered decreasing the dose, for example, in order to assess whether a patient's agitation or pain could be managed so they were less sedated and able to eat and drink. This observation is in the context that people being treated by this unit were often close to the end of their lives.[40]

There were also concerns on other units, including some relating to use of syringe drivers.[41] Given these concerns, about patients not living long, it was no wonder the Commission was anxious about the confusion it found on some units about the concept of palliative care. It aims at relieving symptoms, rather than treating disease or illness, when a patient is close to death. However, the concept was being applied to patients who were not close to death but who instead displayed challenging behaviour that was difficult to manage. On one unit in particular, palliative care was being provided when instead more consideration should have been given to treating the root causes of the patients' behaviour – such as physical

---

39 CQC (Care Quality Commission) (2010) *Investigation into the mental health care for older people provided by Devon Partnership NHS Trust, June 2010.* London: CQC, p.5.

40 CQC (Care Quality Commission) (2010) *Investigation into the mental health care for older people provided by Devon Partnership NHS Trust, June 2010.* London: CQC, p.5.

41 CQC (Care Quality Commission) (2010) *Investigation into the mental health care for older people provided by Devon Partnership NHS Trust, June 2010.* London: CQC, p.9.

illness, depression, psychosis, adverse environmental conditions, fear and disorientation.[42]

CLAIRE RAYNER, FORMER nurse, agony aunt and campaigner for decent, basic health care, died during the writing of this book in October 2010. It turns out that she was a fan of John Stuart Mill.[43] He, as many people know, propounded utilitarianism, which can be characterised as 'the greatest good of the greatest number'.

There is a suspicion, or a danger, that the way the health service is coming to be run (or not run) for the elderly is based – at least in the eyes of central government and NHS trust executives – on a distorted variation of this principle of utility, albeit *unspoken*. Namely, that older people with significant health needs will have to put up with deplorable levels of service, including suffering, pain, degradation and death for the good of everybody else.

This will not do. First, with the increasing age of the population and statistics for health service use, it is far from clear just who comprise the greater number and who 'everybody else' is, especially as we all get old. Second, it is not a policy that has been articulated in public, debated and voted upon in a country that prides itself on being a social democracy.

Third, even were the policy made transparent, it would not be morally acceptable. There may or may not be a case for rationing expensive health care interventions – on the basis of age and the general, likely economic productivity of an individual. Professor Grimley Evans argued certainly not, if we want to avoid valuing people only for their potential as soldiers, workers or breeding females – thereby creating a class, the elderly, 'of *Untermenschen* whose lives and well being are deemed not worth spending money on.' He maintained that we should not discriminate against older people, but instead base treatment on a person's physiological condition and ability to benefit.[44] Such an approach is not, by the way, the same as fuelling the vain pursuit of immortality – as some have suggested.[45]

But in any case, we are dealing with something different here. The greatest good of the greatest number was never meant to be a formula for the State actively to perpetrate degradation on a particular section of the

42 CQC (Care Quality Commission) (2010) *Investigation into the mental health care for older people provided by Devon Partnership NHS Trust, June 2010*. London: CQC, pp.13, 18.
43 'Claire Rayner.' *The Times*, 13 October 2010 (obituary).
44 Grimley Evans, Prof. J. (1997) 'Rationing health care by age: The case against.' *British Medical Journal 314*, p.822.
45 Williams, Prof. A. (1997) 'Rationing health care by age: The case for.' *British Medical Journal 314*, p.820.

population. John Stuart Mill's writing makes this clear when he refers to how the principle of utility is connected with justice. Utility would not, in general, embrace the infliction of a positive hurt in the form of direct suffering or privation on somebody else.[46]

Fourth, any such policy would also have to be tested against the law and would be found to be wanting as, in principle, contrary to human rights, common and even criminal law. (And, fifth, Claire Rayner would never have approved.)

CRUMBLIES, CABBAGES, BED blockers and frequent flyers. The use of such terms in hospitals makes it easier to palm off the old.

In 2007, Professor Ian Philp, the 'national director' for older people appointed by the Department of Health, drew attention to the major mismatch between the needs of older people and the health care being provided. However, he also pointed to deep-seated negative attitudes toward older people:

> Older people are the main users of hospital and residential services. There have been high profile cases of poor treatment of older people in mental health and general hospitals, in care homes and in domiciliary care. It is important that care in all these settings is geared to the needs of older people, especially for those approaching the end of their lives. Our work will seek to challenge deep-seated negative cultural attitudes towards older people, the root cause of failure to treat older people with respect for their dignity and human rights.[47]

In 2009, a report commissioned by the Department of Health concluded that discrimination against older people in health and social care persisted and was importantly due to negative attitudes – and that this contributed to poor quality care.[48]

This then may be an additional, contributory factor to poor and neglectful care. It is not obvious, though, that such attitudes on the front line of health care are necessarily the only or even the main culprit. For every nurse with a suspect attitude to older people, there will be many others who have the right approach but lack time, resources and support from management. More importantly, the Department of Health's rhetoric

46 Mill, J.S. (1962) *Utilitarianism*. Glasgow: William Collins, p.317. (First published in 1861.)

47 Philp, I. (2006) *A new ambition for old age: Next steps in implementing the National Service Framework for older people, a report from Professor Ian Philp, National Director for Older People*. London: Department of Health, p.4.

48 Carruthers, I. and Ormondroyd, J. (2009) *Achieving age equality in health and social care*. London: Department of Health, p.7.

and vague aspiration aside, if the actual effect of its policies were instead used as a yardstick of its attitude to the elderly, then it would appear to be a, if not *the*, major source of the very negativity that it complains about.

One illustration of this relates to conducting inquiries. The evidence of extremely poor treatment of many elderly patients throughout the health service is, and has been, there for all to see for many years. Yet the New Labour government had to be threatened legally before it would appoint an independent inquiry into events at Mid Staffordshire. Even then it flatly refused a public inquiry. This can be contrasted with the setting up of an independent inquiry with a wide remit to report on access to health care of people with learning disabilities.[49] Yet, the trigger for this inquiry was a report by the voluntary body, Mencap. Its report, *Death by indifference*, referred to just six cases of what might have been preventable deaths of people with learning disabilities.[50] The contrast suggests that the Department of Health views older people as very much more expendable than other patients.

As a report prepared for the Mid Staffordshire Public Inquiry pointed out, the sudden death of a younger person is a cause célèbre; the slow decline and death of older people from dehydration, drug errors and neglect are not.[51]

ALL THIS SAID about policy, prejudice and contempt are alive and well on the ground. Some doctors refer to the care of the elderly as akin to 'market gardening' (with reference to cabbages) and to the patients themselves as 'crumblies'.[52] Other pejorative terms include 'bed blocker', a symptom of the unspoken animosity against older people's use of hospital resources. Likewise is the reference to 'frequent flyers' because of regular hospital admissions.[53] The use of such belittling terms may result in the application of therapeutic negativity:

> It isn't just about politically correct language, however. These attitudes affect diagnosis and treatment. The customary diagnostic rigour, which we have been trained to apply as standard, can

49 Michael, J. (Sir) (2008) *Healthcare for all: Report of the Independent Inquiry into access for healthcare for people with learning disabilities.* London: Department of Health.

50 Mencap (2007) *Death by indifference.* London: Mencap.

51 Vincent, C. (2010) *Patient safety in the UK National Health Service: The events in Mid Staffordshire in context*, p.7. Accessed on 20 December 2010 at: www.midstaffspublicinquiry.com/ hearings/s/120/week-two-15-18-nov-2010.

52 Oliver, D. (2008) '"Acopia" and "social admission" are not diagnoses: Why older people deserve better.' *Journal of the Royal Society of Medicine 101*, 168–74.

53 Curtis, P. (2006) '"Frequent flyers" costing NHS £2.3bn a year.' *The Guardian*, 13 February.

be mysteriously replaced in older patients by ageist therapeutic nihilism.[54]

PLAINLY THEN, THE problems of providing treatment, care and rehabilitation are not new. They existed long before *The NHS Plan* was published in 2000. Nevertheless, it would seem in the last decade that some major ingredients of government policy are distinctly unhelpful. To outward appearance, this is odd. If *The NHS Plan* and *National Service Framework for Older People* were taken at face value, this should not have been the case. The former spoke about a debt of honour:

> Older people are the single biggest users of the NHS. They are the generation which built and have supported the NHS all their lives. The commitment to deliver patient-centred care – the right care, in the right place, at the right time – must, above all, be honoured in the delivery of care for older people.[55]

It talked also of autonomy, dignity, privacy, treating the whole person, good nutrition, tissue viability and importantly, good clinical practice recognising the complexities of caring for the elderly.[56]

The *Framework* went on to state, in Standard One, that NHS services would be provided, regardless of age, on the basis of clinical need alone. The second standard stipulated that the NHS should treat patients as individuals.[57] Dignity and privacy would be respected.[58] People's personal hygiene needs, including toileting and bathing, would be met sensitively; other intimate interventions would be carried out in privacy.[59]

Crucially, hospital care would mean attention being paid to all those things, omission of which, arguably lead not just to needs not being met but to neglect. It listed maintaining fluid balance, pain management, pressure sore management, acute confusion, falls and immobility, nutrition, continence, cognitive impairment, rehabilitation potential,

---

54   Oliver, D. (2008) '"Acopia" and "social admission" are not diagnoses: Why older people deserve better.' *Journal of the Royal Society of Medicine 101*, 168–74.

55   Secretary of State for Health (2002) *Delivering The NHS Plan: Next steps on investment, next steps on reform.* Cm 5503. London: The Stationery Office, p.32.

56   Secretary of State for Health (2000) *The NHS Plan: A plan for investment, a plan for reform.* Cm 4818-I. London: The Stationery Office, p.124.

57   DH (Department of Health) (2001) *National Service Framework for Older People.* London: DH, p.12.

58   DH (Department of Health) (2001) *National Service Framework for Older People.* London: DH, p.23.

59   DH (Department of Health) (2001) *National Service Framework for Older People.* London: DH, p.25.

depression, infection control, medicines management and end of life care.[60]

The ten-year plan set out in the *Framework* sounded promising. Many health care professionals genuinely hoped and believed it would represent a turning point. So what happened? It is impossible to avoid the conclusion that whilst the *Framework* was beckoning in one direction, other more powerful elements in health care policy were headed elsewhere. Just where is considered in the following chapter.

---

60 DH (Department of Health) (2001) *National Service Framework for Older People.* London: DH, pp.53–4.

13

Patient Voices, Consumers and Markets

> This site is firstly dedicated to Bella Bailey 16/02/1921 –
> 08/11/2007...and also to the many others who have lost their
> lives needlessly on wards in Staffordshire General Hospital. We
> launched this campaign after witnessing 8 weeks of elderly care
> in this hospital. What we saw after the first few days left us fearing
> for my Mother's life and too frightened to leave her. We stayed by
> her side sleeping on a chair for 8 weeks... What we saw horrified
> us and from the letters we have received, it haunts many others
> who have had relatives/friends on those wards. Some relatives
> have spent longer staying in the hospital than us and have shared
> their experiences. Most of the letters relate to wards 7, 8, 10,
> 11 and 12 and it is ward 11 where my Mother spent her last
> days. After her needless death, who yes was ill but not ready to
> die, we her family felt unable to let the suffering/abuse we saw
> continue... The launch of the campaign with the help of the
> Staffordshire newsletter brought in many similar stories to ours.
> Their loved ones had been neglected or abused on those wards.
> My Mum was lucky she had us to help care for her. Many didn't,
> they died alone. (Cure the NHS: campaigning organisation of
> relatives, 2010)[1]

The content of the quote immediately above is not what *The NHS Plan*, published in 2000, had in mind. It had described a civilised approach to improving health care by giving patients a voice. It did not envisage or explain that relatives (the patients themselves being mostly dead or unable to speak out) would have to fight desperately against NHS managers and evasive politicians who were absolutely determined not to listen to tales of woe.

The NHS Plan, published in 2000, was meant to be the great saviour of the National Health Service (NHS) and to bring about the provision of high quality, equitable services to all. It was to give patients more

---

1   Cure the NHS (2010) *About Cure the NHS*. Accessed on 20 October at: www.curethenhs.co.uk/
     site/content_about.php.

choice and control.[2] In 2004, a review published by the Department of Health looked at progress.[3] A conspicuous element in the review was the idea of choice, a concept of consumerism in health care intended to drive the improvement of health services. This later developed into the policy of 'choose and book', the idea of shopping around for one hospital or another. And the coalition government elected in 2010, for all its concentrated criticism of its predecessor, seems set to follow exactly the same consumerist path, referring to the patient's choice of provider, of a consultant-led team and of general practitioner (GP) practice.[4]

The implications of this approach need to be examined in relation to systemic poor and neglectful care of vulnerable patients, in particular the notion of such patients as consumers, having a strong voice in a health care 'market'. That is, where there are, increasingly, a range of health care providers to choose from, providers who will be competing with each other for the patient's custom.

THE 2004 REVIEW of *The NHS Plan* gave the impression that it viewed patients as consumers or customers, perhaps in a restaurant or a hotel. It talked of the quality and availability of food – and menus – but not of helping people to eat it. Likewise, while the NHS was heading full tilt into a series of scandals involving failure to provide the most basic of care, the review was still talking about the importance of bedside televisions and telephones.[5] And, as we have already seen in the Introduction to this book, the developers of the Queen's Hospital in Essex spoke of it as looking like a hotel. But there the analogy breaks down.

Hotels generally provide guests with decent bedrooms, food and drink, with clean bathrooms and with clean linen. It is remarkable then, six years on from that review, to read of regular use of storerooms to nurse patients because of a shortage of beds, as happened at the Norfolk and Norwich Hospital. Mrs Doris McKeown occupied a small, narrow windowless room, closely surrounded by shelves of hospital supplies. Because she was stowed away, she missed some medication rounds and meals. She referred to it as a broom cupboard; the hospital maintained

---

2   Secretary of State for Health (2000) *The NHS Plan: A plan for investment, a plan for reform.* Cm 4818-I. London: The Stationery Office, Chapter 10.

3   Secretary of State for Health (2004) *The NHS improvement plan: Putting people at the heart of public services.* London: The Stationery Office.

4   Secretary of State for Health (2010) *Equity and excellence: Liberating the NHS.* Cm 7881. London: The Stationery Office, pp.3, 20. Also: DH (Department of Health) (2010) *Liberating the NHS: Greater choice and control, a consultation on proposals.* London: DH.

5   Secretary of State for Health (2004) *The NHS improvement plan: Putting people at the heart of public services.* London: The Stationery Office, p.22.

that it was a treatment room and conceded that 26 other wards had similar rooms. Admitted for a spinal operation for trapped nerves, she had been transferred to the storeroom in the middle of the night because of a shortage of beds.

Mrs McKeown's daughter happened to be a GP and chair of the British Medical Association's community care committee. She summed it succinctly: 'My mother needed emergency surgery and she ended up in a cupboard. Where's the dignity in care?'[6]

She was not alone; another, 85-year-old woman, Mrs Rhoda Talbot, also occupied such a room in the same hospital, surrounded by shelving for stores, green buckets containing dirty needles and oxygen cylinders. Nurses went in and out all night, turning the light on and off. And a third, younger woman, Helen Howes, found herself hemmed in by packs of dressings, bags for catheters and other medical supplies; her handbag was perched on a medical waste bin. During the night, she found her bed being moved, so that nurses could access supplies.[7]

This is a particularly apt example, because the Norfolk and Norwich Hospital was meant to be the epitome of a modernised, dignified NHS. It was built as part of the then government's modernisation initiative, involving the private finance initiative (PFI). Built at a cost of £229 million and opened in 2001, it pays £40 million annual rent. It is run by the Norfolk and Norwich University Hospitals NHS Foundation Trust.[8]

In his *A history of modern Britain*, covering the period from 1940 to 2008, Andrew Marr concludes thus: 'This history has told the story of the defeat of politics by shopping.'[9] There seems to be a danger now that the notion of shopping, applied inappropriately to at least some aspects of the health service, will vanquish both basic care and common sense.

THE IDEA BEHIND developing patient choice and a health care market is simple. It is to drive up the quality of service; the consumer will choose and the good providers will flourish and the bad go to the wall. The difficulty with this is that the notion of the active shopper is by and large an irrelevance to a, perhaps the, key group of patients, older people. Taken to hospital following an acute episode and with other underlying

6   Hope, J. (2010) 'Shocking picture shows how elderly patient was abandoned for two days in hospital store cupboard with little food or medication.' *Daily Mail*, 14 February.

7   Hope, J. (2010) 'Now three MORE female patients "kept in hospital store cupboard" surrounded by blood-stained bins.' *Daily Mail,* 17 February.

8   Hope, J. (2010) 'Shocking picture shows how elderly patient was abandoned for two days in hospital store cupboard with little food or medication.' *Daily Mail*, 14 February.

9   Marr, A. (2009) *A history of modern Britain*. London: Pan, p.597.

problems, they simply wish to be treated well, locally and as near to their families as possible. Shopping around would be the last thing on their mind; desperately sick patients do not make good shoppers. Besides which, even suppose more than one accessible choice, it would still not be straightforward.

For instance, it is striking how so many accounts given by patients acknowledge that the care on one hospital ward may be good, on another poor. How would you know which ward you were going to end up on? Even if you know what you are entering hospital for, this does not mean you will end up on the appropriate ward. Many patients are placed on the 'wrong' one, because of overcrowding. You may start off on a caring ward, but rapidly be transferred to a non-caring one. In addition, unless it is elective treatment, you may not know which consultant you will come under; so talk by a new government of choosing a consultant and his or her team is of limited relevance to many vulnerable patients.

The websites Patient Opinion and NHS Choices record the comments of patients and relatives about local hospitals. A number refer to the fact that if you are not reasonably able, you are in trouble; in other words, if you are not physically and mentally able – as the ideal customer must be – and you cannot help yourself, then nobody else will. For instance, at Hinchingbrooke Hospital, the following comment was made in October 2007:

> …watching elderly patients having food put in front of them, and not being fed was the most distressing thing i have seen. equally listening to them begging for help was heart breaking. if you could not care for your own needs, you were really neglected.[10]

At North Tyneside General Hospital, in 2009, a patient referred to the same issue:

> The ward was not very clean. The ward was understaffed. At one point a lady was chastised for soiling herself after being told she could not go to the toilet yet as they were serving dinners and their was no one to help [sic]. A soiled adult nappy was left on my chair and only removed when I asked and the chair was not cleaned after. I frequently had to ask for my medication as the nurses appeared to overlook me. At no time did anyone introduce themselves or tell me what was happening. At the time I was 48 and able to (most of the time look after myself). The ward was

---

10 NHS Choices. Accessed on 20 September 2010 at: www.nhs.uk/Services/Hospitals/ PatientFeedback/DefaultView.aspx?id=1429&pid=RQQ31&pageNo=5&sort=1&record PP=0.

full of elderly ladies who sadly were not treated with respect or dignity. I know we are in hospital not for luxuries but to simply get better but on several days we did not even get a hot drink.[11]

And in 2010, a relative visiting Basildon pinpointed the inability of dementia or stroke patients to get attention:

Staff need to retrained especially when it comes to bedside manners. Elderly patients deserve to be treated with respect not shouted at or in some cases we saw on visits totally ignored. Management never availble [sic] to discuss concerns with. The elderly patients we saw were mostly unable to make themselves known as they had serious issues such as dementia or many were stroke patients, they deserve to be treated with more respect. Many elderely [sic] patients have no family to fight their corner and this should not be allowed.[12]

'PAYMENT BY RESULTS' is a policy related to the development of a health care market. If a health service is to be operated along market lines, involving both internal competition as well as use of independent providers under contract to the NHS, treatment and care obviously have to be priced up. Introduced during the 2000s, this approach relies in part on mapping out pathways of care and quantifying the input, time, resources and cost for particular types of patient. Essentially it is about measurement, about imposing a tariff cost on episodes of treatment. Younger adults with one discrete condition fit this approach relatively well. It is like labelling and pricing up tins in the supermarket.

However, quantifying what is required for many older people – even with the same condition as a younger person – is by no means as easy. As already outlined, this is because significant numbers of older people suffer from multiple pathology. So the treatment they require for the precipitating condition or event becomes complicated by other factors. They are also not so predictable, and they need more time, more effort and more expertise. In other words, you can't put a price and label on the tin, because you don't know what's inside.

Even worse, this unknown content is likely to be expensive. In short, older people are simply and increasingly commercially unattractive. This is both important and troubling, because the pricing up of care, signified by payment by results, is the necessary prelude to tendering

---

11 Patient Opinion. Accessed on 20 September 2010 at: www.patientopinion.org.uk/opinions/14000.

12 Patient Opinion. Accessed on 20 September 2010 at: www.patientopinion.org.uk/opinions/39422.

out health services to the independent sector. This is a policy adopted by both New Labour and, now, by the coalition government. Obviously you can't sell things very well, or at all, if you are unable to put a sensible price on them. And this is the great problem with the elderly; generally speaking, they have the disadvantage of being that bit more complex and expensive. They are at huge risk of being regarded as shoddy, unsaleable and undesirable in this move to a modern health care market place.

This situation means that not only might complex conditions or needs come to be shunned by hospitals, but there could also be an incentive to operate at 'below tariff', in order to generate a profit. This might create a perverse incentive to reduce the quality of care.[13] Such an incentive may be accentuated by the operating principle of NHS foundation trusts, to which status all NHS trusts are expected to progress. They increasingly are adopting 'service line reporting'; a concept derived from business. It puts a premium on breaking the trust up into business units or service lines, each one analysed in terms of revenues, expenditure, patients, profit and financial surpluses.[14]

In summary, key elements of government policy are premised on a notion of consumerism and relatively simplistic financial measurement, both of which are ill suited to the needs of older people with more complex needs. Although the problem lies with the system, it is older people who are deemed to be problematic, who carry the can for this mismatch – and who, along the way, and as a result, are at higher risk of suffering more or less poor and neglectful care.

THE DEVELOPMENT OF a consumer, patient-driven health service relies, in theory, on giving much more power to the patient and on giving the patient a voice.

If patients are to have more power and more voice, then correspondingly health care professionals should have less. This follows if power implies authority over others, which is one meaning of the word. Thus, health care policy over the last 20 years appears to have been based at least in part on the idea that health care professionals are a self-interested group. And that, in the name of the patient, their power base had to be reduced; the interests of the service provider should be secondary to that of the consumers.

---

13 O'Connor, R. and Neumann, V. (2006) 'Payment by results or payment by outcome? The history of measuring medicine.' *Journal of the Royal Society of Medicine 99*, 226–31.
14 Monitor (2006) *How Service-Line Reporting can improve the productivity and performance of NHS foundation trusts.* London: Monitor.

An attack had to be launched. In the vanguard have been the chief executives of NHS trusts, doing the bidding of central government but ultimately serving the public. To the extent that arrogant professionals were suborning patient welfare to their own nefarious ends, nobody would argue with this policy. If such alleged wickedness ever really was the case in recent or indeed in any times; as Raymond Tallis observed in 2004, it was more a case of the hospital consultant as overworked cog rather than god.[15] To this purported end, the last decade in particular has seen the triumph of managerialism over the clinicians and health care professionals. But, as ever, it is not that simple.

It is one thing to curb excessive power exercised by clinicians; quite another to give untrammelled power to a new generation of chief executives. Checks and balances are required; as, in fact, Florence Nightingale discussed when she wrote about the running of hospitals in the 1860s. She believed that patients were better cared for when there was a 'perpetual rub' in the hospital between, for example, doctors, nurses, governors, treasurers and casual visitors. Patients fared worse when a 'chief' had too much power.[16]

This imbalance between managers and clinicians has had some unfortunate effects. These include the supremacy of political targets over the clinical care, welfare and even life of patients – for instance, at Stoke Mandeville, in Kent and in Mid Staffordshire. In addition, the ascendancy of politicians and of managerialism, both in the supposed name of the patient, has led to an undermining of trust. And this has itself come in two forms.

First, the trust between managers and health professionals may fracture. This is manifest in the ever-increasing bureaucracy and stifling instruction, the sort of currency which managers understand best and which they impose on professionals as a means of seizing and retaining power. And, second, is an erosion of trust between patient and clinician; in a consumer market, the idea is to stoke up tension between the service provider out for what he or she can get, and the consumer seeking to drive the best bargain. It is far from clear that this will lead to an optimum health care system, in which trust between doctor (and nurse) and patient arguably should be fundamental.[17]

Governments of all hues have come to see professionals and clinicians as an obstacle to progress and modernisation in the NHS. The theory

15 Tallis, R. (2004) *Hippocratic oaths: Medicine and its discontents.* London: Atlantic Books, p.76.
16 Nightingale, F. (1863) *Notes on Hospitals.* London: Longman, Green, Longman, Roberts, Green, p.184.
17 Tallis, R. (2004) *Hippocratic oaths: Medicine and its discontents.* London: Atlantic Books, pp.102–108.

is that if non-clinician managers are well paid they will objectively and disinterestedly implement government policy for the greater public good. It has been suggested that this idea has its roots in game theory developed during the 1950s; applied to the NHS, it assumes clinicians are not to be trusted because of their tendency to self-interest.

This is a shameless policy, prosecuted under false pretences. If we are to talk about trust, we can – as the informed consumers which the government believes we are – ask whom we would rather trust: the health professions or the managers bankrolled by the politicians. Indeed, in recent years managers in the health service have come to resemble political myrmidons, with chief executives sometimes acting like latter-day apparatchiks. The answer to our question requires a simple comparison between clinicians and those politicians. It is really no contest. The former have expert knowledge, many years of training, practice scientific medicine and are subject to a legally-enforceable code of ethics. Most are dedicated and take patient care and welfare seriously and personally. Politicians on the other hand usually have no training or education in health care, are bound by no ethical code and will generally say and do anything to get elected and to stay elected.

Whom would we rather trust? The managers (adhering to politically-imposed targets) who refused to isolate highly infectious patients at Stoke Mandeville Hospital; or the professionals of the infection control team who were urging immediate isolation, and the other nurses and doctors who urged the Board to take action?

However, it also appears that the behaviour of non-clinician managers has not turned out to be as disinterested as the theory supposed; they do act out of self-interest and indeed may manipulate the system for their own ends.[18] It is called cheating. They have met priorities and targets but sometimes only doing so at a high cost to other aspects of the health service, including basic, decent care.

The cover for this assault on professionals has been the patient; it is all meant to be for his or her benefit. Much of the ammunition has come from the well publicised cases of individual health care clinicians and professionals who have gone a very long way off the rails. Cases include, for instance, those of the murdering GP, Harold Shipman, and nurses such as Beverley Allitt (murder of children)[19] or Colin Norris (murder of

---

18 Curtis, A. (2007) 'The trap: What happened to our dream of freedom.' BBC Television, shown on BBC2 on 11 March 2007. And see also: Binmore, K. (2007) 'Rules of the game.' *Prospect*, 25 November.

19 Foster, J. and Pillinger, C. (1994) 'Chances to stop killer nurse were missed: Allitt report highlights understaffing.' *The Independent*, 12 February.

non-diabetic patients, in hospital with hip fractures, with insulin).[20] Also the inquiry into children's deaths at Bristol Royal Infirmary attacked the 'club culture' of clinicians.[21] All this has led to more regulation of health care professionals. It has removed local initiative and policymaking from clinicians, but has also distracted attention away from the greater harm that has come in its place. That is, unbridled execution of policies by chief executives, obediently backed by docile trust boards, who understand little about health care or, if they do, are too frightened to say so. And by some senior clinicians and health care professionals who have lost their way in the local hospital corridors of power.

This should not happen of course, according to the theory; the public, the patient as consumer, should be driving the actions of these chief executives so that decisions are made in the patient's interest. Where then, is this patient voice, and why is it not being heard?

In fact the reason is very simple. Government does not really want to hear the patient voice. The term is a cipher; 'choice' is a shorthand to refer to the development of a health care market and the break-up of a State-provided health service. But more than this, the government's idea is that the patient voice should remain fairly compliant, upbeat and resemble the decision to shop, on a Saturday morning, at one supermarket rather than another. What it does not want, like or understand is the voice of the patient driven by fear, anger and – worst of all from central government's point of view – by first-hand experience of some extremely unpleasant and raw aspects of health care policy.

IT IS UNDOUBTEDLY a good idea to listen to patients and their relatives, particularly when they are being subjected to horrendous indignities (emphasis added):

> The principal, if not the sole, purpose of having a National Health Service is the promotion and protection of the health and welfare of those who seek its help. Where those who do so are systematically mistreated and left without care in such numbers, and with the frequency that has been shown by the evidence presented to me, *their voice must be listened to with particular care –* all the more so when those charged with the responsibility of

---

20 Cantrill, P., Foster, E., Lane, P. and Pate, R. (2010) *Report of the Independent Inquiry into the Colin Norris incidents at Leeds Teaching Hospitals NHS Trust in 2002.* Leeds: Yorkshire and Humber Strategic Health Authority.

21 Kennedy, I. (Chair) (2001) *Learning from Bristol. The report of the Public Inquiry into children's heart surgery at the Bristol Royal Infirmary 1984–1995.* Cm 5207(1). London: The Stationery Office, p.68.

ensuring an appropriate standard of care have apparently failed to detect or react to bad standards at virtually all levels of the system.[22]

Health policy is, and has been for some time, apparently premissed on patient choice and control. *The NHS Plan* in 2000 said that the NHS would shape its services around the needs and preferences of individual patients, their families and their carers.[23] It referred to over-centralisation and to disempowerment of patients as matters that would have to be tackled. It went on to say that the NHS would have to be patient centred and offer a personalised service that, by 2010, would be commonplace.[24]

This was not just a New Labour idea. A White Paper published in 2010 by the new coalition government, of Conservatives and Liberal Democrats, has continued the theme:

> ...patients will be at the heart of everything we do. So they will have more choice and control, helped by easy access to the information they need about the best GPs and hospitals. Patients will be in charge of making decisions about their care.[25]

Implementation guidance for *The NHS Plan* of 2000 did concede, in principle, that choice – in terms of the patient shopping around and choosing between different hospitals – had a more limited role to play in the case of some services. The guidance stated that for such services, other mechanisms would ensure patient preference was complied with – through patient surveys. The net result would be that patients would occupy the 'driving seat'.[26]

In line with all of this, guidance from the Care Quality Commission (CQC) states that people should be confident that comments and complaints will be listened to and be acted on effectively – and that they will not be discriminated against because they have complained. Providers should have systems in place for comments and complaints, support people to comment and to complain – and consider fully,

22 Francis, R. (Chair) (2010) *Independent Inquiry into care provided by Mid Staffordshire NHS Foundation Trust January 2005–March 2009.* London: The Stationery Office, p.48.

23 Secretary of State for Health (2002) *Delivering The NHS Plan: Next steps on investment, next steps on reform.* Cm 5503. London: The Stationery Office, p.4.

24 Secretary of State for Health (2000) *The NHS Plan: A plan for investment, a plan for reform.* Cm 4818-I. London: The Stationery Office, pp.10, 17.

25 Secretary of State for Health (2010) *Equity and excellence: Liberating the NHS.* Cm 7881. London: The Stationery Office, p.1.

26 Secretary of State for Health (2002) *Delivering The NHS Plan: Next steps on investment, next steps on reform.* Cm 5503. London: The Stationery Office, pp.23–4.

respond appropriately and resolve, where possible, such comments and complaints.[27]

Thus, there is common political consensus (not necessarily correct) that the solution to achieving good health care – and, by definition, the avoidance and detection of serious lapses – lies in choice and in listening to patients and their relatives. It is equally plain that the politicians, policymakers and their cheer leaders, in the form of managers down the line, find it extraordinarily difficult to listen. And when they are being told things they don't want to hear, it is beyond them altogether.

THE MAIN PURPOSE of the Independent Inquiry in Mid Staffordshire was to record the experiences and views of the patients and their families.[28] It did so remorselessly and with a vengeance, as it relayed the terrible and degrading experiences of patients – in a manner not achieved by any number of Healthcare Commission reports during the 2000s:

> The experience of listening to so many accounts of bad care, denial of dignity and unnecessary suffering made an impact of an entirely different order to that made by reviewing written accounts. It is fair to say that all members of the Inquiry team and advisers who were able to participate in these hearings were deeply affected by what we heard. While it is difficult, if not impossible, to convey this impact by the written word, in my view it is important that staff employed by the Trust, as well as the general public, have access to the accounts I have received, both written and oral, so that they can make their own assessment and be motivated by this material to inform the promotion of good standards of care in the future. This may also help them, individually and collectively, to acknowledge and accept that care given in the past fell far below what was acceptable.[29]

Of all the formal reports and evidence considered in this book, the Mid Staffordshire Independent Inquiry stands out. It is the patient voice *par excellence*. It cut straight to the quick; its chair listened to, and recorded, what patients and relatives said in painstaking and distressing detail. The report blew away the rhetoric and euphemism so often employed to gloss over highly unpleasant unrealities. It is exactly what central government

27 CQC (Care Quality Commission) (2009) *Guidance about compliance: Summary of regulations, outcomes and judgement framework.* London: CQC, p.34.

28 Francis, R. (Chair) (2010) *Independent Inquiry into care provided by Mid Staffordshire NHS Foundation Trust January 2005–March 2009.* London: The Stationery Office, p.34.

29 Francis, R. (Chair) (2010) *Independent Inquiry into care provided by Mid Staffordshire NHS Foundation Trust January 2005–March 2009.* London: The Stationery Office, p.10.

should have wanted – but didn't. It sought to prevent the inquiry taking place and acceded to it only under legal threat from outraged families of patients.[30] Government gave every indication that at most it wanted to hear the patient voice only *sanitised* – not in the raw. It didn't want the horrors.

Even aside from this ambivalence about whether the patient's voice really is valued, it is anyway not necessarily easily come by. For example, one of the Department of Health's own reports into events at Mid Staffordshire stressed the importance of complaints.[31] But, as the Independent Inquiry there recorded, people and their relatives are often afraid to complain – for fear of 'reprisals' by staff:

> He had rung the buzzer. He must have waited nearly an hour. The same thing happened to the gentleman in the opposite bed who was older than my father on a couple of occasions, and I think he ended up soiling the bed linen, and he was very, very distressed. Obviously I overheard and I said I was going to complain. He got very, very agitated and distressed saying: "don't say anything, don't say anything, they will take it out on me".[32]

The Healthcare Commission had made this very point some years earlier. In evidence to a parliamentary committee, it had reported that 'our inspections repeatedly highlighted reluctance by older people to complain due to fear that this would affect the treatment that they or their relatives received'.[33] Whether or not this is a well-founded fear in every case is irrelevant; either way, the patient is not being heard.

In any case, apart from fear, patients may not be in a physical or mental state to complain; and relatives might be too worn down and distressed to do so. Always assuming that there are any relatives or other visitors. Professor Sir George Albert's report, the second of the Department of Health's reports into Mid Staffordshire, also perceived that obtaining patient views is not straightforward. The Trust's system for hand-held electronic devices to gather samples of patients' experiences required

---

30 Leigh Day & Co. (2010) 'Mid Staffordshire report leads to further partial inquiry, 26 February 2010.' Accessed on 12 July 2010 at: www.leighday.co.uk/news/news-archive-2010/mid-staffordshire-report-leads-to-further-partial.

31 Thomé, D.C. (Dr) (2009) *Mid Staffordshire NHS Foundation Trust: A review of lessons learnt for commissioners and performance managers following the Healthcare Commission investigation.* London: Department of Health, p.7.

32 Francis, R. (Chair) (2010) *Independent Inquiry into care provided by Mid Staffordshire NHS Foundation Trust January 2005–March 2009.* London: The Stationery Office, p.54.

33 House of Lords and House of Commons Joint Committee on Human Rights (2007) *The human rights of older people in healthcare. Eighteenth Report of Session 2006–07.* HL 156-I, HC 378-I. London: The Stationery Office, p.68.

the patient to be competent to answer; it thus leaned toward the fitter patients on the wards. He suggested that the Trust think about getting 'real feedback' from patients and, importantly, their families.[34]

Even if complaints are made, responses may be inadequate. One ploy is to give complainants a copy of a policy covering the subject matter of the complaint, as though the existence of a policy on paper equates by definition with reality. A typical example of this might be a complaint – about how long it took nurses to answer a call bell, perhaps 20–30 minutes – which is handled with reference to a policy setting out a three-minute response time.

Of course, the trouble is that the policy doesn't guarantee the practice. For instance, even when a record is kept electronically of call bell response times, hard pressed nurses have in some hospitals contrived to hoodwink the system. They turn off the call bell but then walk away from the patient, only returning, if at all, later. Where there is a will – and enough pressure to undermine patient care, notwithstanding fine sounding policies and apparent monitoring – there is a way.

So at Mid Staffordshire, action plans on paper simply did not translate into practice. Complainants were given, meaninglessly, copies of policies as an answer to complaints brought – even though those policies were simply not being followed.[35]

THE FOLLOWING EXAMPLE, provided by a relative, speaks volumes about the ineffectiveness of complaints systems and the sheer frustration patients and relatives may experience. A complaint was taken against the Northern General Hospital, Sheffield. It was about not giving a patient nutrition and allowing him to develop pressure sores. Both the Healthcare Commission and coroner were involved. The hospital gave assurances about lessons learned and new procedures:

> In August 2007 my father died in the Northern General Hospital. The circumstances of his death lead [sic] to a hospital investigation (which took several months), a Healthcare Commission investigation (which roundly condemned the hospital) and a coroner's inquest (18 months after the event), which found that my father's death was unnatural as a result of the hospital's neglect and failures. My family was sent reams of official documents

34 Alberti, G. (Professor Sir) (2009) *Mid Staffordshire NHS Foundation Trust: A review of the procedures for emergency admissions and treatment, and progress against the recommendation of the March Healthcare Commission report.* London: Department of Health, p.15.
35 Healthcare Commission (2009) *Investigation into Mid Staffordshire NHS Foundation Trust, March 2009.* London: Healthcare Commission, pp.90, 96, 97.

by the hospital purporting to show that new procedures had been put in place to prevent the same thing happening again, and we were given endless assurances to the same effect. One of the issues we had was patients being starved of food because nurses/auxiliary staff could not be bothered to help those too ill, elderly, confused or infirm to feed themselves, (my father lost a stone in weight during a 10-day stay in hospital), another was failure to deal with pressure sores by not using the Waterlow score properly/not providing the appropriate type of mattress for the patient's needs.[36]

The account continued with events two-and-a-half years later, when despite promises at the highest level, nothing seemed to have changed:

Fast-forward 2½ years. A family friend has a 3-week stay on Brearley 1 in the Northern General, and during that time sees exactly the same thing happening time and gain [sic] – patients being served with meals, being unable to eat them, receiving no help (or even an enquiry as to whether they would like help) and the meal being removed untouched at the end of service. She told us this when we visited her, and doesn't know anything about the circumstances of my father's death other than he died in hospital.

This same friend, who has a lot of problems with her legs and circulation, returns home with bed sores on her heels, which the hospital failed to do anything about until the morning of the day she was discharged. The nursing staff failed to even ascertain that she was at risk of developing, or had developed, bed sores, and still discharged her, presumably knowing of her mobility and circulation problems. Our friend is now terrified she will develop leg ulcers, which she has had before and took a very long time to heal…

The lesson learnt according to this observer: don't believe anything you are told and keep your relatives and friends under close observation:

Moral of this story – I now don't believe a word that anyone in the Sheffield Teaching Hospitals NHS Trust tells you (our assurances came from the very top – the Chief Exec) and if you have an infirm, elderly or very sick relative or friend, watch them like a hawk to make sure they are getting enough to eat and drink, that their condition is not deteriorating, and if you have any concerns pester the staff and keep pestering until something is done.

---

36 Patient Opinion. Accessed on 20 September 2010 at: www.patientopinion.org.uk/opinions/29132.

In October 2010, the Patients' Association noted wryly that the 'lessons will be learnt' response is served up now as standard fare – as unerringly as the continuing failure to put those lessons into practice.[37] A month later, it was advocating the setting up of an independent complaints system in order to combat poor care and neglect.[38] But it is doubtful whether complaints can be truly effective in the context of systemic blight within a system. Not only will NHS trusts learn to guard against them, but there is no particular reason to suppose that successful complaints would result in improvements generally in the service. And the conflict, ill feeling, antagonism and added bureaucracy created by large numbers of complaints could easily, in the greater scheme of things, be counter-productive to good patient care. Patients were first encouraged to complain under the Patients' Charter, first published in 1991;[39] we should note that over these last 20 years, this complaints culture has not resulted in the extirpation of neglectful care. Quite the contrary.

UNDUE RELIANCE ON the patient's voice, in order to combat and prevent neglect and abuse, is too simplistic an approach. It could unwittingly lead to a mentality that, if patients do not speak up and shop around, it is their fault if it all goes wrong. In effect the phrase, beloved in the law of contract, *caveat emptor* (buyer beware), the unwise shopper. Indeed, the law of contract assumes, at least in theory, some sort of parity between seller and buyer. But, as the chair of the CQC pointed out in September 2010, there is 'an unequal power base' between, for example, residents of a care home and care home staff,[40] and by implication, patients and hospital staff. It could lead to a distinctly unhealthy situation, whereby professional standards are subsumed totally to the expectations of the consumer.

By way of illustration, the *Weston and Somerset Mercury* reported in 2007 the experiences of three patients at Weston General Hospital. One of these, Mr Stuart Ludlow, was reported by his wife (a qualified psychiatric nurse) to have been given 'degrading and diabolical treatment'. He had been suffering from prostate and bone cancer. Her account detailed how she had not been informed that he had contracted *Clostridium difficile*. In addition, pressure sores and bleeding on her husband's heels, bottom and

---

37 Lister, S. and de Bruxelles, S. (2010) 'Nurse switched off life support by accident.' *The Times*, 26 October.

38 Patients' Association (2010) *Listen to patients, speak up for change.* London: Patients' Association.

39 DH (Department of Health) (1991) *The Patients' Charter.* London: DH.

40 Rose, D. (2010) 'Watchdog closes care homes over fears for "the very basics of life".' *The Times*, 29 September.

genitals had been left untreated and open to infection. He had been left in his own urine and faeces. He did not receive help with personal hygiene, including washing and teeth cleaning, and was refused a commode because of a shortage. The ward toilet was sometimes covered in faeces. He had been left in a corridor, in pain, for three hours. His wife noted that before admission to the hospital, she had provided care by keeping him showered, in clean clothes and free from pressure sores.

She went on to say that she, her husband and visitors had observed patients complaining about being left unwashed, not receiving medication, medication trolleys being left unattended and patients who had fallen on the floor being ignored by nurses. In response to these allegations, the hospital's medical director conceded, with polished euphemism, that because of unprecedented demand and limited resources, 'sometimes we don't meet patients' and relatives' expectations and for that we apologise'.[41]

We should remind ourselves of the implications of the statement by the medical director. Her use of the word 'expectations' infers that standards of basic care hinge on consumer expectation, and that if patients did not expect to receive half decent care, then there would be no need to provide it. It fails to convey the point that such care, irrespective of expectations, is a professional imperative.

NONE OF THIS is to say that listening carefully to patients and their relatives is not essential and necessary, just that it is not sufficient. Indeed, general failure in communication – not talking and listening to patients and their relatives – can lead to catastrophe, if it means you stop treating them as people.

While patients in Kent were dying from infection in overcrowded wards with poor care standards, the Healthcare Commission was clear that numbers trumped the care of individuals: 'Communication between the trust and the PCTs focused on numbers of patients treated and associated costs. There was very little focus on the quality of care.'[42]

Yet at the level of policy, priorities, targets and outcomes, patients seem increasingly to be viewed as financial and political units. At front-line level, it becomes a vicious circle. Once you stop meeting people's basic needs – such as giving them food and drink, taking them to the

41 '"We need extra resources to cope": Dr Tricia Woodhead, acting chief executive.' *Weston, Worle and Somerset Mercury*, 19 January 2007.

42 Healthcare Commission (2007) *Investigation into outbreaks of* Clostridium difficile *at Maidstone and Tunbridge Wells NHS Trust, October 2007.* London: Healthcare Commission, p.103.

toilet, helping them keep clean, and even talking to them – it becomes all the easier to treat them as less than human. And once that happens, it becomes still easier not to give them food and drink and not to take them to the toilet at all.

The Mid Staffordshire Independent Inquiry noted how individual patients were lost from view, and how shocking it was when the Trust board was reminded – in a most unwelcome way – of what it had been actually doing to real people. The Board had become detached from reality and from the people it was meant to be serving. The Inquiry noted that in the end the only thing that should have mattered was individual patients; data star ratings and benchmarks were no substitute:

> A common response to concerns has been to refer to data, often of a very generic type such as star ratings, CNST [Clinical Negligence Scheme for Trusts] levels and so on, rather than to the experiences of patients and their families. This is not to downgrade the importance of a collective and analytical approach to organisational assessment to draw attention to the only thing that really matters in a hospital – namely, individual patients. The story of Stafford, however, shows graphically and sadly that benchmarks, comparative ratings and foundation trust status do not in themselves bring to light serious and systemic failings.[43]

The detachment from patients involved not only decision making about finance and performance but also being cocooned away from subsequent protest about the effects of those decisions. When the Board, too late, finally sat down with relatives, it professed itself shocked. Reality had reasserted itself when the insulation had been stripped away:

> Another aspect of the preference for figures rather than people has been the failure to listen, or to listen properly. Many of the complaints made to the Inquiry had already been made in precisely the same terms to the Trust. Many of them, even if taken on their own as one person's observation, should have been enough to alert a listener to the existence of a serious systemic problem. Often the responses were formulaic. Even where they were not, the action taken as a result was inadequate. Perhaps most importantly, representative stories hardly ever reached directors. Otherwise it is difficult to believe they would have been

---

43   Francis, R. (Chair) (2010) *Independent Inquiry into care provided by Mid Staffordshire NHS Foundation Trust January 2005–March 2009*. London: The Stationery Office, p.398.

as shocked as they were when eventually Cure the NHS members were given a chance to speak to the Board.[44]

The daughter of Mrs Joan Morris, who died at Stafford Hospital, tried to talk to the NHS Trust's chief executive about her mother's care. She put it this way: 'I'd have had more chance of getting in touch with the Lord himself than getting in touch with Martin Yeates.' (Just to fill out the picture a little: the daughter was the manager of a day centre for elderly people and former nursing cadet, her husband a social worker – and their son was a doctor, who also gave evidence to the Mid Staffordshire Public Inquiry. He too related what he had seen when visiting his grandmother at the hospital; but noted that 'career suicide' came to mind when he decided to give evidence to the Inquiry.)[45]

Failure to listen to tales of woe figures large. But sometimes it is even more fundamental than listening to complaints. It may be about no more than communication with patients, day to day, during a hospital stay. At Mid Staffordshire, staffing levels were blamed for the lack of communication with patients and relatives.[46] This comprised lack of reassurance for patients and of information, wrong information being given, not involving patients in decisions, insensitivity, lack of engagement and so on.[47] Some patients found it unusual if somebody actually came to talk to them:

> One elderly but very lively patient who was a retired nurse herself told me: [a member of the nursing staff] who was in training doing the university course, I think, and she was doing a little spell on the ward, and on my first day she came and sat and chatted to me and talked about my experiences and my problem, and I enjoyed that, but that was the only time while I was in there that anybody came and talked to me.[48]

Overall, as one nurse put it in response to a survey by the Royal College of Nursing (RCN):

44   Francis, R. (Chair) (2010) *Independent Inquiry into care provided by Mid Staffordshire NHS Foundation Trust January 2005–March 2009*. London: The Stationery Office, p.399.

45   Sawer, P. (2010) 'Stafford scandal: Doctor speaks out over grandmother's "appalling" treatment.' *Daily Telegraph*, 17 December.

46   Healthcare Commission (2009) *Investigation into Mid Staffordshire NHS Foundation Trust, March 2009*. London: Healthcare Commission, p.5.

47   Francis, R. (Chair) (2010) *Independent Inquiry into care provided by Mid Staffordshire NHS Foundation Trust January 2005–March 2009*. London: The Stationery Office, p.15.

48   Francis, R, (Chair) (2010) *Independent Inquiry into care provided by Mid Staffordshire NHS Foundation Trust January 2005–March 2009*. London: The Stationery Office, p.128.

> Need more money to invest in staff/patient ratio. Please, this would give me time just to sit and talk to my patients without continually being aware of all the tasks I still have to undertake. Patients often don't discuss their fears/anxieties or even something as simple as themselves because they can see how busy we are. Hospitalisation must be an extremely lonely time for some patients![49]

Think of an elderly patient in hospital with a suddenly diagnosed, aggressive terminal illness awaiting, and then recovering from, a surgical procedure. She is moved from ward to ward, mostly as an outlier (that is, on the wrong ward), the nurses therefore not knowing much about her condition, some of them even ignorant as to why she is there at all. Nobody talks to her anyway, with or without that knowledge, because they don't have time and have got out of the habit. She is utterly distressed and frightened; her voice and fears go unheeded.[50]

Being in hospital can, as the nurse quoted above states, be very lonely. And here is the rub. Policymakers talk fondly and ideologically of the patient voice and patient-centred care, and yet they enforce models of 'productivity' which too frequently silence that voice and leave the vulnerable patient to cut the most forlorn and peripheral of figures.

In 1915, DURING World War I, General Kitchener berated Sir John French, the British commander, for wasting artillery shells in the Flanders mud; this was because men could be easily replaced whereas shells could not. The former were expendable.[51]

Somewhere then, in all the talk of a patient-centred health service, the patients have become indistinct, or at least a certain type of patient: the vulnerable and elderly with more complex needs. They seem to have become, more than ever, expendable, pawns in a modern management war game of priorities, targets, finance, unit measurement, care pathways and bed management. Cannon fodder in the machinations and calculations of the politicians, the bureaucrats and the accountants. The human aspect has left the field; suffering, distress, lack of dignity and avoidable mortality lie in wait to take its place.

49 Baillie, L., Gallagher, A. and Wainwright, P. (2008) *Defending dignity: Challenges and opportunities for nursing.* London: Royal College of Nursing, p.7.
50 Personal communication: patient in a London hospital, 1996.
51 Marr, A. (2009) *The making of modern Britain: From Queen Victoria to V.E. Day.* London: Pan, p.132.

14

Staffing Levels, Competence and Attitude

> Several recent [Healthcare Commission] investigations have
> shown in detail how senior managers and Boards have failed in
> their most basic duties as regards patient safety, with disastrous
> consequences. In each of these cases, patient safety was found
> to have been crowded out by other priorities, including the
> meeting of targets, financial issues, service reconfigurations and
> achieving Foundation status. As we have already noted, in these
> cases inadequate staffing levels have been a particular factor in
> compromising patient safety – despite the enormous increase
> in funding and staffing across the NHS as a whole. (House of
> Commons Health Committee, 2009)[1]

In July 2010, a coroner returned a verdict of misadventure, following the
death of a 77-year-old woman at Stoke Mandeville Hospital in January
of that year. For the last 36 hours of Mrs Margaret Brown's life, doctors
and nurses failed to give her the medication she required to keep her
heart rate regular and to avoid fluid retention. She had originally been
admitted following a fall. After coming round from a dose of morphine,
she was bright and chatty. But as the effects of not being given her
medication took hold, she deteriorated rapidly and died. The picture that
emerged was one of near chaos reflecting both bed and staff shortages.

The coroner referred to the haphazard efforts to get her the medicine
she needed and to the lack of urgency shown. The drugs chart had gone
missing from the nursing station and by the time the doctor realised
what had happened it was too late. The staff nurse said that all but one
of the drugs was unavailable on the ward; because of bed shortages, Mrs
Brown had been assigned to a gynaecology ward. The one drug that was
available was, according to the nurse, counter-indicated for this patient.

The ward was under-staffed, which made it more difficult to chase up the
drugs required from the pharmacy. The staff nurse passed the information
on to her relief at 2pm, but the next staff nurse on duty had to deal with

---

1   House of Commons Health Committee (2009) *Patient safety: Sixth report of Session 2008–09.* HC
      151-I. London: The Stationery Office, pp.86–7.

a patient bleeding heavily on a side ward. It was four-and-a-half hours
before she turned her attention to Mrs Brown, only to find the drugs
chart missing. The hospital security team was asked to break into the
pharmacy but this plan was unsuccessful.

Mrs Brown had taken her medication with her to accident and
emergency (A&E) when first admitted. The coroner stated that it had not
been in anyone's contemplation that she was at special risk of dying very
soon, and that:

> The medication she didn't get in the last 36 hours of her life was
> the medication prescribed and deemed appropriate by the doctor
> and registrar. The most obvious thing that was different in the
> last 36 hours was she didn't have the medication. We can't say
> that would have prevented her death, but it seems ridiculous to
> ignore the proximity of that failure to administer that medication
> – and it was a failure – and her death from the very causes the
> medication was designed to prevent… It seems to me to be a
> matter of extreme urgency somebody should be pushing the red
> button and saying "We have a problem", but that didn't happen.
> Not getting medication in a hospital strikes me as fundamentally
> unacceptable.[2]

He had pointed out in effect the absurdity of a patient not being given
their established, life-preserving medication in, of all places, a hospital.
The coroner could also have gone on to say that this was not just any
hospital. It was the one where but a few years earlier chaos, poor standards
of care, unbridled infection – and, yes, staffing and bed shortages (still
obviously an issue at the hospital) – held sway. And where the Healthcare
Commission had at that time found that although the hospital correctly
avoided prescribing broad spectrum antibiotics (which can render people
vulnerable to the infection *Clostridium difficile*), the shortage of nurses
meant there was not always time to wake patients to give them the
antibiotics they had been correctly prescribed.[3]

MANY HANDS MAKE light work. Even so, it would of course be over-
simplistic to suggest that neglect and abuse arises solely from shortage of
staff. Competence and attitude undoubtedly come into it, too.

---

2   Carswell, A. (2010) 'Elderly patient dies after Stoke Mandeville hospital staff fail to give her
    medication.' *Bucks Free Press*, 9 July.

3   Healthcare Commission (2006) *Investigation into outbreaks of* Clostridium difficile *at Stoke
    Mandeville Hospital, Buckinghamshire Hospitals NHS Trust, July 2006.* London: Healthcare
    Commission, p.49.

Nonetheless, whilst adequate staffing may not be a sufficient condition for good care, it is plainly a necessary one. As Frank Dobson, Health Secretary when Dignity on the Ward emerged as a campaign in 1997, put it nine years later: 'I wish ministers would give up the stupid pretence that getting rid of hundreds of staff will not damage patient care.'[4] Just what this family's comments at Hinchingbrooke Hospital were getting at when their relative was not given food and drink:

> My mother, 63, was admitted to HH with a fractured hip due to a fall at home (she suffered from osteoporosis). Due to sepsis after her operation she had to remain in hospital on lime ward where her condition deteriorated and she sadly passed away in Feb 08. The staff were very good and did the best to their ability to make sure she was comfortable although actually they were very stretched (understaffed) and as she was so physically weak she could not water herself or feed herself and we found that she went long periods (usually until visiting time, when we would hold cup or spoon) before anything would pass her lips. She also fractured her other hip as a result of being turned as she was bed ridden. Its a sad last few weeks for an amazing wife and mother to suffer so much pain and indignity…(dressings for pressure sores not changed and smelling, catherta [sic] over flow etc) we really do not blame the nurses as I do know how busy they are but I do blame them for her last sad lonely week.[5]

In 2009, the House of Commons Health Committee put this view on a more formal footing. It linked inadequate staffing levels to the undermining of safe health care in a number of 'notorious' cases. This was quite unacceptable.[6] At its simplest it might be a question of whether a care assistant helps a person go to the toilet or eat but not both; there is no time.[7]

It wasn't meant to be like this. *The NHS Plan* of 2000 stated that staff should not be rushed off their feet:

> Our vision is of an NHS where staff are not rushed off their feet and constantly exhausted; where careers are developed not

4   Carvel, J. (2006) 'NHS hospital redundancies gather pace.' *The Guardian*, 23 March.

5   NHS Choices. Accessed on 20 September 2010 at: www.nhs.uk/Services/Hospitals/PatientFeedback/DefaultView.aspx?id=1429&pid=RQQ31&pageNo=6&sort=1&recordPP=0.

6   House of Commons Health Committee (2009) *Patient safety: Sixth report of Session 2008–09*. HC 151-I. London: The Stationery Office, p.56.

7   House of Lords and House of Commons Joint Committee on Human Rights (2007) *The human rights of older people in healthcare. Eighteenth Report of Session 2006–07*. HL 156-I, HC 378-I. London: The Stationery Office, p.58.

stagnant; where staff are paid properly for good performance; and where childcare is provided in every hospital. Ours is a vision of a renewed public service ethos, a system that values the dedication of staff and believes that trust is still the glue that binds the NHS together.[8]

And guidance from the Care Quality Commission (CQC) – breach of which may indicate contravention of legal regulations – states that people's health and welfare needs should be met by sufficient numbers of appropriate staff with the right knowledge, experience, qualifications and skills.[9]

The almost heartbreaking contrast between the optimistic, visionary nature of *The NHS Plan*, and the high pressure, tumultuous scenes in hospitals, drove a nurse to write up her experience in a newspaper – anonymously:

> Sadly, I have found myself hastening relatives' goodbyes to a deceased loved one as I know that there are seriously ill people waiting to occupy the bed space. And sometimes I have hissed "fuck right off" to a bed manager when asked how long it will take me to wipe the excrement and blood from a dead body. The fundamentals of nursing are to ensure that patients are pain-free, clean, comfortable, well-fed, nourished, valued and respected as human beings. We believe passionately in all these things, but they sit at odds with the current belief that this can be all done at superhuman speed.[10]

For such a practitioner, how hollow all the promises, made in 2000, must have rung. Ten years later, a new government set out its stall in another White Paper. It talked of the need for yet more productivity.[11] Use of such a word does not bode well for a system in which under-staffing and undue haste are already rife and a direct cause of poor and neglectful care.

Forty-two years ago, a forward thinking physician, Dr Monnica Stewart, wrote a book about geriatric medicine called *My brother's keeper?* The introduction refers to the book as being 'a *cri de coeur* from a hard-pressed geriatric department that has been squeezed to its limits and now

---

8   Secretary of State for Health (2000) *The NHS Plan: A plan for investment, a plan for reform.* Cm 4818-I. London: The Stationery Office, p.17.

9   CQC (Care Quality Commission) (2009) *Guidance about compliance: Summary of regulations, outcomes and judgement framework.* London: CQC, p.27.

10 Moffat, M. (a pseudonym) (2006) 'Nurses can't walk away.' *The Guardian,* 28 April.

11 Secretary of State for Health (2010) *Equity and excellence: Liberating the NHS.* Cm 7881. London: The Stationery Office, p.11.

the veritable pips are beginning to squeak'.[12] Now, in some hospitals, the squeaking is replaced by untended patients calling out, moaning or even screaming (in the absence of pain relief) – untended because of shortage of staff.

A survey conducted by the Royal College of Nursing (RCN), published in 2008, entitled *Defending dignity*, recounted how one nurse described the battle to treat patients as people, rather than things, and to maintain professional integrity:

> One respondent vividly described the impact on nurses: "The constant battle of meeting targets in surgery, A&E four-hour waits, reducing length of stay which can at times leave staff feeling harassed in delivering care in a dignified and timely way." Another said: "The organisation needs to understand we are looking after people not things and the most important part of our job is the patient not a four-hour target." There appears to be a paradox here of a government that has declared "zero tolerance" of undignified care, but that persists in allowing mixed sex accommodation and setting management targets that may themselves be inherently undignifying.[13]

The real battle she identified was with paradoxical government policy that leads to short-staffing, as the following case shows.

In 2010, a coroner concluded that Mrs Margot Kennedy had been denied her 'rights to dignity' by Leicester General Hospital. She had been admitted with pneumonia and dehydration; she had previously suffered a stroke but had remained lucid and independent. She died in a filthy and depressing ward. She was not properly washed for six weeks before her death. Nurses had left her sheets covered in faeces. Doctors had failed to tackle her refusal to eat as she rapidly lost weight. This might have been a psychiatric issue but no assessment was made. Staff had made it clear to her four daughters that they were not welcome outside of normal visiting hours, even though they drove hundreds of miles to visit regularly. Her fingernails were often caked with faeces. One of her sisters stated that:

> I never knew we would have to fight the system to get our mother the essential dignity she was entitled to when she had worked her whole life. I believe she ceased to want to exist. I wouldn't have wanted to exist either in the environment where she was.

---

12 Stewart, M. (1968) *My brother's keeper?* London: Health Horizon, p.7.
13 Baillie, L., Gallagher, A. and Wainwright, P. (2008) *Defending dignity: Challenges and opportunities for nursing.* London: Royal College of Nursing, p.6.

The ward sister admitted at the inquest to appalling standards of care, including leaving Mrs Kennedy in bed for a month. She said there was no excuse, *but they were short-staffed*. The coroner could not attribute cause of death to the poor care but stated that it caused distress and removed dignity. The University of Leicester National Health Service (NHS) Trust apologised.[14]

It may be not just hygiene that suffers in the case of short-staffing, but the immediate physical safety of patients. At the Birmingham Heartlands Hospital, there was a policy called the Falls Care Plan. It was to be applied after a person's first fall, in order to help nurses prevent further accidents. However, in the case of Mrs Joyce Dempster, an 84-year-old woman, it was implemented only after the third of her falls within a space of two days, in June 2009. This last fall resulted in a broken leg and necessitated a hip operation. She subsequently died. The consultant pathologist gave the injury as a contributory cause but that death was from bronchopneumonia; the deputy coroner, in a narrative verdict at the inquest, found that she had died after bowel surgery (the reason for her admission) and having three falls. The senior nurse blamed short-staffing for tardy implementation of the plan.[15]

In August 2010, a coroner wrote to the NHS in Gloucestershire following the death in 2007 of an 86-year-old woman, Mrs Ivie Daum, at Cheltenham General Hospital. Terminally ill, she had effectively been left to her own devices because of a shortage of nurses. Her family had become so concerned that they employed private nurses to care for her on the ward, even though she was already a private patient at the NHS hospital. Her family related how she had not been helped to eat her meals, despite being incapable of managing by herself.

The coroner was concerned that she had not been moved sufficiently to prevent the development of pressure sores; and also about shortcomings in record keeping, including nutritional records. On one occasion, she had fallen from her pillows and ended up lying for some time with her head against the bars on her bed; marks were left across her face. The nursing sister conceded that staff shortages had meant a lack of appropriate care for some patients.[16]

---

14 Schlesinger, F. (2010) 'Grandmother "gave up on life" in hospital that stripped her of all dignity.' *Daily Mail*, 15 April.

15 Suart, P. (2010) 'Family considers legal action against Heartlands Hospital.' *Birmingham Post*, 18 May.

16 Casey, G. (2010) 'Hospital criticised after Lechlade pensioner left to own devices before death.' *Wilts and Gloucestershire Standard*, 3 August.

The Patients' Association published an account in 2009 of how Mr Leslie Kirk was prevented from using the call bell when suffering from severe pain in Nottingham City Hospital:

> At one point my father's personal alarm was taken away, making it difficult for him to get help from staff when suffering through the night from severe pain. When we challenged staff as to the reason for the removal we were told that it was because he kept pressing it. This answer we found astonishing particularly as we know it was not in our father's nature to complain unless he had a very good reason for doing so.[17]

AND IT IS doctors, not just nurses or health care assistants, who may be in short supply. In September 2010 a coroner recorded a narrative verdict in the case of Mr Roland Holbrow, an 88-year-old man. He had been admitted with breathing difficulties to Musgrove Park Hospital, Somerset. The coroner heard from the clinical director of the A&E department at the hospital; the latter referred to Mr Holbrow's treatment as 'unacceptable' and 'very poor'. With two doctors on duty, he was one of ten patients waiting to be seen. He was not, until over five hours after admission. By then he was dead. The coroner had already, a few months earlier, queried the death of another patient; she had died in distress at a time when one junior doctor was covering 100 patients.[18]

This had overtones of the death, some years earlier, of Mr Paul Varnum at Leicester Royal Infirmary; it, too, was associated with inadequate medical staffing. Admitted as an emergency with splitting head pains, he remained on a ward trolley for nearly eight hours before he was able to see a doctor. An advanced brain abscess was then diagnosed and an operation performed; he died. A doctor told the inquest that had he been treated promptly, he probably would have survived. Only one registrar was on duty and no consultants, even though four were meant to be available. In reaching a verdict of death by natural causes contributed to by neglect, the coroner condemned the lack of senior staff on duty in the A&E department.[19]

17 Patients' Association (2009) *Patients not numbers, people not statistics*. London: Patients' Association, p.11.
18 de Bruxelles, S. (2010) 'Coroner warns about doctors' hours after fatal hospital delay.' *The Times*, 11 September.
19 Lister, S. (2004) 'Patient died after eight hours of hospital neglect.' *The Times*, 7 May.

INDIVIDUALLY REPORTED CASES aside, regulatory bodies have repeatedly picked up on inadequate staffing as a cause of low standards of care. The message is that if you sufficiently diminish the numbers or competence of staff, then even the best of care on genuinely fine, caring wards will be undermined.

At West London Mental Health NHS Trust, a poor quality of care was reported in 2009 by the CQC; it was associated with low staffing levels. This resulted in staff being moved from ward to ward to fill gaps in shifts. It also meant locking off parts of wards to patients, to make things easier to manage for the staff. The consequence was that staff would be separated from patients by locked doors; this was putting everybody at risk. Sometimes doors were padlocked in response to the staff shortage. There were high sickness levels in existing staff, patients received inadequate physical health care, and medicines were not sufficiently monitored.[20]

Such a report indicates that once staffing levels dip too far, a domino effect takes hold. In 2010, the Commission published an investigation into inpatient provision at Totnes Hospital for older mental health patients. Staffing levels seemed to be a major factor. The Commission reported various deficiencies in relation to the use of syringe drivers, care plans, monitoring of patients, and the inappropriate application of palliative care approaches to patients who were not close to death but whose behaviour was difficult to manage. The CQC noted that staffing levels were the focus for savings in the Trust's financial recovery plan; that staffing costs had fallen but the costs of management had risen; and that at ward level it was repeatedly told that staff numbers were insufficient.[21] The Commission observed:

> Our impression as we visited the older people's mental health inpatient units was of highly dedicated ward managers, nurses and nursing assistants working under constant pressure. On more than one occasion, we came across ward managers who were trying to do their best for their patients with too little resource and fearful that they had not covered every aspect of patient care and the management of their ward. The message from members of staff we spoke to on all the units was a need to have more staff on the wards. Several members of staff told us that they did not feel that the staffing levels were sufficient, and were not safe

---

20 CQC (Care Quality Commission) (2009) *Investigation into West London Mental Health NHS Trust.* London: CQC, pp.37–41.

21 CQC (Care Quality Commission) (2010) *Investigation into the mental health care for older people provided by Devon Partnership NHS Trust, June 2010.* London: CQC, p.28.

given the unpredictable behaviour and potential for violence and aggression of the particular group of patients.[22]

At Maidstone and Tunbridge Wells NHS Trust, the effects identified by the Healthcare Commission of staffing shortages illustrated not so much a domino effect as a major chain reaction. Elements associated with too few staff included an inability to practise cohort nursing (isolation nursing) effectively, to give patients their medication, to complete fluid balance and food charts, to ensure patients took their food and nutritional supplements, to supervise confused patients who wandered in and out of isolation areas, to practise good hand hygiene, to answer call bells and empty commodes promptly, to change soiled bedding quickly and to use new or cleaned equipment for each patient.[23] An overwhelming catalogue of rudimentary failure.

In Mid Cheshire, too, low staffing levels led to poor standards of patient care, including the very basics. Nurses, patients and relatives believed the safety of patients was compromised. The Healthcare Commission noted that an independent inquiry had already 'described a culture of nurses who were rushed, short staffed, stretched and not delivering basic standards of care'.[24]

Nurses failed to attend training as a result. On one shift, a nursing sister, a student and a health care assistant had to deal with ten emergency admissions, eight transfers to other wards, three discharges and one emergency transfer to another hospital – with serious problems resulting. Health care assistants generally did not have time to shave patients or answer buzzers, drug rounds were late, tablets were just left on lockers.[25]

At Stoke Mandeville hospital, the Commission concluded in 2006 that a shortage of nurses probably contributed to the lethal outbreak of infection. Staff were too rushed to follow basic procedures such as washing their hands, wearing aprons and gloves consistently, emptying commodes promptly – and cleaning mattresses and equipment properly. Compromised also was the answering of call bells, using new or properly cleaned equipment for each patient, waking patients to give them

---

22 CQC (Care Quality Commission) (2010) *Investigation into the mental health care for older people provided by Devon Partnership NHS Trust, June 2010.* London: CQC, p.30.

23 Healthcare Commission (2007) *Investigation into outbreaks of* Clostridium difficile *at Maidstone and Tunbridge Wells NHS Trust, October 2007.* London: Healthcare Commission, p.66.

24 Healthcare Commission. *Investigation into Mid Cheshire Hospitals NHS Trust, January 2006.* London: Healthcare Commission, p.30.

25 Healthcare Commission (2006) *Investigation into Mid Cheshire Hospitals NHS Trust, January 2006.* London: Healthcare Commission, pp.6, 29–31.

antibiotics, completing fluid balance charts and supervision of confused patients wandering in and out of isolation areas.[26]

MID STAFFORDSHIRE NHS Foundation Trust supplies the further account, if one were really needed, of what can happen when staff numbers are systematically and crudely curbed in order to hit financial targets. The detail repays study; some of it is distinctly hair raising.

Even if Stafford Hospital represents the extreme end of failure, it would be a complacent and dim sighted NHS trust that dismissed it as irrelevant. Nobody associated with Mid Staffordshire – the Board, Monitor, the strategic health authority (SHA), primary care trust (PCT) – set out to provide the care they ended up with, but they all connived at the reduction in staffing.

Reporting in 2009, the Healthcare Commission related how the A&E department was so under-staffed that receptionists had to carry out patient assessments – although patients in the waiting room could not be seen from the reception area. This happened because there were too few nurses. Receptionists categorised people as major or minor. None of the receptionists was clinically qualified.[27]

Patients had to wait for medication, pain relief and wound dressings. There were delays in scanning patients out of normal hours. The fact that there were too few doctors resulted in junior doctors having to rush decisions to avoid breaching the target of everybody having to be seen within four hours. For the same reason, patients would be rushed out of A&E to the 'emergency assessment unit'. However, this unit was deficient. Patients were not monitored properly; it was busy, chaotic and under-staffed.[28]

Epidurals were wrongly sited, morphine prescribed but not given; patients were visited and found by relatives screaming with pain.[29] This might have been from lack of pain-relieving medication:

> She went on to document that when her husband "desperately needed pain relief towards the end of his life, I had to keep asking

---

26 Healthcare Commission (2006) *Investigation into outbreaks of* Clostridium difficile *at Stoke Mandeville Hospital, Buckinghamshire Hospitals NHS Trust, July 2006.* London: Healthcare Commission, pp.5–6.

27 Healthcare Commission (2009) *Investigation into Mid Staffordshire NHS Foundation Trust, March 2009.* London: Healthcare Commission, p.43.

28 Healthcare Commission (2009) *Investigation into Mid Staffordshire NHS Foundation Trust, March 2009.* London: Healthcare Commission, p.5.

29 Healthcare Commission (2009) *Investigation into Mid Staffordshire NHS Foundation Trust, March 2009.* London: Healthcare Commission, p.79.

for his syringe-drivers to be refilled when they emptied. It just didn't seem to be a priority. On two occasions, I waited for over an hour for a reply to the call-button and eventually I just had to go and find a nurse and insist that they left the patient they were with to come and help... He was crying by that time and in great distress due to the pain he was experiencing."[30]

Or screaming for some other reason; it didn't seem to make any difference:

And as I walked in my Mum was on the bed, on a bed pan, and she was falling off and she was in agony. She had been left like that for over an hour. The nurses' button which, if you read in the notes, my Mum had said before, please don't put it out of reach, was left on top of a drip. I struggled to reach the nurses' button. My Mum was in absolute agony, I can hear her screams now, as I walked into the ward. I slammed the nurses' button, the emergency button. Nobody came and I ran out and said: please, somebody come and help my Mum. As we went back in with the nurse, they went: ooh, we'd forgotten about her. I said: can't you hear. And at that point she grabbed my hand and said: please don't let me die in here...the nurse came that came [sic] in said: I am so sorry, we had forgotten about her; yes, she has been there for some considerable time...[31]

A&E nurses described, to the Healthcare Commission, the staffing situation as 'abysmal' and 'horrendous'.[32] The emergency assessment unit should have had one nurse to every six patients; instead it had one to every fifteen. Visitors reported how an elderly patient was left unattended on a commode and fell to the floor. As a result of the shortage of staff on this unit, patients failed to receive basic care. They were not washed or escorted to the toilet. Patients were not helped to eat, including opening up food containers and cutting up food. The unit was generally chaotic and filthy.[33]

On the medical wards, patients might be left in their soiled nightwear during the afternoon after lunch; relatives would help other patients to get to the toilet or to eat their food. A patient might be told to use the buzzer if she needed help even if she could not reach it; and when

30 Francis, R. (Chair) (2010) *Independent Inquiry into care provided by Mid Staffordshire NHS Foundation Trust January 2005–March 2009*. London: The Stationery Office, p.394.

31 Francis, R. (Chair) (2010) *Independent Inquiry into care provided by Mid Staffordshire NHS Foundation Trust January 2005–March 2009*. London: The Stationery Office, pp.56–7.

32 Healthcare Commission (2009) *Investigation into Mid Staffordshire NHS Foundation Trust, March 2009*. London: Healthcare Commission, p.47.

33 Healthcare Commission (2009) *Investigation into Mid Staffordshire NHS Foundation Trust, March 2009*. London: Healthcare Commission, p.58.

somebody else would press it for that patient, no nurse would come anyway. Poor care was endemic, including lack of nutritional assessment and care, falls, poor communication and pressure sores.[34]

One senior sister was left to cover 78 beds on the medical wards. It was also reported that two nurses were covering 40 medical beds.[35] At one point, there were only three matrons in Mid Staffordshire NHS Foundation Trust, and the loss of confidence and morale as a result of this state of affairs led to further loss of skilled and experienced nurses.[36]

Telephones would not be answered for 20 minutes; a patient with dementia might eventually pick up the phone. Percutaneous gastrostomy feeds were not being recorded or monitored. A nurse found several patients who had been left a long time, lying in bed in their own faeces. Patients did not always have help to take their medication.[37]

The Mid Staffordshire Independent Inquiry concluded that the failure to take people to the toilet, to help them on the commode and to clean up soiled bedding promptly was in a small number of cases due to an uncaring attitude of staff – but was mostly due to 'inadequate staff on duty to deal with the challenge presented by a population of elderly, confused patients'.[38]

DESPITE THIS BOND between too few nurses and decent care, it is not just about numbers. Competence and attitude plainly matter. As the family of a dying patient at Hinchingbrooke Hospital observed of nurses who were screaming, laughing and having a water fight, whilst their mother lay dying:

> The ward was closed due to a vomitting [sic] bug and we were not allowed to see our mum (even tough [sic] we are all fit and healthy) and even though they had put her on pallative care we were not informed till she had passed into a coma. we never got to see her concious and she must have thought we had deserted her to die alone. Even her consultant who ran through her post mortem results with us was mortified that we were not allowed to

34 Healthcare Commission (2009) *Investigation into Mid Staffordshire NHS Foundation Trust, March 2009.* London: Healthcare Commission, p.63.

35 Healthcare Commission (2009) *Investigation into Mid Staffordshire NHS Foundation Trust, March 2009.* London: Healthcare Commission, p.92.

36 Healthcare Commission (2009) *Investigation into Mid Staffordshire NHS Foundation Trust, March 2009.* London: Healthcare Commission, p.132.

37 Healthcare Commission (2009) *Investigation into Mid Staffordshire NHS Foundation Trust, March 2009.* London: Healthcare Commission, pp.64–5.

38 Francis, R. (Chair) (2010) *Independent Inquiry into care provided by Mid Staffordshire NHS Foundation Trust January 2005–March 2009.* London: The Stationery Office, p.61.

visit her when they knew she was dying. To top it all off, when she was in her coma with six grieving members round her bedside on the main ward, the nurses decided to have a water fight to celebrate a student doctor leaving…the laughter and screams of excitment [sic] are all very well but not next to someone who is dying. There is a time and a place.[39]

That said, for obvious reasons, it will not do to blame poor care solely on these two factors. Even highly skilled, dedicated health care professionals can only do so much when the odds against them are stacked too high. Furthermore, whilst there will always be some staff with the wrong attitude, they and others will tacitly be encouraged in the wrong way if they receive an unspoken message from senior management that basic care does not matter, and that other things, such as patient throughput, finance, statistics and plausible and good looking paperwork count for more.

It has all been said before. The *National Service Framework for Older People*, published in 2001, recognised the importance of staff competency, particularly for older people. It contains a standard stating that older people's care in hospital should be 'delivered through appropriate specialist care and by hospital staff who have the right set of skills to meet their needs'. In particular, it recognises that older people may have a pre-existing illness or disabilities, and be vulnerable to problems arising during a hospital stay. It notes that the care of older people in hospital is complex and that it depends not just on health care but also respect for the person as an individual.[40]

CQC guidance states that staff should be fit, appropriately qualified and physically and mentally able to do their job.[41]

The Standing Nursing and Midwifery Advisory Committee had stated, also in 2001, that 'the nursing care of older people is highly skilled and physically and emotionally taxing'. Yet many nurses felt they worked in conditions that obstructed high quality care. The Committee noted that 'skilled senior nurses must be re-engaged in the fundamental skills of nursing to improve standards of care'. Also, that older patients tended to require more skilled, specialised and intense nursing than younger

39 NHS Choices. Accessed on 20 September 2010 at: www.nhs.uk/Services/Hospitals/PatientFeedback/DefaultView.aspx?id=1429&pid=RQQ31&pageNo=6&sort=1&recordPP=0.

40 DH (Department of Health) (2001) *National Service Framework for Older People*. London: DH, p.51.

41 CQC (Care Quality Commission) (2009) *Guidance about compliance: Summary of regulations, outcomes and judgement framework*. London: CQC, p.26.

adults. In reality, it reported that significant problems existed including deficiencies not just in staff numbers, but also in specific nursing skills relating to basics such as incontinence, nutrition, skin integrity – as well as staff numbers.[42]

CLAIRE RAYNER, THEN President of the Patients' Association and herself a former nurse, wrote in 2009 that those nurses who were responsible for terrible care should be struck off their professional register. Her comments reflect the view that not all poor care is due to inadequate staffing or even skills. There comes a point when individual health care professionals must be held accountable for their actions:

> By a sad coincidence I trained as a nurse with one of the patients who suffered so much, and I know that she, like me, was horrified by the appalling care she had before she died. We both came from a generation of nurses who were trained at the bedside and in whom the core values of nursing were deeply inculcated. I am sickened by what has happened to some parts of my profession of which I was so proud. These bad, cruel nurses may be – probably are – a tiny proportion of the nursing work force, but even if they are only one or two percent of the whole they should be identified and struck off the Register.[43]

So, despite clear evidence that inadequate staffing levels and competence causes or contributes to poor care, there is another strand of evidence suggesting that staff attitude is an additional, significant factor. For instance, the Association recorded a striking account – given by Julie Bailey, daughter of Bella Bailey who was a patient at Stafford Hospital – not just of unanswered call bells and of falling and crying patients, but of the squealing and giggling of nurses overlaying this:

> We found some staff cared for the patients but most were uncaring. Confused patients often wandered around semi naked and some staff passed them by in the corridor without a care. Night time and weekends were the worst. Night time was often the most busiest and noisiest. Staff squealed and giggled whilst patients tried to grab a bit of sleep in between their discomforts. The staff disturbed confused patients, who then wandered the wards looking for attention. Buzzers often rang for 40–50 minutes whilst patients waited for the commode then they sat for

---

42 Standing Nursing and Midwifery Advisory Committee (2001) *Caring for older people: A nursing priority integrating knowledge, practice and values: A report*. London: Department of Health, pp.3, 6, 13.

43 Patients' Association (2009) *Patients not numbers, people not statistics*. London: Patients' Association, p.4.

another 40 minutes waiting to be hauled back into bed. Some struggled alone and sounds of patients falling and crying, was not uncommon.[44]

In 2008, a relative criticised the care her mother had received at Wexham Park Hospital, calling into question the attitude of nurses who appeared not to treat patients as human beings, regarding them instead as 'lumps of meat and bone':

> I do not think it is acceptable to leave a 90 year old on a bed pan, unable to support herself because of problems with her arms, with the bed pan edge digging into a back sore, originally started 11 months earlier at WPH, for 30 minutes. Another patient timed the length of time and told me. My mother confirmed this. She said she had been in agony. None of bell pushs [sic] appear to work and other patients would get out of bed to get someone to aid each other. Patients should be treated like people and not as lumps of meat and bone that need to be processed. Somewhere along the line nurses' training has stopped teaching them about patients being human beings. Computers and clever equipment to aid recovery is a very good thing. A balance needs to be achieved with nurses actually interacting with the patients more. Nursing is no longer a vocation![45]

In 2010, a relative, a nurse herself, felt there came a point where a basic failure to care at Tameside General Hospital, even given the pressures on staff, was simply *wrong*:

> As a registered nurse myself I was extremely disappointed to see a supposedly qualified nurse taking a BP [blood pressure] with an inappropriate cuff, it was too small and the nurse asked my relative to hold it on with her hand thus making the BP reading completely useless, Call bell inoperable making it difficult for my relative to inform staff that she needed pain relief… Staff completely disinterested abpout [sic] basic nursing care wound dressing changes hygiene needs etc… As I trained at TGH many years ago and was pround of the standard of care delivered to my patients I ma [sic] extremely disappointed with the level of care offered to my relative. I understand the pressures on the nursing staff but to just not care is wrong.[46]

---

44 Patients' Association (2009) *Patients not numbers, people not statistics*. London: Patients' Association, p.27.

45 Patient Opinion. Accessed on 20 October 2010 at: www.patientopinion.org.uk/opinions/12712.

46 Patient Opinion. Accessed on 20 September 2010 at: www.patientopinion.org.uk/opinions/31302.

In the following case, related by a patient at the Royal Oldham Hospital in 2009, things went awry, whether due to attitude or under-staffing or a bit of both:

> My experience of a recent stay on ward 3 at Royal Oldham Hospital was one I would not want to repeat. After undergoing surgery on my Achilles tendon (tendon transfer) I was confined to my bed. Due to me having a bad reaction to the general anaesthetic I was vomiting profusely and in need of assistance from the nursing staff. I had no buzzer to summon help, so another patient rang hers for me. She rang & rang, nobody came. Oops, no container, I soiled the bed. When eventualy [sic] a nurse arrived at my bedside and surveyed my vomit-soiled bedclothes, she was very rude and said I would have to stay in this dirty state until she had time to change my bedclothes, as she was busy with another patient. I asked if another nurse couldn't do it? Her answer: "No, you are my patient." And with that she walked off. One hour later she returned to clean me up.[47]

The Independent Inquiry at Mid Staffordshire reported many problems arising from poor staffing levels and management, but also that it had received reports of staff who were simply uncaring, for example, staff who did not attend to people's need to go the toilet to the prompt changing of soiled bedding.[48] It reported evidence of an A&E admission:

> ...when I was told I was to be admitted, I was left in a small cubicle for several hours on a trolley, no pillows, no blankets, and when I rang to tell my wife, I was admonished quite sharply by someone who told me to "get a life" and not use the phone in hospital. Eventually I got a pillow and then an hour later, a blanket arrived which I refused because it was covered in someone else's blood.[49]

Likewise the account about a nurse reacting to the need of a person needing to urinate:

> ...he said: I need to go to the toilet...he said she seemed quite angry that he wanted to go to the toilet. So she flounced out and went to get a bottle and she came back in and – yes, the urinal wasn't on the bed...and she came back in and he had done it

47 Patient Opinion. Accessed on 20 September 2010 at: www.patientopinion.org.uk/opinions/18576.

48 Francis, R. (Chair) (2010) *Independent Inquiry into care provided by Mid Staffordshire NHS Foundation Trust January 2005–March 2009*. London: The Stationery Office, p.11.

49 Francis, R. (Chair) (2010) *Independent Inquiry into care provided by Mid Staffordshire NHS Foundation Trust January 2005–March 2009*. London: The Stationery Office, p.154.

because she took quite a while to get the bottle and she was due to go on a break, and he said to her: I'm really sorry but I have done it, and with that she exploded. She threw the urinal down on to the bed and she pushed his trolley up against where he was with his dinner and she went out and she never came back.[50]

Similar was the response of a nurse to a patient who had complained because of a shortage of water jugs and his being left with nothing to drink:

There simply wasn't sufficient water jugs to go round. So he was left totally without any drink. He had actually complained, hadn't he, about the treatment he had received from one nurse whilst there? And as a result this nurse totally ignored him for the rest of his stay; like she would walk by the bottom of his bed, he would ask for help or a drink and she just totally ignored him.[51]

It seems that patients may feel abandoned by staff who are more interested in other things, as noted by a relative at Basildon Hospital:

My elderly relative has been in hospital for over 9 weeks some of the staff are lovely but the majority have an attitude problem, you try to talk to them and they ignore you, or give you incorrect information, they spend most of their time in the staff room discussing what they did last night or where they are going on holiday. Staff need to retrained [sic] especially when it comes to bedside manners. Elderly patients deserve to be treated with respect not shouted at or in some cases we saw on visits totally ignored. Management never availble to discuss concerns with. The elderly patients we saw were mostly unable to make themselves known as they had serious issues such as dementia or many were stroke patients, they deserve to be treated with more respect. Many elderely [sic] patients have no family to fight their corner and this should not be allowed.[52]

A patient at Cheltenham General Hospital in 2009 related how detached and uninterested the nurses were, rarely speaking to patients. They:

...seemed more animated and chatty when standing at the nurse's station talking to each other rather than bothering to go around the ward. One nurse was an exception, she was incredibly caring,

50 Francis, R. (Chair) (2010) *Independent Inquiry into care provided by Mid Staffordshire NHS Foundation Trust January 2005–March 2009*. London: The Stationery Office, p.154.

51 Francis, R. (Chair) (2010) *Independent Inquiry into care provided by Mid Staffordshire NHS Foundation Trust January 2005–March 2009*. London: The Stationery Office, p.158.

52 NHS Choices. Accessed on 18 October 2010 at: www.nhs.uk/services/hospitals/patientfeedback/defaultview.aspx?id=744&pid=rddh0&sort=4&pageno=5.

kind, and actually spoke to me as if I was a person. Well done, that nurse…a credit to your profession. Please remember, going into hospital is a pretty frightening/un-nerving experience for most people, hospitals are not factories, those are real people in the beds and your job is to care for them psychologically as well as physically. Yes, you may not have the time anymore to sit at the bedside chatting, I appreciate you are sometimes incredibly busy, but being human instead of looking indifferent and totally avoiding eye contact just in case a patient asks you for something is not exactly being part of a "caring" profession, is it?[53]

Professor Tallis observes that a new generation of more academically-trained nurses may, whatever their good intentions, emerge 'dumbed up'; that is, without the understanding and skills to undertake the profoundly humane activity of hands-on care. And that whilst health care assistants instead step in, it may well be detrimental to patients – lonely, afraid, thirsty and left in pools of their own urine – for their nursing care to be separated from the nurses responsible for it.[54]

A CULTURE OF poor attitude and indifference to patients can take hold in smaller units as well.

Ford Ward is a self-contained unit that provides rehabilitation and palliative care at Fordingbridge Hospital in Hampshire. Following complaints about the attitude of staff and their care and treatment of patients, an Independent Inquiry was appointed. It reported in August 2008. The ward was closed for nine months to new admissions in 2007 because of the levels of concern; it reopened after a £130,000 refurbishment that, amongst other things, ensured adequate call bells.[55]

The final report has never been revealed in full, although a severely edited version is in the public domain. From this, the key issues seem to have included the following. A lack of bell cords in the lounge meant that patients had to shout for help or bang on tables. And although further details of complaints were excised from the report, the problems can be gleaned indirectly from the recommendations. These included the need for the adequate supervision of patients, palliative care to a reasonable standard, individual care plans covering all areas of need (including falls,

53 NHS Choices. Accessed on 15 October 2010 at: www.nhs.uk/Services/Hospitals/PatientFeedback/DefaultView.aspx?id=2231&pid=RTE01&pageNo=5&sort=1&recordPP=0.

54 Tallis, R. (2009) 'How will a degree help a frightened patient?' *The Times*, 13 November.

55 Fordingbridge Hospital. Accessed on 23 August 2010 at: www.hchc.nhs.uk/component/content/article/24-fordingbridge-hospital/42-fordingbridge-hospital.

infection and hydration) – and for the reporting of undignified treatment of patients and visitors.[56]

The Inquiry also found that staff did not attend patients promptly when the latter called for assistance; this had been a particular problem when staff were taking a break together. The Inquiry itself had observed four unsupervised patients, whilst nurses were chatting together out of sight.[57] In addition, many people interviewed gave evidence that staff sometimes spoke to patients and to visitors in an abrupt and aggressive manner – shouting, being intimidating and rude to them. More generally, the Inquiry believed that staff were thoughtless, casual, off-hand and lacked awareness about their practices and interactions with patients.[58]

Staff sometimes ordered for the patients, food which in fact the staff intended to eat themselves. The Inquiry was clear that these shortcomings in staff behaviour and attitude developed because of management failure over a long period to provide effective leadership.[59]

IT WOULD SEEM that the overwhelming reason for poor care provided by health care staff in hospitals is under-staffing. But lack of competence and uncaring attitudes feature strongly as well. It is also likely that some staff may appear to be uncaring when in fact this is only because – downtrodden, demoralised, overworked and set entirely the wrong example by management – they have succumbed.

What then, overall, is to be made of the hospital staff involved; are they overworked angels, fallen angels through little fault of their own or, as one journalist put it provocatively, simply 'devil nurses'?[60]

56 Lampard, K. and Brougham, C. (2008) *An investigation into the quality and care of patients at Fordingbridge Hospital: A report for Hampshire Primary Care Trust.* London: Verita, pp.12, 19–20.

57 Lampard, K. and Brougham, C. (2008) *An investigation into the quality and care of patients at Fordingbridge Hospital: A report for Hampshire Primary Care Trust.* London: Verita, p.38.

58 Lampard, K. and Brougham, C. (2008) *An investigation into the quality and care of patients at Fordingbridge Hospital: A report for Hampshire Primary Care Trust.* London: Verita, p.47.

59 Lampard, K. and Brougham, C. (2008) *An investigation into the quality and care of patients at Fordingbridge Hospital: A report for Hampshire Primary Care Trust.* London: Verita, pp.48, 66.

60 Marrin, M. (2010) 'Fallen angels – the nightmare nurses protected by silence.' *The Sunday Times*, 30 August.

15

Priorities, Targets, Fear and Bullying

A senior manager told us "if anyone says that the top priorities aren't money and targets, they're lying". (Maidstone and Tumbridge Wells NHS Trust: evidence to the Healthcare Commission, 2007)[1]

The achievement of the Government's targets was seen as more important than the management of the clinical risk inherent in the outbreaks of *C. Difficile*. (Healthcare Commission: Stoke Mandeville Hospital, 2006)[2]

Basic care is very simple and fundamentally important. If it is abandoned, with barely a whisper from so many health care managers and staff, then an explanation is undoubtedly called for. Something most odd must be going on.

The Care Quality Commission (CQC) observed in 2010 that the House of Commons Health Committee had recently called for safe care to be 'the top priority' for National Health Service (NHS) managers.[3] It is extraordinary, one might think, that either the Committee or the Commission should have to stress this point to the NHS – an organisation whose primary and indeed only role should be to treat and care for people competently and safely. But the observation is unsurprising, because the evidence is clear that NHS policymakers and managers have been focusing on other things.

A new government in 2010 has promised to remove at least some of the targets that have been fingered as the villains of the piece, though the suggestion is that some may remain. But, in any case, if one set of priorities (targets) is substituted by another set of priorities (albeit not

---

1   Healthcare Commission (2007) *Investigation into outbreaks of* Clostridium difficile *at Maidstone and Tunbridge Wells NHS Trust, October 2007*. London: Healthcare Commission, p.92.

2   Healthcare Commission (2006) *Investigation into outbreaks of* Clostridium difficile *at Stoke Mandeville Hospital, Buckinghamshire Hospitals NHS Trust, July 2006*. London: Healthcare Commission, p.6.

3   CQC (Care Quality Commission) (2010) *The state of health care and adult social care in England: Key themes and quality of services in 2009*. HC 343. London: CQC, p.77.

called 'targets'), there is no guarantee that neglectful and abusive care will suddenly be rooted out. Besides which, underpinning all is the financial stringency the government has stated must be imposed from 2010 onward.

And it is financial, not just performance, targets which, even during the past decade, have exacerbated poor care because of the resulting shortage of beds and of front-line staff. In other words, arguably the reason why targets – in themselves potentially useful – have had a detrimental effect is that lack of resources has meant that the achievement of those targets has come only at the expense of other parts of the service, which have been left to rack and ruin. For instance, adherence to a four-hour accident and emergency (A&E) target has often led to chaos and substandard care elsewhere in a hospital. In other words, targets are meant to enhance one particular aspect of health care, but not at the same time quietly destroy another. Frequently politicians and NHS chief executives beguile the public about this.

There is another variable that must be factored into the equation. Policies and dictates from above, resulting in poor care, have sometimes removed from many managers and staff the cardinal virtue of questioning and initiative. They sometimes act as though they have been wiped quite clean of any independent thought. As the evidence reveals, this is not an exaggeration. Others have retained the virtue, but have been afraid to exercise it because of two key lubricants needed to ensure that priorities and targets are hit, come what may and no matter how detrimental: fear and bullying.

IN MARCH 2009, *The Sunday Times* published an article about three reports commissioned by the government from organisations in the United States. They contained severe criticism of the way in which targets had been framed and implemented in the NHS. All three reports were suppressed.

One of the reports noted how managers had crowded patients into beds in order to meet waiting targets, but in doing so, they had lost sight of fundamental hygiene requirements. This was at Maidstone and Tunbridge Wells NHS Trust where many patients died of *Clostridium difficile*. It went on to refer to the lack of prominent focus on patient needs as constituting a serious obstacle to improvement in the NHS; the patient appeared barely to be in the picture.[4]

---

4   Rogers, L. (2010) 'Labour hid ugly truth about the National Health Service (NHS).' *The Sunday Times*, 7 March.

The reported observations and conclusions of these suppressed reports were less than startling, but more notable was a continuing refusal of central government to exercise introspection and to own up, especially as the Healthcare Commission had already consistently identified, in the case of severe lapses in care, a preoccupation with centrally imposed finance and performance targets.

The NHS is a pyramidal, command and control structure. Targets and other imperatives emanate from the centre. The expectation is that they will be rigidly adhered to. If targets consistently skew care at local level, it is inevitably a function of the system higher up.

Astonishingly, given that it would push the target culture for the next four years, even the Department of Health acknowledged in 2006 the detrimental effect on safety caused by targets:

> Championing at a national level has raised the profile of patient safety. However, patient safety is too often seen by NHS boards and managers as not having the same priority as achieving financial and access targets.[5]

But this report fell short of making the obvious inference; it was the Department of Health itself that was determining how boards operated – with a mixture of incentive and threat which put targets and finance first, and everything else second. In fact, the 'everything else' could sink from sight altogether.

HAS THE CORROSIVE effect of finance and performance targets been exaggerated by inveterate whingers, doom mongers and nay sayers to change? After all, performance targets were introduced with the best of intentions; for instance, to overcome the scandal during the 1990s of patients left on trolleys for hours in A&E departments.

The difficulty with this notion is that a neutral onlooker may be struck by the way in which NHS trusts seek to hit targets and make financial savings. The purpose is to improve certain aspects of care, such as A&E waits, not to jeopardise other parts of the service. The outcome has sometimes been quite the opposite and more akin to the famous three card trick. Narrow imperatives are obeyed, but the overall facts get spirited away in the blur of a sleight of hand, and so too do the patients. Then it is not just 'find the lady' but also find the patient, who turns

---

5   DH (Department of Health) (2006) *Safety first: A report for patients, clinicians and healthcare managers.* London: DH, p.19.

up in a store room, mop cupboard or hospital kitchen,[6] if not already inappropriately discharged from the hospital.

Alternatively, the patients may be found in corridors, the very type of unofficial ward the targets were trying to eradicate. In early March 2010, Gloucestershire Hospitals NHS Foundation Trust denied that patients were treated in corridors. Later that month a nurse had anonymously passed a rota to the local newspaper, which revealed that nurses were indeed being allocated to specific hallways, or corridors, in which to care for patients. This happened when there was no room for a patient to get into the A&E department. The hospital denied it was a corridor, referring instead to a 'small area' in which three to four trolleys could be held – and open only to clinical and to ambulance staff, not the public.[7]

People may still end up in trolleys but after, rather than before, they have had some sort of assessment within the four-hour A&E target. In the introduction to this book, an example of two 19-hour waits on trolleys by the same patient was described, together with the fatal consequences. Another example is that of Mrs Doris Murgatroyd, 83 years old and in the final stages of a terminal illness, who, having received an assessment from a doctor within ten minutes, was then left on a trolley for seven hours, waiting for a bed at Pinderfields Hospital. She died six days later.[8] In such cases, the target has flattened one mole hill only for it to rise again, almost immediately, somewhere else.

AT STAFFORD HOSPITAL, a major reconfiguration of the medical wards, which led to drastic reductions in staff and a drop in standards of care, was decided without an apparent evidence base. The Independent Inquiry noted that the 'attraction of the advantages – the financial savings – discouraged proper attention being paid to the disadvantages'. There was no evidence of the Board having discussed the changes to staffing numbers, skills and mix.[9]

A separate report commissioned by the Department of Health into events at Mid Staffordshire echoed this concern, stating that all the NHS

6   Ramesh, R. (2010) 'Hospital patients routinely treated in storerooms, survey shows.' *The Guardian*, 9 March.

7   Morris, S. (2010) 'Nurse rotas show A&E patients held in hospital corridors.' *The Guardian*, 25 March.

8   'Woman left for seven hours on trolley dies.' *Yorkshire Post*, 27 January 2002.

9   Francis, R. (Chair) (2010) *Independent Inquiry into care provided by Mid Staffordshire NHS Foundation Trust January 2005–March 2009*. London: The Stationery Office, pp.17–18.

organisations involved should focus on high quality care – and that targets should not distract from this bigger picture.[10]

The Healthcare Commission had already concluded that the Trust's top priority was the achievement of foundation status – and that this had led to disastrous cuts in staffing. But governance issues were not discussed in connection with how this prize was to be seized, nor were the poor standards of nursing care.[11] For instance, staff and managers told the Healthcare Commission that the four-hour target, for treatment in the A&E department, was given a higher priority than the control of infection. This led to patients being moved from ward to ward and often to inappropriate areas. There was increased risk of infection and poor handovers of patients. In short, as one senior manager related, the target had led directly to chaos in the rest of the system.[12]

Thus, the minutes of Board meetings at Mid Staffordshire NHS Foundation Trust were dominated by discussion of finance, targets and achieving foundation trust status. While patients were enduring the most terrible care, the Board was not in fact talking about this; it spent its time instead discussing how to divest itself of the hospital laundry service.[13] The Independent Inquiry indicated that finance had disastrously become the master, dominant over even the most basic standards of care:

> If one lesson is to be learned from the Stafford experience, it is that changes made or demanded in haste can be inimical to good patient care. This is not to exempt the NHS from the prioritisation and re-allocation of resources that any government must consider. However, safe and consistent care cannot be delivered unless change is properly planned and risk assessed, with proper engagement of the staff whose duty it is to deliver that care. Finance, in the sense of the resource made available to the Trust, must always be the servant of the Trust's purpose – the delivery of good and safe care – and not the master which dictates the standard of delivery, however poor.[14]

10 Thomé, D.C. (Dr) (2009) *Mid Staffordshire NHS Foundation Trust: A review of lessons learnt for commissioners and performance managers following the Healthcare Commission investigation*. London: Department of Health, p.3.

11 Healthcare Commission (2009) *Investigation into Mid Staffordshire NHS Foundation Trust, March 2009*. London: Healthcare Commission, p.106.

12 Healthcare Commission (2007) *Investigation into outbreaks of* Clostridium difficile *at Maidstone and Tunbridge Wells NHS Trust, October 2007*. London: Healthcare Commission, p.93.

13 Healthcare Commission (2009) *Investigation into Mid Staffordshire NHS Foundation Trust, March 2009*. London: Healthcare Commission, p.106.

14 Francis, R. (Chair) (2010) *Independent Inquiry into care provided by Mid Staffordshire NHS Foundation Trust January 2005–March 2009*. London: The Stationery Office, p.229.

Under-staffing, a consequence of financial performance targets, surfaces elsewhere. Three years earlier, at Mid Cheshire NHS Hospitals Trust, the Healthcare Commission had reported on an organisation that, by common consensus, was dominated by finance and targets to the point of being 'stifling'.[15]

And, as long as seven years before that, in 1999, at the North Lakeland NHS Trust, the Commission for Health Improvement (CHI) had identified seriously abusive practice toward older people; staff were in no doubt that numbers and quality of staff had been reduced to meet financial targets.[16]

AN UNFORTUNATE EFFECT of targets, or other narrowly defined priorities, is to make everything else invisible, no matter how serious. At the most basic level, NHS chief executives have tended not to lose sleep over whether older people are helped to eat and drink, are taken to the toilet, are spoken to civilly (or at all) or helped to keep clean. The directives to which they work, achievement of which determines their job security, are not aimed at such mundane matters as humane care. At times it appears that centrally set targets and priorities have literally removed the power of independent thought and initiative from senior management and staff at local level. As the following instances show, this is not to over-state the case.

At Stoke Mandeville Hospital, the strategic health authority (SHA) had regional oversight over the hospital. Nonetheless, because control of MRSA, but not *Clostridium difficile*, was a government target, the SHA focused only on the former, until asked belatedly to do so by the Department of Health.[17] On paper *Clostridium* was invisible because there was no target or priority, yet it was from *Clostridium* that scores of patients were dying.

Similarly, at Maidstone and Tunbridge Wells NHS Trust, where even more people died of infection than at Stoke Mandeville, the chief executive pleaded in her defence that the government was focusing on MRSA and not *Clostridium*.[18] Effectively, notwithstanding scores of her

15 Healthcare Commission (2006) *Investigation into Mid Cheshire Hospitals NHS Trust, January 2006*. London: Healthcare Commission, p.50.

16 CHI (Commission for Health Improvement) (2000) *Investigation into the North Lakeland NHS Trust*. November. London: CHI, pp.1, 25.

17 Healthcare Commission (2006) *Investigation into outbreaks of* Clostridium difficile *at Stoke Mandeville Hospital, Buckinghamshire Hospitals NHS Trust, July 2006*. London: Healthcare Commission, p.8.

18 Graham, M. (2009) 'Rose Gibb: I was victimised, demonised.' *Kent Online*, 27 January. Accessed on 5 August 2010 at: www.kentonline.co.uk/kentonline/newsarchive.aspx?articleid=55860.

patients dying, she seemed to be implying that if it was not a government focus, it did not exist – or at least did not qualify as a priority.

The totally preposterous nature of such arguments put forward by NHS trusts is an indictment of a system that has removed local initiative and judgement and created a culture of dangerous, indiscriminate obsequiousness and servility. This mindlessness can spread to front-line staff as well. Commenting that infection control had improved at Peterborough General Hospital, a patient noted that nurses were doing the right thing but not for the right reason. They were more interested in staying out of trouble than keeping patients safe:

> All this was in December 2005 and I think that things have improved since then because I was recently a patient in the same hospital and staff take much more care about infection control now. But from what I saw this was because staff are worried about getting into trouble, not because they know it's the right thing to do. So there are "clean hands" notices everywhere but I still heard staff saying "Oh I'd better not come in the kitchen with my apron on because I'll get into trouble" – not because they realised that they shouldn't go into the kitchen with an apron straight after dealing with a patient.[19]

An investigation into the West London Mental Health NHS Trust also revealed tension between hitting targets and providing safe care. The CQC's 2009 report referred to competing priorities and nationally set performance targets to be achieved. But it pointed out that fundamentally, the Trust had to make sure its patients were safe. The Commission had doubts whether it had done so. A number of suicides seemed to be associated with an ineffective approach to the assessment and removal of ligature points. Although the old buildings made removal of all such points difficult, the Trust did not have a dedicated programme to manage to remove or reduce the number of such points. Because of insufficient beds, patients sometimes slept on sofas or remained too long in the intensive care unit – practices that posed significant safety risks. Patient areas suffered outbreaks of infestation by mice and cockroaches.[20]

In the same vein, following the abuse of elderly, mental health patients on Rowan Ward in Manchester, the CHI considered the lack of external scrutiny of Manchester Mental Health and Social Care Trust.

19 Patient Opinion. Accessed on 20 September 2010 at: www.patientopinion.org.uk/opinions/18274.

20 CQC (Care Quality Commission) (2009) *Investigation into West London Mental Health NHS Trust.* London: CQC, pp.3–4.

This failure in scrutiny had allowed the latter to gain 'care trust' status, on the basis that it was providing high quality clinical services. The Commission wanted to know why the Greater Manchester SHA, together with the NHS North West Regional Office and the Directorate of Health and Social Care (North), had all failed in their role of performance management and scrutiny of the Trust. It concluded that all these bodies had been concentrating on government-set activity times and targets for acute services.[21] And not much else.

Effectively, mental health was therefore of little interest to these supervisory bodies. Not only did this mean that eyes had been taken off the ball; the ball had effectively vanished altogether.

THINKING AND CONSCIENTIOUS senior managers and staff should be valued. But for an NHS trust under pressure, they can pose a problem. The difficulty is how to keep them on board, even when the world has turned upside down and the trust is pursuing sometimes disingenuous and ruthless policies detrimental to the dignity and welfare of patients. To solve it, two special ingredients are required: fear and bullying. They are of course ingredients that should not be in the pot at all. The *Code of conduct for NHS managers* states that:

> I will seek to ensure that…NHS staff are valued as colleagues, properly informed about the management of the NHS, given appropriate opportunities to take part in decision-making, given all reasonable protection from harassment and bullying.[22]

It may seem outlandish to suggest that a national institution, the NHS, full of caring professionals should be afflicted with a culture of bullying, in particular when it comes from above. However, in 2009, the Healthcare Commission's chairman referred to a serious problem of bullying in the NHS, in line with the results of annual survey, showing 12 per cent of staff felt bullied, with 8 per cent identifying it as coming from managers and team leaders.[23]

And in 2010, the Secretary of State for Health openly referred to the culture of secrecy, fear and bullying that had taken hold at Mid

---

21 CHI (Commission for Health Improvement) (2003) *Investigation into matters arising from care on Rowan Ward, Manchester Mental Health and Social Care Trust, September 2003.* London: CHI, p.41.

22 DH (Department of Health) (2002) *Code of conduct for NHS managers.* London: DH, p.4.

23 Santry, C. (2009) 'Bullying: the "corrosive" problem the NHS must address.' *Health Service Journal,* 23 April.

Staffordshire NHS Foundation Trust.[24] A management style had existed, giving all the appearance of bullying. The director of human resources (HR) referred to staff being scared of raising issues and concerns, for fear of repercussions. A manager referred to a 'downward spiral of bullying and inexperience'. Staff were afraid of the nursing director, who was perceived to have an abrasive and bullying style.[25]

Nurses reported leaving meetings in tears and being threatened that their jobs were at stake because of breaches of the four-hour target. Staff believed that patient care had become secondary to the hitting of targets and avoiding breaches.[26] Thus from a manager at Mid Staffordshire who spoke of staff quaking in their boots and emerging from meetings, crying:

> I came from a meeting one day and one of the staff nurses was crying in the department and I said: what on earth is the matter? And she said: I have had a breach. I went: right, and? And she was literally quaking in her boots because she thought I was going to shout from the rooftops. And I said, it is not a problem. We haven't got to be like this at all…on occasion you would expect patients to breach for clinical need… An emergency physician told me: The nurses would go into that meeting and they were told in the meeting that [if] there were any breaches to – that is breaches of the four-hour rule – they would be in danger of losing their jobs. On a regular basis, and I mean a number of times per week, when I was on day shifts, I would see nurses coming out of that meeting crying.[27]

Mid Staffordshire has not been alone. At the West London Mental Health NHS Trust a number of consultant psychiatrists had held meetings with the Healthcare Commission. The concerns raised by some (but not all) consultants included fear of staff in coming forward about quality of care issues, about an authoritarian and bullying style of management within the Trust, some aggression in management – and a wish not to hear about problems, so long as budgets were adhered to.[28]

24 Lansley, A. (Secretary of State for Health) (2010) *Hansard.* House of Commons Debates, 9 June, col. 334.

25 Francis, R. (Chair) (2010) *Independent Inquiry into care provided by Mid Staffordshire NHS Foundation Trust January 2005–March 2009.* London: The Stationery Office, pp.159–62.

26 Healthcare Commission (2009) *Investigation into Mid Staffordshire NHS Foundation Trust, March 2009.* London: Healthcare Commission, p.49.

27 Francis, R. (Chair) (2010) *Independent Inquiry into care provided by Mid Staffordshire NHS Foundation Trust January 2005–March 2009.* London: The Stationery Office, p.165.

28 CQC (Care Quality Commission) (2009) *Investigation into West London Mental Health NHS Trust.* London: CQC, p.60.

At Maidstone and Tunbridge Wells NHS Trust, many staff, including senior managers, described the approach of the chief executive as autocratic and dictatorial. She controlled what went to the Board. Non-executives felt unable to challenge her on patient care matters, not least because relevant information – including low staffing and the hygiene code – was not given to the Board in a timely fashion. As a result, quality of care, as opposed to finance, was rarely discussed. Senior management confessed that they were dealing with a group of stressed managers, who were in fear of losing their jobs if targets were not achieved. Both senior nurses and managers described ward staff as exhausted and downtrodden.[29] A subsequent independent report referred to the chief executive's style as combative, inflexible and demanding, making it difficult for the rest of the Board, executive and non-executive members, to make constructive criticism and indeed to do their jobs.[30]

Deaf to advice about how to manage lethal infection, as well as oppressive and intolerant of failure: this was how management at Stoke Mandeville Hospital was viewed by staff. The executive team did not want to hear adverse messages. Staff were frightened to speak openly. The culture was of stressed and distressed managers, of everything being a 'top priority' and of failure not being an option. Managers were regularly in tears and others on medication.[31]

And the perception at Mid Cheshire Hospitals NHS Trust was not only of an organisation driven by finance and targets – but also of a chief executive whose 'span of control was so wide, and power was so centralised, that it undermined the formal management and accountability structure at the trust'.[32]

THAT PEOPLE'S JOBS may come under threat in NHS trusts if priorities, finance and performance, are not met, seems plain. And the fear is passed down from the top layer in the NHS hierarchy. At Mid Staffordshire, the chair of the Trust reported how the current chief executive of the NHS in 2010, previously in post at an SHA, was in the process of removing

29 Healthcare Commission (2007) *Investigation into outbreaks of* Clostridium difficile *at Maidstone and Tunbridge Wells NHS Trust, October 2007.* London: Healthcare Commission, pp.91–2.

30 Marsden, E. and Mechen, D. (2008) *An independent review into the board leadership of Maidstone and Tunbridge Wells NHS Trust: A report for NHS South East Coast.* London: Verita, pp.20–3.

31 Healthcare Commission (2006) *Investigation into outbreaks of* Clostridium difficile *at Stoke Mandeville Hospital, Buckinghamshire Hospitals NHS Trust, July 2006.* London: Healthcare Commission, pp.7, 70.

32 Healthcare Commission. *Investigation into Mid Cheshire Hospitals NHS Trust, January 2006.* London: Healthcare Commission, p.38.

an entire non-executive team at another NHS trust for failing to break even financially:

> I can give you an example. On December 22 2005 and it is in my mind because that was the day that we had our first strategic board interview with the strategic health authority to go for foundation trust, and that was conducted by David Nicholson who is currently chair of the NHS and Antony Sumara, who is actually chief executive here now. They were very preoccupied during our board interview and spent a lot of time getting up and going out and taking phone calls and that was because the North Staffs had said that it had refused to break even at the end of the financial year and the entire non-executive team and chair were being removed that afternoon. So those are the consequences. If you don't break even you get removed and somebody that will break even is put in.[33]

Allegations were made by David Bowles, chair of the United Lincolnshire Hospitals Trust, who resigned, citing bullying by the East Midland SHA in relation to the hitting of targets. He was supported by other non-executive members of the Trust's Board. His position was that he was not prepared to guarantee the hitting of non-urgent targets at a time when emergency admissions were very high. He wanted to know from the chief executive of the NHS (David Nicholson) 'whether he thinks it is fair and reasonable to ask for that guarantee… I would like to know whether this is a renegade SHA or do ministers agree with unconditional guarantees on non-urgent targets.' His stance was that, were he to offer such a guarantee, this would be at the expense of patient safety.[34]

David Nicholson then set up an inquiry, chaired by an independent consultant, a former SHA chief executive. It exonerated East Midlands SHA of harassment and bullying. However, it did note that: 'Given the increasing pressures on NHS leadership and management that will result from the impact of the economic downturn on public services there is the possibility of firm performance management being interpreted as bullying or harassment.' It refers also to the importance of good relationships and collaborative behaviour.[35]

33 Francis, R. (Chair) (2010) *Independent Inquiry into care provided by Mid Staffordshire NHS Foundation Trust January 2005–March 2009*. London: The Stationery Office, p.225.

34 Moore, A. (2009) 'Resigning trust chair calls for David Nicholson to investigate "SHA pressure".' *Health Service Journal*, 27 July.

35 DH (Department of Health) (2009) *Review of allegations of bullying and harassment of the United Lincolnshire Hospitals NHS Trust by the East Midlands Strategic Health Authority: Summary of findings, 28th October 2009*. London: DH.

This cries out for a reading between the lines; the power and pressure wielded by SHAs is well known within the NHS. It would be sensible therefore to give equal weight to the observation of the local Member for Parliament, Mark Simmonds, who, before the Inquiry reported, referred to what appeared to him to be 'a substitution of bullying for performance management and an obsession with targets rather than safety.'[36] It is arguable that the Inquiry's findings almost certainly imply the existence of bullying – in all but name.

36   Moore, A. (2009) 'Resigning trust chair calls for David Nicholson to investigate "SHA pressure".' *Health Service Journal*, 27 July.

16

Misinformation, Concealment and Spin

In the chief executive's letter to the [Health Protection Unit] on 12 June 2006 it was claimed that the outbreak in the trust "has now gone" and "current *Clostridium difficile* levels are less than the usual background levels." The first of these statements was premature and the second was inaccurate…

Some senior clinicians and managers, and external stakeholders however, remarked upon the degree of "positive spin" used by the trust and in particular the chief executive. The Healthcare Commission's own experience of the trust's approach to the investigation underlined some of the concerns expressed about the extent of openness in the trust, the accuracy of statements made and of information provided. (Healthcare Commission: Maidstone and Tunbridge Wells NHS Trust, 2007)[1]

In the midst of chaos, overcrowding, filth, infection, lack of basic care and dignity, a nursing report was submitted to the Board of the Maidstone and Tunbridge Wells NHS Trust.

The report assured the Board that every patient had received 'the best care in the best place on the ward' – a claim dismissed as pure fabrication by the Healthcare Commission.[2] Leaving aside the departure from the facts, this claim is devoid, if one thinks about it, of any real meaning. Because of the relative and superlative nature of the word 'best', its use was a logical nonsense, as well as grotesque in the midst of demeaning care and death. It is, by definition, simply not possible for everybody to enjoy the best.

However, this type of phrase is used within the health service by managers as incontinently as it is frequently. And, as misleading euphemism, it does immense harm. The report was using language derived from a mantra in *The NHS Plan* (which is discussed later in this

---

1 Healthcare Commission (2007) *Investigation into outbreaks of* Clostridium difficile *at Maidstone and Tunbridge Wells NHS Trust, October 2007*. London: Healthcare Commission, p.94.

2 Healthcare Commission (2007) *Investigation into outbreaks of Clostridium difficile at Maidstone and Tunbridge Wells NHS Trust, October 2007*. London: Healthcare Commission, p.87.

chapter). No self-respecting health care professional should have dreamt of making such a claim. Likewise no board member, worthy of his or her status, should have stood for it.

WITH THE BEST will in the world, things sometimes fundamentally go wrong which are politically unacceptable at both a central and local level. When this happens, politicians and NHS trust managers look for face-saving measures. Concealment is one such.

It comes in many forms. It can include outright lies and deception, withholding of information from the public, giving of partial information – and the operating of systems of clinical governance or incident reporting which have the effect of suppressing the evidence of substandard care, including neglect and abuse. It also comes in the form of euphemism, wishful thinking, and what, without exaggeration, sometimes qualifies as Orwellian doublethink. Or maybe spin. These types of concealment are located above all in management circles and are rife throughout the hierarchy – local, regional, central – of the National Health Service (NHS).

All this may sound like rash assertion or wild accusation; not so.

IT WOULD BE tedious and repetitious to refer to the following codes and guidance were it not for the fact that they are so frequently disregarded when it comes to the giving of full and accurate information about what happens within the health service. We need to get an idea of how polished the veneer is, before seeing how rotten the wood beneath can sometimes be.

The *Code of conduct for NHS managers* states that the public should be properly informed and misleading statements should not be made:

> I will also seek to ensure that the public are properly informed and are able to influence services... I will be honest and will act with integrity and probity at all times. I will not make, permit or knowingly allow to be made, any untrue or misleading statement relating to my own duties or the functions of my employer.[3]

A code of governance for NHS foundation trusts states that the chair is responsible for 'ensuring the provision of accurate, timely and clear information to directors [and] ensuring effective communication with staff, patients and the public'.[4] More generally, it states that the 'NHS

3   DH (Department of Health) (2002) *Code of conduct for NHS managers*. London: DH, p.4.
4   DH (Department of Health) and NHS Appointments Board (2003) *Governing the NHS: A guide for NHS boards*. London: DH, p.16.

has a fundamental obligation to provide timely and accurate information about plans and performance'.[5]

For NHS foundation trusts, another code states that non-executive directors on the board:

> ...should satisfy themselves as to the integrity of financial, clinical and other information, and that financial and clinical quality controls and systems of risk management and governance are robust and implemented.[6]

The chair of a foundation trust should ensure that the board receives accurate information; the board should not be passive, though, and:

> ...is responsible for ensuring that the directors and governors receive accurate, timely and clear information. Management has an obligation to provide such information but directors and governors should seek clarification or amplification where necessary.[7]

The codes are not enforceable in law by any regulatory body.

PAPERWORK, TOGETHER WITH its electronic equivalent, plays a key role in facilitating concealment, deliberate or otherwise. A closed and secretive culture of leadership and senior management tends to build up a parallel universe, in which everybody pretends that all is well. Ultimately, everybody comes to believe it. Boxes are ticked, soothing and selective and anaemic reports are written. Overall, reassurance is stamped.

In support of its application to become an elite, foundation trust, the Mid Staffordshire NHS Foundation Trust declared on paper to the overseeing organisation, Monitor, that it provided high quality care for patients. There could be no better, or rather worse, example of the gap between rhetoric and reality. The Healthcare Commission pointed out that it is not enough that a system of clinical governance looks good on paper; it actually has to work in practice.[8] The Independent Inquiry, too, noted that patients were being moved from accident and emergency (A&E) 'on paper but not in reality'.[9] The journalist Melanie Reid summed this up as 'death by empty words':

---

5   DH (Department of Health) and NHS Appointments Board (2003) *Governing the NHS: A guide for NHS boards.* London: DH, p.18.

6   Monitor (2010) *The NHS foundation trust code of governance.* London: Monitor, p.10.

7   Monitor (2010) *The NHS foundation trust code of governance.* London: Monitor, p.20.

8   Healthcare Commission (2009) *Investigation into Mid Staffordshire NHS Foundation Trust, March 2009.* London: Healthcare Commission, p.11.

9   Francis, R. (Chair) (2010) *Independent Inquiry into care provided by Mid Staffordshire NHS Foundation Trust January 2005–March 2009.* London: The Stationery Office, p.289.

> What killed hundreds of people in Mid Staffordshire was
> semantics; the first big case of death by empty words. It won't
> be the last. Incompetence was an accomplice – it always is – but
> the main culprit was the cloak of evasive language. The entire
> health service floats on an Orwellian sea of newspeak strategies,
> policies, stakeholders, parameters, benchmarking, outcomes,
> actioning, pathfinding. Third-rate jargon, that great weapon of
> the inadequate, has become the accepted way to con the public
> – sorry, service users. And create jobs too – because someone
> spends a lot of time writing the bloody stuff.[10]

The Care Quality Commission (CQC) found serious problems with
patient care in the West London Mental Health NHS Trust. However, the
Trust had previously declared itself compliant with all 24 core standards.
A reading of the Commission's report suggests that the Trust declared
this on the basis of a mixture of reassurance from managers, ignorance
about what was going on (for example bed occupancy and staffing levels
were discussed only occasionally) and wishful thinking.[11]

Maidstone and Tunbridge Wells NHS Trust was in the throes of a
lethal outbreak of *Clostridium difficile* and providing care at such a poor
level that manslaughter charges were considered, though never brought.[12]
Yet at the time this was going on, the NHS Trust had declared itself
in compliance with the core national standard for infection control.[13]
Which it clearly wasn't.

The flimsiness of paper claims is also found at national level. For
instance, in 2004, the Department of Health published an upbeat
report detailing progress with *The NHS Plan* and 'putting people at the
heart of public services'. One of its claims was that hospital cleanliness
had improved; whereas in 2000 over 200 hospitals had been judged
as unacceptable, by 2001 all hospitals had met or exceeded minimum
standards.[14] This was an extremely ill judged statement for a Secretary
of State for Health, backed up by a Prime Ministerial foreword, to make.
Its utter vacuity was exposed in the next few years by constant reports of
filthy wards up and down the country – and the harrowing conditions of

10 Reid, M. (2009) 'Mid Staffs: the first big case of death by empty words.' *The Times*, 19 March.

11 CQC (Care Quality Commission) (2009) *Investigation into West London Mental Health NHS Trust.*
    London: CQC, pp.58–9.

12 Hawkes, N. (2008) 'No-one to be prosecuted over 90 C-difficile deaths at Kent hospitals.' *The
    Times*, 30 July.

13 Healthcare Commission (2007) *Investigation into outbreaks of Clostridium difficile at Maidstone and
    Tunbridge Wells NHS Trust, October 2007.* London: Healthcare Commission, p.7.

14 Secretary of State for Health (2004) *The NHS improvement plan: Putting people at the heart of public
    services.* London: The Stationery Office, p.23.

hygiene at Maidstone and Tunbridge Wells NHS Trust, Stoke Mandeville and Mid Staffordshire.

The first verse of an old, nonsense, nursery rhyme runs thus: *If all the world were paper, And all the sea were ink, If all the trees were bread and cheese, What would we do for drink?* This imaginary existence lacks drink. In parallel, as the above examples demonstrate, the illusionary world depicted by NHS policymakers and management may, extraordinarily, leave one looking in vain for any actual health care.

To MUDDY THE waters, concealment by NHS trusts of the true picture may not be confined to declarations made to external regulatory bodies, but extend to internal and local dealings as well. Thus, the non-executive members of the board of Maidstone and Tunbridge Wells NHS Trust had access only to incomplete or inaccurate information. They, together with the public, were consistently denied, or given inaccurate, information by the executive. The second outbreak of infection that occurred was not made public for two months until a Press enquiry had been received, and even then the number of relevant deaths was under-stated.[15]

The extent of this reported concealment and manipulation of information in Kent warrants spelling out in further detail, not least because of the remorseless exposure of it by the Healthcare Commission. It is a noteworthy example of systematic obscuration which delayed the taking of steps to protect patients from undignified care and potential death from infection. At worst, this detail suggests wilful concealment. At best, it signifies a veiling of the facts through collective wishful thinking, selective information provision and perhaps incompetence – a combination almost as alarming as deliberate dissimulation.

First, in May 2006, the outbreak was discussed in the Board meeting – but only in the private, not the public, part. Even in private, a fiction was being played out; the nursing report claimed (absurdly) that every patient had received superlative care – a claim directly contradicted by the evidence unearthed by the Healthcare Commission.

Second, the explanation given to the public, as to why part of the Board meeting about infection was held in private, stated that individual patients were to be named; yet there was no evidence that this was the case. The private part of the meeting conceded that the infection was at outbreak level; the public part of the meeting was told that the infection was under control. The Board was assured in the private part of the

---

15 Healthcare Commission (2007) *Investigation into outbreaks of* Clostridium difficile *at Maidstone and Tunbridge Wells NHS Trust, October 2007*. London: Healthcare Commission, p.30.

meeting that the regional Health Protection Unit was happy with the Trust's handling of the outbreak; in fact the Unit had expressed its formal concerns and unease to the Trust.

Third, the Board was informed that a comprehensive training programme had been put in place for staff working with infected patients; yet there was no evidence of any such programme. The Board stated that the advice of the Trust's infection control team was central to its decisions – but in reality the team's advice was not always followed. This meant, for instance, four months' delay in setting up an isolation ward. The Board was also told in a nursing report submitted to it that no other NHS trust in England had done as much to manage infection. This was another striking incongruity; the evidence was quite to the contrary.

In addition, the director of infection control told a member of the public that new commodes were available on the wards; months later, there were still no new commodes and condemned commodes were still in use. The Board was told, and Press releases stated it later, that the Trust had requested that the strategic health authority (SHA) investigate the infection outbreak; in fact it was the other way around.[16]

To crown it all, there was even a track record of culpable concealment at the Trust. Back in 2003, an external report into goings on at the Trust had concluded that waiting times figures had been misrepresented by the Trust – and that managers, stressed and under extreme pressure to hit targets, had been complicit. This report had referred to deliberate, serious and unacceptable misrepresentation.[17] This is about as near to the words lying and deception as one can get.

CONCEALMENT HAS BEEN exposed elsewhere. At Stoke Mandeville hospital, hit by two serious outbreaks of *Clostridium difficile*, the public was not told what was going on until a leak to the Press triggered national publicity. Furthermore, the Healthcare Commission found that either the outbreaks had not been discussed at Board level or they had not been minuted. Either way it was a matter of concern. The Board was unable to explain why it had not discussed the second outbreak before it was reported in the national Press.[18]

16 Healthcare Commission (2007) *Investigation into outbreaks of* Clostridium difficile *at Maidstone and Tunbridge Wells NHS Trust, October 2007.* London: Healthcare Commission, pp.87–9.

17 Healthcare Commission (2007) *Investigation into outbreaks of* Clostridium difficile *at Maidstone and Tunbridge Wells NHS Trust, October 2007.* London: Healthcare Commission, p.19.

18 Healthcare Commission (2006) *Investigation into outbreaks of* Clostridium difficile *at Stoke Mandeville Hospital, Buckinghamshire Hospitals NHS Trust, July 2006.* London: Healthcare Commission, pp.7, 63.

The Healthcare Commission, with characteristic under-statement, recorded that its own experience of the NHS Trust underlined the concerns generally felt about the Trust's approach to openness, the accuracy of statements made and of information provided.[19]

The sensitivity of NHS trusts about untoward information concerning patient care getting into the public domain was illustrated by a particular incident at Stafford Hospital. A member of the Patient and Public Involvement Forum (PPIF) attached to the Trust believed that information about the *Clostridium difficile* incidence and outbreak should be in the public domain.

He obtained a copy of minutes of an infection control meeting which referred to 341 cases, averaging 36 new cases a month. The minutes were not marked as confidential. He released them to a newspaper. He was consequently expelled from the forum. The chair of the Trust said confidential documents would no longer be shown to the PPIF. These events at Mid Staffordshire occurred after the Healthcare Commission's report into infection at Stoke Mandeville and its criticism of that Trust's lack of openness.[20]

This particular episode was part of a wider picture in Mid Stafford. The Healthcare Commission found that the leadership operated a closed culture.[21] The Board was averse to criticism about services. It did not discuss in public poor results from patient or staff surveys. The Trust had a good relationship with the chair of the PPIF, but did not welcome individual members of the forum raising concerns. Information about escalating levels of *Clostridium difficile* infection was released neither to the Board nor the public; likewise information about the high mortality rate. The audit committee continued to report to the public part of Board meetings; the governance, risk and finance committees were heard only in private.[22]

A report, internal to the Trust, about *Clostridium* infection listed lack of isolation of patients, inadequate cleaning of commodes and bedpan holders, delay in sending samples for testing, poor communication between health professionals and delay in commencing treatment for

19 Healthcare Commission (2007) *Investigation into outbreaks of* Clostridium difficile *at Maidstone and Tunbridge Wells NHS Trust, October 2007.* London: Healthcare Commission, p.94.

20 Healthcare Commission (2009) *Investigation into Mid Staffordshire NHS Foundation Trust, March 2009.* London: Healthcare Commission, p.89.

21 Healthcare Commission (2009) *Investigation into Mid Staffordshire NHS Foundation Trust, March 2009.* London: Healthcare Commission, p.133.

22 Healthcare Commission (2009) *Investigation into Mid Staffordshire NHS Foundation Trust, March 2009.* London: Healthcare Commission, pp.106–7.

symptomatic patients. This was not drawn to the attention of the Board.[23] The Inquiry also found evidence of fabrication of records to conceal breach of the A&E waiting time target.[24]

What constitutes concealment amounting to deception? At Mid Staffordshire, complacent and cocooned from all that happened around it, the Board had applied for foundation status for the Trust by self-declaring the quality of its care. The Independent Inquiry did not believe that Board members deliberately deceived anyone; however, the declarations about quality of care 'revealed a profound misunderstanding of their responsibilities'.[25] The Inquiry was at pains to reject allegations that the Board had been duplicitous. Yet its conclusions were equally damning, referring to the Board's alarming lack of insight, lack of focus on patient welfare, pervasive attitude of denial, complacency and absence of reflection.[26]

EVEN WHEN EVASIVE action fails, and embarrassing disclosure breaks the surface, some NHS trusts still cling to the wreckage tenaciously and wage a damage limitation exercise to the bitter end.

Fordingbridge Hospital is a case in point. Driven to commission an Independent Inquiry into the treatment and care of inpatients in a rehabilitation and palliative care unit, Hampshire Primary Care Trust (PCT) issued a short summary but not the report itself. The newspaper, the *Southern Daily Echo*, appealed to the Information Commissioner under the *Freedom of Information Act 2000*. The PCT was then obliged to release the report but only after it had blanked out large parts of it, ostensibly to protect patient and staff confidentiality and avoid distress. The surviving part of the report points to unacceptable staff behaviour but gives no real insight into the detail of what went on and how serious it was.[27]

It is difficult to believe that quite so much had to be removed from the report, in order to achieve this degree of confidentiality. The PCT had obviously wanted the report buried. The assiduousness with which

23 Healthcare Commission (2009) *Investigation into Mid Staffordshire NHS Foundation Trust, March 2009*. London: Healthcare Commission, p.130.

24 Francis, R. (Chair) (2010) *Independent Inquiry into care provided by Mid Staffordshire NHS Foundation Trust January 2005–March 2009*. London: The Stationery Office, p.174.

25 Francis, R. (Chair) (2010) *Independent Inquiry into care provided by Mid Staffordshire NHS Foundation Trust January 2005–March 2009*. London: The Stationery Office, p.22.

26 Francis, R. (Chair) (2010) *Independent Inquiry into care provided by Mid Staffordshire NHS Foundation Trust January 2005–March 2009*. London: The Stationery Office, p.338.

27 Yandell, C. (2009) 'NHS asked for full report after "unacceptable behaviour" at Fordingbridge Hospital.' *Southern Daily Echo*, 18 January. Also: Yandell, C. (2009) 'Report details appalling treatment of elderly Fordingbridge Hospital patients.' *Southern Daily Echo*, 10 December.

it sought to obscure the findings seemed to be in proportion with its own failings, which had allowed the problems to develop in the first place. One surviving part of the report noted that, over a long period of time, management had failed to provide effective leadership.[28]

EUPHEMISM HAS BECOME something of an art form in the language of the NHS. In fact, use of the term to describe some of what is uttered is itself euphemistic; the more extreme 'Orwellian doublethink' seems sometimes to be a more apt description. Or, perhaps, 'outrageous spin'. One can heap ridicule on it, but it can be highly damaging to patients.

At a conference in March 2010, a consultant nurse on secondment to the Department of Health, Lynne Phair, put her finger on this use of language and the difficulty that the health service has with straight talk. By such means, the seriousness of inadequate care can be concealed; for instance, use of the term 'sub-optimal care' instead of neglect, 'systems failure' instead of recklessness, 'clinical error' instead of clinical incompetence, 'busy ward' instead of dangerous practice, 'learning collective lessons' instead of acceptance of personal responsibility and 'isolated incident' instead of pattern of behaviour.[29] We have also the storerooms or cupboards at the Norfolk and Norwich Hospital, reportedly utilised routinely for patients under the nomenclature of 'treatment rooms'.[30]

In 2000, the nearest The NHS Plan got to referring to the fact that older people were being routinely subjected to poor care and neglect on acute hospital wards was to state that: 'Standards of care for patients are often good in the NHS. Sometimes, however, they need to be better'.[31]

The Mid Staffordshire NHS Foundation Trust displayed unawareness and unconcern about its dying and degraded patients, but it at least recognised that it had to safeguard and promote its reputation. It took on the services of a public relations company:

> It was clear from the minutes of the trust's board that it became
> focused on promoting itself as an organisation, with considerable

28 Lampard, K. and Brougham, C. (2008) *An investigation into the quality and care of patients at Fordingbridge Hospital: A report for Hampshire Primary Care Trust.* London: Verita, p.66.
29 Phair, L. (2010) 'The Vetting and Barring Scheme and its role in safeguarding.' Presentation notes at a 'Safeguarding vulnerable adults: empowerment through implementation of "No secrets"' Conference held on 17 March at 4 Hamilton Place, London.
30 Hope, J. (2010) 'Shocking picture shows how elderly patient was abandoned for two days in hospital store cupboard with little food or medication.' *Daily Mail*, 14 February.
31 Secretary of State for Health (2000) *The NHS Plan: A plan for investment, a plan for reform.* Cm 4818-I. London: The Stationery Office, p.89.

attention given to marketing and public relations. It lost sight of its responsibilities to deliver acceptable standards of care to all patients admitted to its facilities. It failed to pay sufficient regard to clinical leadership and to the experience and sensibilities of patients and their families.[32]

Put another way, as long as the media – tame, seduced or duped – was on board, it didn't matter too much about the anarchy behind the scenes. A year or so later, when figures emerged pointing to the hospital having the fifth highest mortality rate in the country, the Trust was able euphemistically to put this down to problems with 'data capture'. The Healthcare Commission found no evidence that this was the explanation.[33]

At the same Trust, the Trust secretary and head of legal services persuaded a consultant to delete sections of a report concluding that the death of a young man had been avoidable – after he had been sent home with a ruptured spleen, following a bicycle accident, undiagnosed. He died. Clearly anxious to stave off any hint of negligence, she justified concealment from both the inquest and the family as follows, impermissibly mixing up defence of the Trust with sparing the family the details: 'As reports are generally read out in full at the inquest and the press and family will be present, with a view to avoiding further distress to the family and adverse publicity, I would wish to avoid stressing possible failures on the part of the Trust.'[34]

Following the Healthcare Commission's report on Mid Staffordshire, the government issued a House of Commons paper, entitled *NHS 2010–2015: From good to great.* It remained coy. The nearest it got to acknowledging a decade of scandal and neglect was to say: 'And, in places, care has fallen below the standards all patients have a right to expect.'[35]

'World class commissioning' is the morale-boosting mantra within the NHS and has been since 2007. To put such a phrase in the context of the care described in this book is incongruous if not outrageous. In the midst of significant misery, total loss of dignity, pain, malnutrition and starvation, filth and infection, the policy talks of 'driving unprecedented

32 Healthcare Commission (2009) *Investigation into Mid Staffordshire NHS Foundation Trust, March 2009.* London: Healthcare Commission, p.10.

33 Healthcare Commission (2009) *Investigation into Mid Staffordshire NHS Foundation Trust, March 2009.* London: Healthcare Commission, pp.10, 109–10.

34 Ellicot, C. (2010) 'Hospital boss tried to cover up details of patient's death after bungling doctors sent him home with painkillers.' *Daily Mail,* 30 September 2010.

35 Secretary of State for Health (2009) *NHS 2010–2015: From good to great, preventative, people-centred, productive.* HC 7775. London: The Stationery Office, p.3.

improvements in patient outcomes, and ensuring the NHS remains one of the most progressive and high-performing health systems in the world'.[36]

To the outsider, looking in on the closed circle of NHS policy and management, such policies and mantras have all the credibility of a *nostrum*, the bread and butter of quack medicine.

Through much of the 2000s, just such a cure-all came in the form of a particular chant which came to be used insidiously and irresponsibly. It was employed extensively to suppress rational debate and to reject clinical arguments against wholesale closure of acute and community hospital beds. It emerged from *The NHS Plan* which stated that, under the policy of intermediate care, older people should 'receive the right care at the right time in the right place'.[37] Instead of adopting the balanced and heterogeneous approach to care of the elderly implicit in *The NHS Plan*, chief executives seized on the mantra with abandon. From their point of view, it was a godsend indeed: meaningless or alternatively capable of meaning anything at all.

Nor must we forget the initial response of North Lakeland NHS Trust to the student whistleblowing which, as already noted, had revealed elderly patients being tied up on commodes, fed while on commodes and denied, deliberately, pullovers and blankets. Its report, with audacious under-statement, referred to 'issues that are open to misunderstanding... departures from accepted practice, but with good intent...issues that require review to ensure that the best approach is being used'. Astonishingly, it even managed to denigrate, albeit in patronising and soothing language, the students who had performed such a public service; it observed 'the type of patient in this ward leads to a marked difference between theory and its application...some of the difficulties encountered between students and staff may have been created by the students' understanding of the relationship between theory and practice'.[38]

When large hospital staff and bed cuts were announced for Southampton in June 2006, following similar cuts the year before, the chief executive stated that not only was it all about improving services for patients but that it would be 'exciting' for staff.[39] By 2010, it was reported that non-clinically justified transfers of patients in Southampton were high, with the clear potential for clinical detriment (whether infection

---

36 DH (Department of Health) (2009) *World class commissioning: An introduction*. London: DH, p.2.

37 Secretary of State for Health (2000) *The NHS Plan: A plan for investment, a plan for reform*. Cm 4818-I. London: The Stationery Office, p.71.

38 CHI (Commission for Health Improvement) (2000) *Investigation into the North Lakeland NHS Trust, November*. London: CHI, p.9.

39 Makin, J. (2006) 'Job cuts will lead to a better service.' *Southern Daily Echo*, 28 June.

or other matters). For instance, between July 2008 and July 2010, an average of 5922 patients were admitted monthly, and of these, 703 would be transferred for non-clinical reasons, that is, 12 per cent of admitted patients.[40] And to bring it all down to an individual in Southampton General Hospital, moved from ward to ward only to develop pressure sores and MRSA and then to die in a nursing home from the latter, a relative gave this account in 2009:

> My Mother was admitted following a fall at home last November. She recovered from the fall with no injuries within 24 hours but was kept in the hospital because of a urine infection. She was moved to 4 different wards for no obvious reason and after a few weeks she developed pressure sores which became infected with MRSA. This was not diagnosed by the hospital while she was in their care. After 8 weeks in hospital she was declared medically fit and released to a Nursing Home where she died 6 weeks later. The principal cause of death on her death certificate was MRSA.[41]

AT THE BEGINNING of this chapter we considered the outlandish nursing report that maintained patients were receiving the best care in the best place on the ward: the exact opposite of what was actually happening. The nursing report puts one in mind of Dr Pangloss. He believed that things were not just well with the world, but that everything was always for the best in this best of all possible worlds. He maintained this in the midst of disease, death, slaughter, cruelty and torture. He remained unshaken in his beliefs. He was absurd; but then he was a fictional figure, in satire.[42] Absurd, we say? But no more so than some senior figures in the health service who do indeed make Panglossian utterance in the midst of real suffering, neglect and avoidable death.

And at least Dr Pangloss was a superior breed of optimist; his views were based on learning and on a deep-seated, if eccentric, philosophy. Whereas the modern chief executive, by comparison, tends to fly a flag of convenience, beholden to the most recent political whim, no matter how ill-informed or unwise, of the Secretary of State. As one chief executive put it: if the Secretary of State tells him one day that hospital beds for elderly people are bad, he will support this cause – and believe in it. If the next day, beds are back in favour, he will support this as well – and

---

40 West, D. (2010) 'Hospital bed transfers put thousands of patients at risk of infection.' *Nursing Times*, 5 October.

41 Patient Opinion. Accessed on 20 October 2010 at: www.patientopinion.org.uk/opinions/14654.

42 Voltaire, R. (2005) *Candide*. London: Penguin. (First published in 1759.)

believe in it, irrespective of what his clinicians tell him and of what the consequences for patients will be.

Dr Pangloss goes on to note that private misfortunes make up the general good, and that the more there are of them, so the greater is the general good.[43] This characterises with unfortunate accuracy how the abject suffering of patients can nonetheless still be wedded to congratulations all round for NHS boards; they achieve financial and performance goals and announce just how marvellous is their world of make believe.

The origin, we should note, of the name Pangloss derives from Greek. It means 'all talk'.[44]

WE MAY LAUGH, therefore, on one level at the smart and even cocky use of language even if, stripped down, it is pure inanity. And we really wouldn't mind even this, if those who deployed it also provided the care they purport to. But more sinister is when such language is used to persuade managers, staff and public to believe the words but not their own eyes; when it is used to create a rarefied, managerial, verbal and essentially 'virtual' world of health care – rather than the actual thing itself.

The wife of Mr John David Drake reported how, dying, he was left unwashed, dehydrated and allowed to fall at the Princess Royal University Hospital in Bromley. Etched on her memory was the hospital's motto:

> The…Guarantee in which your Trust promises is delivered through getting the basics right. The…Guarantee is about high quality care, delivered by caring people, in safe and clean hospitals.[45]

43 Voltaire, R. (2005) *Candide*. London: Penguin, p.12. (First published in 1759.)

44 Voltaire, R. (2005) *Candide*. London: Penguin, p.xxxvi. (First published in 1759.)

45 Patients' Association (2009) *Patients not numbers, people not statistics*. London: Patients' Association, p.48.

17

Muted Voices: Clinical and Professional Integrity

> I heard from a very lively 90-year-old woman who was admitted to Stafford Hospital for 10 days in 2008. She was in good health and had even undertaken a parachute jump on her 90th birthday in order to raise money for soldiers returning home from conflict. During her working life she had practised as a qualified nurse for about 20 years, while raising her two sons…
>
> This lady told me of her great concern for other patients on the ward. She said "So many old people lying dependent on too few staff was for me frightening. For them, many of whom were deaf, partially blind or crippled, they must have felt that they had been completely abandoned. *I cannot believe that supposedly fully trained nurses with vocation, care and compassion gain any satisfaction from such an abysmal situation.*" (Mid Staffordshire NHS Foundation Trust: evidence to the Independent Inquiry, 2009; emphasis added)[1]

Odd mistakes, lapses and accidents will always happen. An error is made by a doctor here, a nurse there, a technician or a manager somewhere else. Somebody forgets to do something, a professional makes an error of judgement. The consequences may be trivial or substantial. When they occur, managers and professionals normally seek to ensure that they are not repeated.

But the care focused on in this book is of a different order. It is of a nature that does not just involve the odd mistake; instead it forms a pattern that has been repeated over and over for at least the last 14 years, comprising the same elements – again and again and again. Furthermore, it does not involve complex, difficult medical or nursing judgements or interventions; on the whole it is of the very simplest order. Therefore, where it occurs, it signifies by definition clinical and professional failure, because it takes place when patients are in the specific care of hospital doctors, nurses, therapists and health care assistants.

---

1   Francis, R. (Chair) (2010) *Independent Inquiry into care provided by Mid Staffordshire NHS Foundation Trust January 2005–March 2009.* London: The Stationery Office, p.293.

There are a number of reasons and safeguards which in principle should mean that this doesn't happen. The first is that front-line professionals should ensure that it doesn't – because it is contrary to everything they should stand for. Second, if they fail, their managers should step in. Third, if together professionals and managers fail, then NHS trust boards have a responsibility to ensure the integrity of clinical care through what is called 'clinical governance' of an National Health Service (NHS) trust. Fourth, part of this last safeguard is to have a system of reporting of serious untoward incidents. Fifth, if all this fails, there remains the remedy of whistleblowing.

All this should in principle involve the right people, the professionals, the managers and board members opening their eyes, listening and above all fighting the cause of basic, humane care. What we have instead, when things go off the rails, is a health care world of mostly muted, not raised, voices. And, too often, silence.

DR DAVID COLIN Thomé's 2009 report endorsed the view that events at Mid Staffordshire NHS Foundation Trust were 'appalling'. He also expressed himself disturbed, disappointed and shocked that the poor care went undetected by any other NHS organisation – and that no individual clinicians, other staff, NHS organisations or public representatives raised serious concerns. He implicates not just staff at the Trust, but also the commissioning body – the primary care trust (PCT) – and also the strategic health authority (SHA) that had oversight and management responsibilities.[2]

The author was shocked; but should he have been? A harsh judgement would be that such a reaction was naïve. For instance, in 2006, the Prime Minister had a meeting with 'captains of industry'. It was suggested, by the chair of Cable and Wireless, that anybody on an NHS board who was 'sympathetic to the whingers among the staff' opposing change should be sacked. The same fate should also befall the one third of managers who were opposed to change; the Prime Minister concurred that this was 'absolutely right'.[3] This sort of attitude has permeated the NHS; the problem being that at least some of those whingers and opponents of certain types of change would actually have been expressing informed concern about their patients.

---

2   Thomé, D.C. (Dr) (2009) *Mid Staffordshire NHS Foundation Trust: A review of lessons learnt for commissioners and performance managers following the Healthcare Commission investigation.* London: Department of Health, pp.3–6.

3   Carvel, J. (2006) 'Blundering ministers are making NHS patients suffer say consultants' leader.' *The Guardian*, 7 June.

In practice therefore, some front-line professionals may speak up, but many do not for various reasons. They may have become numb to poor care, may lack confidence, may be intimidated and may be, justifiably or not, afraid. Managers without a background in clinical care are unhampered by professional and ethical codes. They unthinkingly, in good faith, pay homage to the bureaucracy in which they serve, to finance and to uncritical obedience. Of perhaps greater concern are those (but not all) senior managers *with a clinical background* who are to be found supporting policies which will clearly be harmful to patients – but who crucially fail even to speak up, let alone boldly try to block the policy. Such uncritical assent arguably betrays not just patients but professional integrity.

Whatever the reasons for professionals and managers not collectively putting their foot down, the outcome should not be fatal. Where they are not doing so, NHS trust boards should anyway be intervening. And so it is to these boards that we must turn our attention; it is they who at local NHS trust level have overall and collective responsibility for the maintenance of decent clinical standards of care.

INESCAPABLY, A SYSTEMIC distortion and undermining of clinical priorities could only take place in an organisation if there is a problem in its higher reaches.

NHS boards are specifically told in a code of practice that operational demands should not displace quality and safety of care:

> The duty of an NHS Board is to add value to the organisation, enabling it to deliver healthcare and health improvement within the law and without causing harm… It is the duty of the Board to ensure through Clinical Governance that the quality and safety of patient care is not pushed from the agenda by immediate operational issues.[4]

Additional guidance published in 2006 talks of quality assurance:

> Managerial and clinical leadership and accountability, as well as the organisation's culture, systems and working practices ensure that probity, quality assurance, quality improvement and patient safety are central components of all the activities of the health care organisation. This should entail sound clinical and corporate governance, promotion of openness, honesty, probity and accountability.[5]

---

4 DH (Department of Health) (2003) *Governing the NHS: A guide for boards*. London: DH, p.9.
5 DH (Department of Health) (2006) *Standards for better health*. London: DH, p.12.

Fine sounding but empty when one considers a simple example. *The NHS Plan* in 2000 had stated that senior nursing sisters would turn the clock back to ensure the basics of care and cleanliness:

> Senior sisters – "modern matrons" – will have the authority to make sure wards are kept clean and that the basics of care are right for the patient.[6]

Add these to the code of practice for boards, and the nurses at Stoke Mandeville Hospital a few years later might have thought that they would be listened to. How wrong they were. They had become concerned about standards of infection control. They were desperate to safeguard patients in the light of rampant infection and the refusal of the Trust Board to take the necessary, recommended infection control measures. Patients were dying. Their words fell on deaf ears. So much so that, admirably sticking to their professional guns, they invoked a grievance procedure via the Royal College of Nursing (RCN). It didn't work. The Trust Board still didn't react.[7] The Healthcare Commission noted that professional standards were being plainly compromised:

> Levels of nursing staff, particularly in areas opened when other wards were full, continued to be inadequate to provide acceptable care and to control infection. Staff were required to work in situations that compromised their professional standards.[8]

In 2009, the Healthcare Commission published a study of how NHS boards dealt with safety in terms of treating it as a priority, its place on the agenda of meetings and consideration of information about safety matters.

The study involved 30 to 35 trusts. Key findings were that infection control was now (following scandals such as Stoke Mandeville, and Maidstone and Tunbridge Wells) being given more attention but took disproportionate priority over other safety issues. Most boards received reports about serious incidents, infection and complaints; however, they did not receive a range of information on other areas of safety – and targets and finance tended to dominate priorities. Most non-executive

---

6   Secretary of State for Health (2000) *The NHS Plan: A plan for investment, a plan for reform.* Cm 4818-I. London: The Stationery Office, p.20.

7   Healthcare Commission (2006) *Investigation into outbreaks of* Clostridium difficile *at Stoke Mandeville Hospital, Buckinghamshire Hospitals NHS Trust, July 2006.* London: Healthcare Commission, p.50.

8   Healthcare Commission (2006) *Investigation into outbreaks of* Clostridium difficile *at Stoke Mandeville Hospital, Buckinghamshire Hospitals NHS Trust, July 2006.* London: Healthcare Commission, p.8.

directors regarded themselves as passive recipients of information about safety with too limited an understanding to challenge.[9]

A PATTERN HAS emerged of boards being closeted – or closeting themselves – from what actually goes on and then expressing denial or shock when daylight floods in.

At North Lakeland NHS Trust, the Commission for Health Improvement (CHI) was in no doubt that the Trust Board – both executive and non-executive members – bore responsibility for the degrading and abusive practices perpetrated by staff against patients.[10]

In response to student nurses' concerns that patients were being cared for abusively, the Trust's original investigation concluded that the nurses were struggling to bridge the gap between theory and practice, given the difficult type of patient on the ward. It would take a further external investigation and then the CHI to expose fully what had been going on in North Lakeland. The Board was not told that an investigation had taken place, and the locality manager sent a note to the chief executive, expressing his confidence in the quality of care being given.[11]

Messages may come from below and be ignored or accorded little priority. Alternatively they may never make it to the board at all. NHS boards may end up in a parallel universe, a comfortable place to be, reassured by the lack of accurate feedback by management about reality on the front line. At Airedale General Hospital, where nurses were routinely and unlawfully prescribing powerful drugs – and police investigated several deaths – this was exactly what happened:

> Equally significant, the management structure in place below the Board did not always reflect back the reality of what was actually taking place at the "coalface". Reasonable assurance requires a close match between "top down" policy dissemination and "bottom up" feedback, otherwise there is a danger that the Board can find itself inhabiting a parallel universe to that of staff.[12]

A 'mortality review group' at Stafford Hospital considered that there were no 'care issues' in the case of a patient who had died from *Clostridium*

---

9   House of Commons Health Committee (2009) *Patient safety: Sixth report of Session 2008–09*. HC 151-I. London: The Stationery Office, p.87.

10   CHI (Commission for Health Improvement) (2000) *Investigation into the North Lakeland NHS Trust, November*. London: CHI, p.2.

11   CHI (Commission for Health Improvement) (2000) *Investigation into the North Lakeland NHS Trust, November*. London: CHI, p.9.

12   Thirlwall, K., Kinsella, E. and Mullanhe, A. (2010) *Airedale Inquiry: Report to the Yorkshire and the Humber Strategic Health Authority*. Leeds: Yorkshire and Humberside SHA, p.129.

difficile – even though he had been left in soiled sheets for four hours.[13] This sort of judgement no doubt set the tone. So, when cases of *Clostridium difficile* rose to the point of being an outbreak, the minutes of the Trust's Board meetings contained no reference to discussion of this.

Similarly, the Healthcare Commission published, during this period of time, an investigation of what had gone wrong at Stoke Mandeville in relation to management of *Clostridium*. It explicitly stated its relevance to all NHS trusts, yet the Mid Staffordshire Board did not even discuss the report.

Thus, on the ground, patients were subject to infection, food was not being given, call bells were being left unanswered, patients were left in soiled bedding and charts remained uncompleted. There was poor hygiene, whilst privacy and dignity were generally disregarded. Despite all this, the Trust's Board remained largely unaware. In relevant reports seen by the Board, to the extent that such matters were included at all, they were grouped into, and lost within, categories such as communication or quality of care.[14]

At the same Trust, the Board – no doubt in good faith – recited the mantra that care of patients had always been a priority. The Healthcare Commission disagreed. It was not until nearly mid-2007, when concerns had been raised externally about mortality rates, that information on clinical outcomes finally went to the Board.[15]

Non-executive members of the Mid Staffordshire Board did not get to see the details of individual complaints and so were unaware of their nature. As a result, the Board expressed itself as shocked when it finally heard from *an organisation of relatives*, Cure the NHS, about what had been happening within the Trust. The Independent Inquiry could only conclude that the Board might have interpreted the distinction between strategic and operational issues too rigidly; to understand the issues, the non-executive directors would have needed to know about operational detail.[16]

13 Healthcare Commission (2009) *Investigation into Mid Staffordshire NHS Foundation Trust, March 2009*. London: Healthcare Commission, p.31.

14 Healthcare Commission (2009) *Investigation into Mid Staffordshire NHS Foundation Trust, March 2009*. London: Healthcare Commission, p.8.

15 Healthcare Commission (2009) *Investigation into Mid Staffordshire NHS Foundation Trust, March 2009*. London: Healthcare Commission, p.9.

16 Francis, R, (Chair) (2010) *Independent Inquiry into care provided by Mid Staffordshire NHS Foundation Trust January 2005–March 2009*. London: The Stationery Office, p.21.

The dividing line, not to mention convenience, for the Board was clear. It disclaimed responsibility for all that went wrong on the operational side.[17]

It would be reassuring to dismiss the findings about the Mid Staffordshire Board as unusual and unrepresentative of the way in which boards operate, but the evidence points the other way. Boards may not like to see it this way, but in reality some of them are up to their elbows and beyond in filth, pain, human excrement, malnourishment and the degradation of their patients.

At Maidstone and Tunbridge Wells NHS Trust, where scores of people died in hospital from *Clostridium difficile*, the Healthcare Commission had in 2007 noted that responsibilities about accountability for risk and serious incidents were confused. Staff concerns about poor care and management of infection were rarely considered by the Trust Board, which 'appeared to be insulated from the realities and problems on the general wards'.[18]

The Board unambiguously and instinctively protested to the Commission that its top priority had always been the safety of patients. Yet the Trust had not even recognised the first outbreak of infection and that there were serious problems with high bed occupancy, the movement of patients and infected patients being cared for on open wards. The Commission found the Board had in reality failed in its responsibilities to protect patients.[19]

In Mid Cheshire, the Trust Board and clinical governance committee had received inadequate information about patient complaints, which related to basic nursing services such as giving patients food, answering call bells, ensuring privacy and dignity and communication.[20]

Likewise, at the University Hospitals of Leicester NHS Trust, the Healthcare Commission found a significant delay, between September 2005 and July 2006, before rising levels of the *Clostridium* infection were brought to the Board's attention. And when this did happen, the Board was told that the increased figures were due to a different system of

17 Francis, R. (Chair) (2010) *Independent Inquiry into care provided by Mid Staffordshire NHS Foundation Trust January 2005–March 2009*. London: The Stationery Office, p.24.

18 Healthcare Commission (2007) *Investigation into outbreaks of* Clostridium difficile *at Maidstone and Tunbridge Wells NHS Trust, October 2007*. London: Healthcare Commission, p.6.

19 Healthcare Commission (2007) *Investigation into outbreaks of* Clostridium difficile *at Maidstone and Tunbridge Wells NHS Trust, October 2007*. London: Healthcare Commission, p.7.

20 Healthcare Commission (2006) *Investigation into Mid Cheshire Hospitals NHS Trust, January 2006*. London: Healthcare Commission, p.5.

reporting; on this basis, it drew erroneous conclusions and the problem was further masked.[21]

At Stoke Mandeville, staff saw the unrelenting 'can do' approach as high risk. It swept aside clinical concerns, disregarded the pressure on front-line staff and the effect on patients. It involved a relentless 'good news' culture. The 'top team' talked only of success. Unsurprisingly, information given to non-executive members of the Board was limited; they remained unaware of the concerns of the RCN and of the Trust's senior nurses, the missing annual reports about infection control and the worries of medical consultants and other clinical staff.[22]

The lack of attention and concern at board level to patient welfare is reflected not just within the NHS trusts and NHS foundation trust boards, which deliver acute care, but also within the NHS PCT boards that commission it. The House of Commons Health Committee expressed its concern in 2009 that:

> …the perception that many PCTs have failed to assess adequately the quality of services they have purchased is reinforced by the fact that in none of the cases of disastrously unsafe care that have recently come to light had commissioners detected and addressed that unsafe care.[23]

Overall, the Committee, referring to 'catastrophic' failure at board level in cases such as Mid Staffordshire, criticised boards generally for 'addressing governance and regulatory processes, when they should actually be promoting tangible improvements in services'. It suggests training in patient safety for board members, so that they are in a position to challenge executive members of the board.[24]

A pastiche of decision making in NHS trusts would depict the Secretary of State for Health, together with senior civil servants, hand picking chief executives of PCTs and NHS trusts for their devotion to the cause and ruthlessness. A type of health care hired gun, they are expected to obey orders at all costs. They are clothed in the legitimacy of a board of directors, including non-executives, who are meant to put a brake

21 Healthcare Commission (2007) *The management of* Clostridium difficile: *The University Hospitals of Leicester NHS Trust*. London: Healthcare Commission, p.4.

22 Healthcare Commission (2006) *Investigation into outbreaks of* Clostridium difficile *at Stoke Mandeville Hospital, Buckinghamshire Hospitals NHS Trust, July 2006*. London: Healthcare Commission, p.47.

23 House of Commons Health Committee (2009) *Patient safety: Sixth report of Session 2008–09*. HC 151-I. London: The Stationery Office, p.67.

24 House of Commons Health Committee (2009) *Patient safety: Sixth report of Session 2008–09*. HC 151-I. London: The Stationery Office, p.6.

on unbridled executive power – but who are, in fact, mere decoration and along for the ride. They also gain false credibility from supportive reports provided by health care professionals who have made their way into management posts, and whose professional knowledge and integrity sometimes become compromised in their eagerness to please.

The final comment on this should go to a non-executive director of an NHS trust, talking after having recently stepped down from a trust board. He explained that he had understood very little of what was going on, nodded sagely, agreed to budget cuts, refrained from posing awkward questions and maintained a consensus from a sense of honour. Disagreement would have been seen as bad behaviour. It was about being part of a happy family, whilst supervising an ongoing worsening of services. He likened it to a child playing with a toy steering wheel in the backseat of a car, tooting, signalling and flashing lights on an imaginary journey. As the child (the non-executive director) plays in the back, the parents (the executive directors) are in control in the front.[25]

BUILDING UP A picture of bad practice and neglect – in order to remedy it – relies partly on the reporting of incidents. Unsurprisingly, in trusts where care is poor and neither the board, nor the commissioners (PCTs), nor the overseers (SHAs) nor central government really want to know about it, such reporting may be sparse. Or, if it does take place, there may be little effective response – itself a discouragement to staff from further reporting.

In 2007, the Healthcare Commission published its investigation into deaths from infection at Maidstone and Tunbridge Wells NHS Trust. It found a muddled system of reporting and then managing serious clinical incidents, and that fear of bad publicity was a contributory factor to allowing this state of affairs to subsist:

> The minutes of the risk and governance committee in June 2006 noted a concern over the lack of clarity on reporting and managing serious untoward incidents. We were told that the likelihood of unwelcome publicity was the major factor...[26]

Ultimately legally enforceable guidance from the Care Quality Commission (CQC) states that providers should monitor the quality of service that people receive, identify risks and get professional advice about safe running of the service. They should take account of comments

25 Barker, P. (2006) 'All work and no say.' *The Guardian*, 5 July.

26 Healthcare Commission (2007) *Investigation into outbreaks of* Clostridium difficile *at Maidstone and Tunbridge Wells NHS Trust*, London: Healthcare Commission, p.79.

and complaints, investigations into poor practice, records held by the service – and advice from and reports by the CQC. They should learn from adverse events, incidents, errors and near misses – and also from the outcomes from comments and complaints, and the advice of other expert bodies.[27]

Under regulations health care providers also have a duty to report certain types of incident to the Commission or to the National Patient Safety Agency.[28]

In 2010, the Department of Health issued further guidance, aimed specifically at the NHS, entitled *Clinical governance and adult safeguarding: An integrated process.*[29] The major gist of the guidance is that when NHS trusts report serious incidents as clinical governance matters they must also be alive to categorising some of those incidents as safeguarding matters. This will then mean informing the local social services authority (i.e. the local council), which has overall responsibility for coordinating local safeguarding activity. The guidance makes no direct reference to the fact that systemic neglect in hospitals poses a large-scale safeguarding problem.

It does include an interesting example of a patient who develops a grade three pressure sore. Interesting because it appears to illustrate how the Department of Health is hamstrung, nervous and ambivalent about equating safeguarding and neglect with hospital policies, bed numbers and staffing – in effect, with resource issues:

> The investigation showed that the initial risk assessment of pressure areas highlighted the "high" level of risk. The patient was moved from ward to ward three times within the first week. A pressure-relieving mattress was identified as part of the care plan but was not applied until day 4 of the admission. The patient had a broken area by day 4. The mattress had been ordered but due to the numerous moves, and shift changes inadequate information had been passed on and reviewed. The equipment was therefore delayed in getting to the patient.[30]

---

27 CQC (Care Quality Commission) (2009) *Guidance about compliance: Summary of regulations, outcomes and judgement framework.* London: CQC, p.32.

28 CQC (Care Quality Commission) (2009) *Guidance about compliance: Summary of regulations, outcomes and judgement framework.* London: CQC, p.41.

29 DH (Department of Health) (2010) *Clinical governance and adult safeguarding: An integrated process.* London: DH.

30 DH (Department of Health) (2010) *Clinical governance and adult safeguarding: An integrated process.* London: DH, p.11.

A conclusion is reached in the example that, effectively because of the shortage of beds and associated chaos, there was no intentional harm or neglect. The inference appears to be, according to the guidance, that there would then be no safeguarding issue to report, as such a report would be triggered only by neglect.[31] The guidance is clearly hesitant; it flirts with the suggestion that the neglect of patients is a venial sin, as long as it occurs in the higher cause of finance, performance and patient throughput.

In this sense, the tone of the guidance has, therefore, arguably evolved little beyond the approach of *The NHS Plan* in 2000, which seemed to acknowledge the need to protect patients from individual rogue clinicians and health professionals, but not from systemic failings.[32] This way of looking at things echoes guidance issued in 2001 about the need to protect patients from a small number of 'problem doctors';[33] institutional mistreatment of patients was not highlighted.

In short, the 2010 guidance does not grasp the nettle. Indeed on this score, it represented an apt swan song for the New Labour government, which was to be deposed shortly after the guidance was published. Throughout its tenure, it had failed to take seriously, let alone tackle, the problem of systemic, neglectful care in the health service.

THE GUIDANCE ON safeguarding presupposes that incidents are recognised in the first place. In 2009, the House of Commons Health Committee noted that a National Audit Office survey showed 22 per cent of incidents and 39 per cent of 'near misses' going unreported – and that in fact the figures of non-reporting might be significantly higher.[34]

At Mid Staffordshire, staff became reluctant to file incident reports because of the lack of feedback and the perception that such reporting was discouraged. There was in any case uncertainty about making serious incident reports; for instance, a number of deaths that led to inquests were not filed as serious incidents.[35]

---

31 DH (Department of Health) (2010) *Clinical governance and adult safeguarding: An integrated process.* London: DH, p.11.

32 Secretary of State for Health (2000) *The NHS Plan: A plan for investment, a plan for reform.* Cm 4818-I. London: The Stationery Office, p.90.

33 DH (Department of Health) (2001) *A commitment to quality, a quest for excellence: A statement on behalf of the Government, the medical profession and the NHS, 27 June 2001.* London: DH, p.1.

34 House of Commons Health Committee (2009) *Patient safety: Sixth report of Session 2008–09.* HC 151-I. London: The Stationery Office, p.39.

35 Francis, R. (Chair) (2010) *Independent Inquiry into care provided by Mid Staffordshire NHS Foundation Trust January 2005–March 2009.* London: The Stationery Office, pp.19–20.

On Rowan Ward in Manchester, apart from the abusive practices taking place against elderly patients, there was generally poor recording, and learning from, untoward incidents. For instance, scald injuries or unexplained bruises were not being assessed, categorised appropriately or reported.[36]

At a drug dependency unit in the North West, the Healthcare Commission investigated because of concerns about medication. It found poor reporting of errors, and that this was associated with a shortage of experienced and qualified nursing staff and under-developed systems for reporting incidents. Although there was no direct evidence that senior managers tried to conceal the problem, the Commission suggested that the culture might have been such that clinical staff would not always have felt able to report errors.[37]

More generally, it would appear that not giving food and drink to patients has not been regarded as an issue – let alone as neglect – in many hospitals. In which case, it will not be reported. Had it been, reporting systems would probably have been overwhelmed.

And if it is reported, there is the further question as to whether anybody will do anything about it. In Mid Cheshire, incident reporting *was* taking place, in particular about shortages of nursing staff, lack of equipment, falls and medication errors. However, feedback was in short supply. Attempts at remedies, such as a system of yellow wrist bands, to identify patients at risk and to prevent falls, were ineffective. The patients who continued to fall were wearing the wrist bands. And the shortage of staff, for example, also led to the death of a patient with diabetes; the Trust stated at the inquest that it would increase staffing levels. Incredibly, or perhaps not, the staffing contingent subsequently decreased on the relevant ward.[38]

Perhaps though there is a bigger point, beyond the huffing, puffing and recriminating about how good reporting is or isn't. There is more than a suspicion that central government has laid increasing emphasis on reporting, precisely because of worrying trends that have developed and become built into the health care system. It cleaves to the hope that bringing to light a blitz of incidents will remedy defects; as if this would then excuse government from attempting to remedy underlying

---

36 CHI (Commission for Health Improvement) (2003) *Investigation into matters arising from care on Rowan Ward, Manchester Mental Health and Social Care Trust, September 2003.* London: CHI, p.12.

37 Healthcare Commission (2005) *Investigation into drug dependency services provided by Bolton, Salford and Trafford Mental Health NHS Trust.* London: Healthcare Commission, p.29.

38 Healthcare Commission (2006) *Investigation into Mid Cheshire Hospitals NHS Trust, January 2006.* London: Healthcare Commission, p.22.

problems. If this is so, it seems to be a vain longing. This is because evidence suggests that incident reporting systems in health care are very poor at detecting adverse events; it is therefore over emphasised as a means of enhancing safety.[39]

IF ALL ELSE fails, whistles are meant to be blown. That is, health care professionals are meant to raise concerns within their employing organisation and beyond if necessary. As Claire Rayner of the Patients' Association put it:

> If only the majority of good caring nurses...would stand up for their patients and their own profession, and blow whistles it would make a difference and bring back to them the sense of pride in the provision of good, safe care that used to be enjoyed by the whole population of this country.[40]

Fear and bullying, weapons of last moral resort but employed all too frequently, are designed to make sure that health professionals go with the flow, and also to deter them from spilling the beans, that is, from blowing the whistle.

The story of the nurse, Margaret Haywood, speaks volumes about whistleblowing in our health services. In 2005, she participated in a BBC Panorama programme about care at the Royal Sussex Hospital. Undercover filming took place. It revealed dreadful care for which Sussex University Hospitals NHS Trust apologised, admitting to serious lapses in the quality of care.[41] Patients were not helped to the toilet and nurses were filmed eating patients' food.[42]

In particular, the programme showed a woman literally gasping with thirst, cancer patients not receiving their pain relief medication in time and crying out in pain, a patient waiting two hours to be helped to the toilet, a nurse speaking harshly to a patient who had called for help, people not getting help with food and drink (including a blind woman), staff eating food intended for patients, fluid and food and weight charts not being kept, missing care plans, medication not being given, a low

39   Vincent, C. (2010) *Patient safety in the UK National Health Service: The events in Mid Staffordshire in context*. London: Imperial College, p.18.

40   Patients' Association (2009) *Patients not numbers, people not statistics*. London: Patients' Association, p.4.

41   Rose, D. (2009) '"Whistleblower" nurse Margaret Haywood struck off over Panorama film.' *The Times*, 17 April.

42   'Whistle blower charges dropped.' BBC News, 27 November 2008. Accessed on 5 August 2010 at: http://news.bbc.co.uk/1/hi/programmes/panorama/7752691.stm.

grade albeit experienced nurse being left in charge of a ward, and people wearing split back gowns for ease of nursing and so losing dignity.[43]

Margaret Haywood received no thanks, from her employer or her regulatory body, for the public service she had performed. By 2009 she was working in a nursing home; then, in April of that year the Nursing and Midwifery Council (NMC) struck her off the nursing register. This was for the breach of patient confidentiality that occurred in the filming of the programme, although no patients or relatives complained about *this*. In fact they had been complaining, previously and without success, about something else: the poor care being provided. The Council stated that what she had done was fundamentally incompatible with being a nurse, as she had filmed elderly, vulnerable patients in the last stages of their lives who could not meaningfully give consent 'in circumstances where their dignity was most compromised'.[44] The Council appeared unconcerned about all those nurses involved in depriving those patients of that dignity.

The NMC was out of step with nurses, the public and, as it turned out, the law. Within a month, a petition launched by the RCN attracted 40,000 signatures.[45] Later that year she won the *Nursing Standard*'s nurse of the year award.[46] In October 2009, the High Court overturned her striking off; she received a one-year caution instead.[47]

Lurking in the background, the Department of Health had responded to her striking off by effectively condoning it, implying she should simply have talked to her managers: 'We expect that any member of staff who reports concerns about the safety or quality of care to be listened to by their managers and action taken to address their concerns.'[48]

Such a statement, given the systemic nature of poor and neglectful care at the behest of managers enslaved by finance and performance

43 'Margaret Haywood interview.' BBC News, 20 July 2005. Accessed on 5 August 2010 at: http://news.bbc.co.uk/1/hi/programmes/panorama/4701521.stm. Also: 'Interview with Peter Coles.' BBC News, 20 July 2005. Accessed on 20 August 2010 at: http://news.bbc. co.uk/1/hi/programmes/panorama/4701921.stm.

44 Plunkett, J. (2009) 'Nurse who secretly filmed for Panorama is struck off the Register.' *The Guardian*, 16 April.

45 Laurance, J. (2009) '40,000 names on petition for sacked NHS whistle blower.' *The Independent*, 11 May.

46 'Whistleblowing nurse Margaret Haywood wins patient award.' *Nursingtimes.net*, 10 November 2009. Accessed on 5 August at: www.nursingtimes.net/whats-new-in-nursing/news-topics/whistleblowing/whistleblowing-nurse-margaret-haywood-wins-patient-award/5008374. article.

47 Smith, L. (2009) 'High Court reinstates nurse who exposed neglect.' *The Independent*, 13 October.

48 'Secret filming nurse struck off.' BBC News, 16 April 2009. Accessed on 30 July 2010 at: http://news.bbc.co.uk/1/hi/england/sussex/8002559.stm.

priorities, was thoroughly disingenuous. Indeed, a few months later, the Department's own chief nursing officer played a different tune. She called for the striking off of nurses involved in the sort of neglectful care outlined by the Patients' Association – exactly the sort of care exposed by Margaret Haywood. In making this statement, she remained silent about the undoubted link between such neglectful care and her Department's own policies.[49]

AT ONE END of the spectrum, whistleblowing is simply about raising a matter of concern with the employer, through management. This is what one would expect health care staff, witnessing poor or neglectful care, to be engaging in frequently. At the other extreme, it may involve going to the Press. Somewhere in the middle, it might be about getting in touch with a regulatory body. These are the three levels of whistleblowing envisaged by legislation which in principle protects whistleblowing staff from subsequent victimisation by the employer.[50]

The evidence suggests that professional, clinical staff are regularly either more or less active in, or at least witness to, totally unacceptable care being provided to significant numbers of patients. Some staff protest to no avail; others become ground down and inured to such care; still others remain unhappy but are reluctant, or fear, to speak out. This is particularly so in those NHS trusts where boards and senior management wish to hear only good news.

Understandable though professional quiescence may be, it is not consonant with professional codes of practice and other guidance. For instance, the British Medical Association (BMA) has issued specific guidance to hospital doctors about whistleblowing. It states that speaking up is a professional responsibility and an 'act of conscience'.

> Raising concerns with your manager is an integral part of a doctor's duty to maintain a professional attitude to colleagues and patients. Sometimes it has been seen in a negative way, but in fact it is a professional responsibility. Every doctor has an obligation to protect fellow colleagues, patients and themselves from unprofessional conduct or acts of clinical negligence. Speaking up is an act of conscience, knowing that inaction, while an easier option, may lead to harm to others.[51]

---

49 Smith, R. (2009) 'Cruel nurses should be struck off: chief nursing officer.' *Daily Telegraph*, 27 August.

50 *Public Interest Disclosure Act 1998*, as it amended the *Employment Rights Act 1996*.

51 BMA (British Medical Association) (2009) *Whistleblowing advice for BMA members working in NHS secondary care about raising concerns in the workplace*. London: BMA, p.5.

The General Medical Council (GMC) has issued guidance to doctors, stating that if the employer does not take action, doctors should take independent advice in order to take the matter further:

> If you have good reason to think that patient safety is or may be seriously compromised by inadequate premises, equipment, or other resources, policies or systems, you should put the matter right if that is possible. In all other cases you should draw the matter to the attention of your employing or contracting body. If they do not take adequate action, you should take independent advice on how to take the matter further. You must record your concerns and the steps you have taken to try to resolve them.

The guidance emphasises that the doctor's duty to raise such matters extends to situations in which patient safety is being compromised by inadequate resources or policies:

> You must give priority to the investigation and treatment of patients on the basis of clinical need, when such decisions are within your power. If inadequate resources, policies or systems prevent you from doing this, and patient safety is or may be seriously compromised, you must follow the guidance.

In other words, such guidance is clearly and highly relevant to the systemic undermining of the basics of good patient care – as illustrated throughout this book.[52] Medical doctors should, according to their own professional guidance, have been whistleblowing in significant numbers.

The Health Professions Council's (HPC) *Standards of conduct* state that protection of patients comes before other loyalties:

> You must protect service users if you believe that any situation puts them in danger. This includes the conduct, performance or health of a colleague. The safety of service users must come before any personal or professional loyalties at all times. As soon as you become aware of a situation that puts a service user in danger, you should discuss the matter with a senior colleague or another appropriate person.[53]

The NMC is equally emphatic, perhaps more so. It is impossible to reconcile the evidence in this book, of poor care involving nurses, with the standards demanded of those nurses – in terms both of providing adequate, or at least reporting inadequate, care. It states:

---

52 GMC (General Medical Council) (2006) *Good medical practice.* London: GMC, pp.9, 11.
53 HPC (Health Professions Council) (2008) *Standards of conduct, performance and ethics.* London: HPC, p.8.

You must disclose information if you believe someone may be at risk of harm, in line with the law of the country in which you are practising.

You must act without delay if you believe that you, a colleague or anyone else may be putting someone at risk.

You must inform someone in authority if you experience problems that prevent you working within this Code or other nationally agreed standards.

You must report your concerns in writing if problems in the environment of care are putting people at risk.[54]

Hospital social workers, too, are meant to adhere to a code of conduct. Part of this states that they should promote the independence of service users, challenge and report dangerous or abusive or discriminatory behaviour, report obstacles to the delivery of safe care – and inform an 'employer or an appropriate authority where the practice of colleagues may be unsafe or adversely affecting standards of care'.[55] Hospital social workers see vulnerable hospital patients all the time and must be accustomed to seeing patients being subjected to poor and neglectful care. It is unclear why they, too, are not shouting from the rooftops.

In addition to these professional codes and guidance documents, standards on better health care issued by the Department of Health in 2006 stated that staff should be able to 'raise, in confidence and without prejudicing their position, concerns over any aspect of service delivery, treatment or management that they consider to have a detrimental effect on patient care or on the delivery of services'.[56]

In 2010, the Secretary of State for Health put a foreword into guidance published by Public Concern at Work, also advocating good practice.[57] The foreword is a most modest gesture. So modest as to suggest that the Department of Health is two faced, or at least ambivalent about, whistleblowing. It cuts an altogether unconvincing figure. On the one hand, it doesn't want too much of it – for obvious reasons – when the subject matter concerns poor care resulting from its own policies. On the other hand, when it talks about the importance of whistleblowing it is in danger of transferring to staff – unfairly, unreasonably and

54 NMC (Nursing and Midwifery Council) (2008) *The Code: Standards of conduct, performance and ethics for nurses and midwives.* London: NMC, pp.2–3.
55 GSCC (General Social Care Council) (2008) *Code of practice: Social care workers.* London: GSCC, paras 3.1–3.8.
56 DH (Department of Health) (2006) *Standards for better health.* London: DH, p.12.
57 Public Concern at Work and Social Partnership Forum (2010) *Speak for a health NHS: How to implement and review whistle blowing arrangements in your organisation.* London: Public Concern at Work and Social Partnership Forum.

unrealistically – the burden of fighting against systemic faults of the government's own making.

The message in principle is unequivocal about the value and importance of whistleblowing. In practice, it is frequently neither encouraged nor welcomed. If you've got any sense, you will keep quiet.

IN THE LATE 1990s, at North Lakeland NHS Trust, it took two sets of student whistleblowers – subsequently praised for their bravery – to raise the alarm about the shocking treatment of elderly patients. However, in contrast, the hospital consultant, in charge of the patients who had been abused, denied all knowledge, saying that he had felt he was a stranger on the ward. The CHI expressed itself greatly disturbed at his passive role – compounded by the fact that he was associate medical director of the Trust with joint responsibility for clinical governance.[58] Nonetheless, the whistleblowers were subsequently intimidated and pilloried by other staff – and things had only got a little better when an external review was published. Even then they still experienced hostility.[59]

So, if other staff members do not recognise that something is awry, the whistleblower is not only up against it, but obstacles to change will be all the greater. The CHI had reported on 'unprofessional, counter-therapeutic and degrading, even cruel, practices' relating to elderly patients. It noted, however, that even during its investigation, following the external review, some staff still failed to recognise that abuse had taken place and that it represented unacceptable practice. The Commission had no confidence that further abuse would be reported or that the Trust would respond to it.[60]

On Rowan Ward in Manchester, the ball was only got rolling, culminating in a CHI report, through whistleblowing. Concerns had grown about the care and abuse – including potential criminal offences – of elderly patients suffering from dementia. During a training event, staff had expressed their disquiet. One nurse agreed to use the whistleblowing procedure; other staff later supported the allegations the nurse had made.[61]

58 CHI (Commission for Health Improvement) (2000) *Investigation into the North Lakeland NHS Trust, November.* London: CHI, p.15.

59 CHI (Commission for Health Improvement) (2000) *Investigation into the North Lakeland NHS Trust, November.* London: CHI, p.16.

60 CHI (Commission for Health Improvement) (2000) *Investigation into the North Lakeland NHS Trust, November.* London: CHI, p.1.

61 CHI (Commission for Health Improvement) (2003) *Investigation into matters arising from care on Rowan Ward, Manchester Mental Health and Social Care Trust, September 2003.* London: CHI, p.8.

It may take a lot of lip pursing for anything to happen. At Stoke Mandeville Hospital, nurses were extremely worried and reported their concerns about infection control and the deaths occurring from *Clostridium difficile* These were not, however, acted on. The nurses then contacted (three times) the RCN, which took a grievance against the Trust – but even this led to no real or sustained improvement.

Likewise, clinical staff at the hospital, including doctors, were worried about patient movement between wards, failure to isolate patients, number of patients on inappropriate wards and the consequent degree of clinical risk. Many senior staff wrote to the executive team; the response was that nothing would change unless a disaster occurred.[62] The nurses felt professionally compromised and helpless.[63] In the end, Buckinghamshire Hospitals NHS Trust only took action when details of the infection outbreak and deaths were leaked to the national Press.[64]

Leaking, anonymously or otherwise, is a big step to take, particularly if staff know that even ordinary reporting within the organisation – without the added embarrassment of publicity – is not welcome. For instance, one of the Department of Health's own reports into events in Mid Staffordshire recognised that:

> Many staff members did raise concerns, individually and collectively, but none experienced a satisfactory response. This discouraged persistent reporting of concerns. In the case of the medical staff, many appear to have been disengaged from the management process…[65]

The formal whistleblowing procedure was barely used.[66] One nurse did raise concerns, to little effect, with senior managers in 2007. A woman with a bowel condition had been brought into accident and emergency (A&E) with acute abdominal pain. A junior doctor wished to examine her but was told to get on and discharge her. She waited seven hours for an

62 Healthcare Commission (2006) *Investigation into outbreaks of* Clostridium difficile *at Stoke Mandeville Hospital, Buckinghamshire Hospitals NHS Trust, July 2006.* London: Healthcare Commission, p.28.

63 Healthcare Commission (2006) *Investigation into outbreaks of* Clostridium difficile *at Stoke Mandeville Hospital, Buckinghamshire Hospitals NHS Trust, July 2006.* London: Healthcare Commission, p.50.

64 Healthcare Commission (2006) *Investigation into outbreaks of* Clostridium difficile *at Stoke Mandeville Hospital, Buckinghamshire Hospitals NHS Trust, July 2006.* London: Healthcare Commission, p.28.

65 Francis, R. (Chair) (2010) *Independent Inquiry into care provided by Mid Staffordshire NHS Foundation Trust January 2005–March 2009.* London: The Stationery Office, p.186.

66 CHI (Commission for Health Improvement) (2000) *Investigation into the North Lakeland NHS Trust, November.* London: CHI, p.1; Francis, R. (Chair) (2010) *Independent Inquiry into care provided by Mid Staffordshire NHS Foundation Trust January 2005–March 2009.* London: The Stationery Office, p.281.

ambulance to take her home; she died the next day of a perforated bowel. The nurse recounted also how she had been ordered to lie about how long people had waited in the A&E department and how:

> Patients were left for hours, unable to reach the buzzer, shouting for help, medication, soiling themselves because no one would assist them. It was completely horrific… I kept thinking what if that patient was my mother, or my grandmother? The way people were being treated was shocking.[67]

IN 2010, IN what was regarded as a perhaps unusual and even landmark case, a hospital consultant, Dr Ramon Niekrash, won damages in an employment tribunal case, for the bullying and harassment he suffered from his employer. He had criticised the Queen Elizabeth Hospital in Woolwich for reducing the number of specialist nurses and closing a specialist urology ward, both of which he argued were detrimental to patients. The hospital responded by excluding him from the hospital and suspending him. The judge noted that there was a clear nexus between the consultant's actions and political and financial stipulations made by the Department of Health:

> What is immediately apparent is that there has been a tension between the professional desire of the claimant and his consultant colleagues to provide a good quality urology service for the patients and the requirement of management to reduce or limit costs and also comply with varying targets laid down by the Department of Health from time to time.[68]

Others before him have not fared well. In 2000, a junior doctor, Dr Rita Pal, decided to raise issues with the GMC and the Press about what she considered to be neglectful treatment of elderly patients on Ward 87 at the City General Hospital in Stoke-on-Trent, North Staffordshire. She had originally raised these matters within the hospital in 1998. Her concerns included lack of basic equipment such as drip sets, lack of support for junior doctors, lack of basic care for patients, inappropriate use of 'do not resuscitate' instructions and gross staffing shortages.[69]

---

67 Donnelly, L. (2009) 'Nurse warned about Stafford scandal: a nurse warned managers about the abuse and neglect of patients at Stafford Hospital more than a year before one of the worst scandals in NHS history was publically exposed, it can be revealed.' *Daily Telegraph*, 16 May.

68 Verkaik, R. (2010) 'Damages win for consultant who criticised cost-cutting.' *The Independent*, 3 February.

69 See: Marsh, P. (2000) 'Doctor quit nightmare of the ward; people put their trust in hospitals and that trust is sometimes being abused.' *Birmingham Post*, 18 February. Also: *North Staffordshire NHS Trust Ward 87: The evidence*. Accessed on 20 October 2010 at: http://sites.google.com/site/ward87whistleblower/home.

An internal report produced in 2001 for the NHS Trust found a substantial core of Dr Pal's concerns justified. Failings within the hospital identified by this investigation related to, for example, patient care, nursing, monitoring, care plans, adequate equipment, induction, supervision, staffing levels and allocation of patients to appropriate wards. There was also an inappropriate response to Dr Pal's concerns; the report noted that, although other medical and nursing staff were worried, only Dr Pal spoke up. This seemed to be because either they had become accepting of what was happening or they felt unable to raise their concerns.[70]

By 2003, she discovered that the Council was investigating *her*, rather than her allegations, and was questioning her mental stability and fitness to practise. She eventually took it to court, alleging breaches of data protection law, human rights breaches and defamation. The Council attempted to have the case dismissed early, by arguing that summary judgment should be given in its favour. The judge refused, holding that a defamation case could succeed. Before the case went to full hearing, the Council settled out of court.[71]

During the course of this hearing, the judge linked the GMC's reaction to that of a totalitarian state:

> For myself I don't really see why somebody complaining about the behaviour of doctors or the GMC, if that is what they are doing, why that should raise a question about their mental stability, unless anybody who wishes to criticise "the party" is automatically showing themselves to be mentally unstable because they don't agree with the point of view put forward on behalf of the GMC or the party... It is like a totalitarian regime: anybody who criticises it is said to be prima facie mentally ill what used to happen in Russia.[72]

In 1999, by the time Dr (later Professor) Steve Bolsin was giving evidence to the Public Inquiry into children's heart surgery in Bristol, he had been reportedly hounded out of medicine in this country and was working in Australia.[73] He had whistleblown and his concerns were fully

---

70 North Staffordshire Hospital NHS Trust (2010) *Report of the extended investigation into the allegations made by Dr R. Pal in November 1998. June 2001, 4th Draft.* Accessed on 20 October 2010 at: http://sites.google.com/site/ward87whistleblower/home.

71 Wells, T. (2005) 'Pay-out victory for doc.' *Sunday Mercury,* 2 October. See also: *Dr Rita Pal v General Medical Council* [2004] EWHC 1485 (QB), High Court, Queen's Bench Division.

72 Transcript, day 2: *Dr Rita Pal v General Medical Council* [2004] EWHC 1485 (QB), High Court, Queen's Bench Division.

73 'Bolsin: the Bristol whistle blower.' BBC News, 22 November 1999. Accessed on 20 September 2010 at: http://news.bbc.co.uk/1/hi/health/532006.stm.

vindicated, but the Public Inquiry noted that he had not been heeded and that the 'difficulties he encountered reveal both the territorial loyalties and boundaries within the culture of medicine and of the NHS, and also the realities of power and influence'.[74]

PREDICTABLY, THE HOUSE of Commons Health Committee concluded in 2009 that NHS workers were fearful of being blamed or victimised if they blew the whistle, that the NHS generally was unsupportive of whistleblowing and that the Department of Health should develop proposals to improve the situation.[75]

In 2010, the Health Secretary of the new coalition government referred to the need to protect whistleblowers and to tackle a culture of secrecy, fear and bullying within the NHS. Linked to the events at Mid Staffordshire, there was a need to give teeth to existing whistleblowing legislation:

> The previous reports are clear that the following existed: a culture of fear in which staff did not feel able to report concerns; a culture of secrecy in which the trust board shut itself off from what was happening in its hospital and ignored its patients; and a culture of bullying, which prevented people from doing their jobs properly.[76]

The Secretary of State for Health's new White Paper on the NHS, published a month later in July 2010, was silent about neglect, dignity – and whistleblowing.[77]

However, a consultation document issued by the government three months later did tackle the subject. It conceded that 'all too often staff who have spoken up for patients have found themselves punished rather than celebrated'. It proposed to highlight the importance of whistleblowing in *The NHS Constitution* and to talk to trades unions about terms and conditions of NHS staff including a contractual right to raise concerns in the public interest.[78]

---

74 Kennedy, I. (Chair) (2001) *Learning from Bristol. The report of the Public Inquiry into children's heart surgery at the Bristol Royal Infirmary 1984–1995*. Cm 5207(1). London: The Stationery Office, p.161.

75 House of Commons Health Committee (2009) *Patient safety: Sixth report of Session 2008–09*. HC 151-I. London: The Stationery Office, p.92.

76 Lansley, A. (Secretary of State for Health) (2010) *Hansard*. House of Commons Debates, 9 June, col. 334.

77 Secretary of State for Health (2010) *Equity and excellence: Liberating the NHS*. Cm 7881. London: The Stationery Office.

78 Suthern, K. (2010) *The NHS Constitution and whistle blowing: A paper for consultation*. London: Department of Health, p.6.

But no suggestion was made about amending legislation; *The NHS Constitution* creates no new legal rights. Furthermore, the government was silent about the consequences for chief executives and NHS trust boards which persecute whistleblowers – or indeed run such an intimidating system of management that people are unlikely to blow the whistle anyway. It is by no means clear that what is proposed will put in place the sort of heavy weight sanctions and protection that will make a significant difference.

The irony is best summed up by the consultation document's reference to Mid Staffordshire, and the fact that there were relatively few protests from staff about what was going on. It also states that 'the clinical instincts and professional ethos of NHS staff are the most effective guardians of safe, effective and respectful care'.[79] In case of systemic poor and neglectful care, associated so often with government policy and constraints, it would be a great deal simpler and more effective to change the policies and to stop NHS trust boards acting as they do.

In other words, to put the burden on overworked and sometimes frightened staff, to prevent systemic problems, is probably unfair and will not be effective. As the journalist, Beatrix Campbell, noted:

> Whistleblowers do what they do because the system silences them. It humiliates them, scares them and often sacks them. These whistleblowers have lost money, time, sleep and self-esteem; they endured nightmares not only about their own future but the safety of patients.[80]

---

79 Suthern, K. (2010) *The NHS Constitution and whistle blowing: A paper for consultation.* London: Department of Health, p.5.

80 Campbell, B. (2009) 'The persecution of NHS whistle blowers.' *The Guardian,* 11 December.

18

Denial, Accountability and Blame

> It is very clear, that whilst still representing a small proportion of the care being given by the NHS the numbers of people receiving substandard care are not small. The NHS treats millions of patients each year. Even if 2% of these are given substandard care this equates to tens of thousands of people. We feel the immense response we have had from the public is the best answer to continual rebuttals by NHS leaders and the Department of Health as they insist on ignoring the scale of the problem. (Patients' Association, 2009)[1]

Good or bad care is not the result of a law of physics. Such care is therefore not inevitable, because it is about human affairs and stems from human agency. This is why morality comes into it. Morality does not attach to scientific laws; it is about goodness or badness of human character or about accepted rules or standards of human behaviour.

In particular, neglectful care, unlike the law of gravity, is not immutable. This means that it is possible not only to improve matters, but also to hold individuals and organisations responsible and accountable for particular actions, omissions and decisions. Nonetheless, few within the health service step up voluntarily to accept responsibility for systemic failure; worse, those with the power to impose it seem reluctant to hold perpetrators to account.

Unthinking obedience to policy and priorities – just following orders – has undoubtedly led to some managers and staff crossing a moral Rubicon. There is no need to spell out where the blind following of orders can lead. Especially deleterious is the suspension by individuals of any independent critical moral sense. Instead, a hollow substitute comes in the form of deference to those higher up; if they are saying it is 'ok' and necessary, then it must be. Once people stop thinking for

---

1   'Patients' Association receives overwhelming public response.' Press Release. Patients' Association, 27 August 2009. Accessed on 2 August 2010 at: www.patients-association.org.uk/ News/289.

themselves and suspend moral and value judgements, it is fatal not just in the metaphorical sense, but also, for some patients, literally so.

There is a sense surely in which we must stop being so 'nice' about it all. What is happening to some patients is nasty, pitiless and brutal, we have to ask ourselves why we are so understanding of, and afraid to confront, the architects and perpetrators of this care. It may seem unfair to start to blame politicians, managers and staff; they will protest that they are merely trying to do their best. But if accountability is not imposed on somebody, how much greater is the iniquity to the suffering patient?

In 2009, Dr Thomé had been commissioned by the Department of Health to review events at Mid Staffordshire National Health Service (NHS) Foundation Trust. His report's conclusion about whether blame should attach seems to show muddled thinking about accountability. Certainly, the report condemns the care at the Trust but then bolts for the exit. Responsibility, it maintains, did lie with the management board and staff, including clinicians. Yet it concludes by saying that blame should not be apportioned, because NHS staff do not come to work to do harm.[2]

Such reasoning would appear to involve a major *non sequitur*. The fact that people do not, at the outset, go to work to harm patients, but then proceed to do so, does not, in any sense – moral, professional or legal – necessarily preclude the attachment of blame. Not least, it ignores the concept of recklessness which does not entail specific intent to do harm but which can still form the basis of criminal legal liability. The report is almost saying that everybody was too 'nice' to be fixed with blame.

If one is not careful, this approach is akin to the case of the nursing home manager, who provided the most awful care for a resident before the latter died from pressure sores. A colleague, who had blown the whistle, remarked that the manager 'wasn't an evil man... He was highly respected in the profession and the residents loved him – their eyes lit up as he walked into the room.' A nice man, just misguided? Maybe. However, there the parallel with Stafford Hospital pulls up short; the manager was convicted of wilful neglect and sent to prison.[3]

By refusing to blame anybody either within the Trust or further up the NHS organisational and regulatory hierarchy, the Thomé report

---

2   Thomé, D.C. (Dr) (2009) *Mid Staffordshire NHS Foundation Trust: A review of lessons learnt for commissioners and performance managers following the Healthcare Commission investigation.* London: Department of Health, pp.3, 14.

3   Hill, A. (2001) 'Tide of cruelty sweeps through our care homes.' *The Observer,* 18 February.

takes a deterministic and fatalistic approach. It fails to recognise the vital quality of human agency; this is unhealthy.

The seeds of such passivity may have been sown, in part at least, by the Department of Health itself, some nine years earlier.

IN HINDSIGHT, THE effect of *An organisation with a memory*, published in 2000,[4] may have diverted people away from pointing the finger of blame – and instead steered them toward looking at wider systemic issues. Such an approach is understandable if it means that individuals are not made scapegoats of unfairly; furthermore, the document did state that this did not preclude the imposition of accountability in case of criminality. However, it did suggest that most of the time this would not be appropriate:

> When things go wrong, whether in health care or in another environment, the response has often been an attempt to identify an individual or individuals who must carry the blame. The focus of incident analysis has tended to be on the events immediately surrounding an adverse event, and in particular on the human acts or omissions immediately preceding the event itself. It is of course right, in health care as in any other field, that individuals must sometimes be held to account for their actions – in particular if there is evidence of gross negligence or recklessness, or of criminal behaviour. Yet in the great majority of cases, the causes of serious failures stretch far beyond the actions of the individuals immediately involved. Safety is a dynamic, not a static situation. In a socially and technically complex field such as health care, a huge number of factors are at work at any one time which influence the likelihood of failure.[5]

This approach may be less than helpful in making politicians, managers and front-line staff think about the consequences of their individual actions. It seems to have knocked regulatory and criminal justice bodies off the ball, and rendered personal – and even organisational – accountability and blame a rare occurrence in cases of systematic neglectful and inhumane care within the health service. Nobody is left to carry the can.

This is illustrated in the case of Mr David Game, 87 years old, who died in Warwick Hospital following a hip replacement operation in 2009. The reason for his death was dehydration which had caused renal and associated multi-organ failure. Staff on the ward had not given him

4   DH (Department of Health) (2000) *An organisation with a memory*. London: DH.
5   DH (Department of Health) (2000) *An organisation with a memory*. London: DH, pp.xiii–xiv.

enough to drink and failed to monitor his fluid intake. Many of the nurses on the ward were from an agency because of staff shortages.

The coroner identified a management failure to identify the shortcomings of the nurses, failure by senior nurses to check the patient's condition and inadequate patient notes. He gave a narrative verdict that neglect either contributed to or caused Mr Game's death. The hospital's response was that it 'was not down to an individual', *but a systemic fault*; therefore no disciplinary action was taken against any staff members.[6]

Which, if we think about it, is a worrying statement; the hospital was in effect claiming that its system operated independently, free of human agency. The absurdity of this was immediately underlined by the information that the hospital decided, following Mr Game's death, that it might just be a good idea to do the absolute obvious: monitor orthopaedic patients with renal problems on a daily basis. Which it was now doing.[7] But if the system could be so easily modified by human adjustment afterwards, why not before? The further implication of the hospital's explanation, more concerning still, is that nurses, including senior nurses, are no longer expected to provide basic care on their own initiative, but only if the system directs them to do so. It is as if hospitals and all their staff have become so mesmerised by political direction, priorities and rigid systems that they have forgotten to think for themselves.

THE STORY OF prescribing practices at Gosport War Memorial Hospital illustrates the difficulty in establishing what happened and then holding anybody accountable. This is despite considerable effort and protest by relatives.

Concern about allegedly excessive prescribing practices for older people from 1998 onward led to a police investigation into a number of deaths at the hospital. By 2002, the Commission for Health Improvement (CHI) had reported its concerns.

Subsequently, however, the Crown Prosecution Service (CPS) declined to proceed with any prosecution. By 2007, not only relatives of the dead, but also a coroner and senior police officer had called for a public inquiry to be held. There were concerns about a possible 92 deaths. The Department of Health rejected these requests.

Unhappy relatives pointed to piecemeal investigations since 1998 by the police, the CPS, the local NHS Trust, the General Medical Council (GMC) and the CHI – all of whom, in their view, had failed adequately

---

6   'Warwick Hospital patient's death down to neglect.' *Warwick Courier*, 17 December 2010.

7   'Warwick Hospital patient's death down to neglect.' *Warwick Courier*, 17 December 2010.

to explain the large number of deaths. The patients concerned had been given doses of painkillers and other sedative drugs usually associated with terminal care, even though they were not terminally ill.[8]

Finally, an inquest was held into the deaths of ten selected patients; in the event, the jury stated that strong painkillers contributed to the deaths of five. However, the coroner excluded from consideration by the jury some or the whole of each of five independent, expert reports into prescribing at the hospital.[9]

Then, in January 2010, the doctor at the heart of the suspect prescribing practices was found guilty of serious professional misconduct by the GMC. This was on the basis of her potentially hazardous prescribing. She was not struck off, but allowed to continue to practise under certain conditions.[10] The doctor referred to unreasonable pressure and an increasing and excessive burden in relation to the patients in her care at the time.[11] At the end of August 2010, relatives were still protesting outside Downing Street.[12]

The case reveals the competing considerations. On the one hand, the General Medical Council disagreed with its own fitness to practice panel's decision merely to impose conditions of practice; the Council believed the doctor should have been removed from the medical register. On the other hand, it appears that the doctor was working at the time in circumstances beyond her control that were not conducive to safe patient care; and that since those events she had practised safely for ten years and produced 200 testimonials from colleagues and patients.[13]

POLITICS MAY BE the art of getting things done but it is also the art of denial. And the health service is plainly political. Which means that denial – and accusation – is employed in plenty.

In January 2002, allegations were made that Mrs Rose Addis had been left unwashed in blood-soaked clothing at the Whittington Hospital in London because no bed was available. Was it neglect or more a case

---

8   Lakhani, N. (2009) 'Gosport deaths "not important" enough to justify public inquiry.' *Independent on Sunday*, 26 April.

9   Semke, C. (2009) 'Gosport inquest evidence nobody heard.' *The News (Portsmouth)*, 22 April.

10 'Misconduct doctor Jane Barton escapes being struck off.' BBC News, 29 January 2010. Accessed on 1 September 2010 at: http://news.bbc.co.uk/1/hi/england/hampshire/8486936.stm.

11 'No manslaughter charges for misconduct GP Jane Barton.' BBC News, 18 August 2010. Accessed on 1 September 2010 at: www.bbc.co.uk/news/uk-england-hampshire-11008943.

12 'Gosport hospital deaths relatives want change in law.' BBC News, 1 September 2010. Accessed on 2 September 2010 at: www.bbc.co.uk/news/uk-england-hampshire-11151196.

13 Dyer, C. (2010) 'Relatives are furious that GP can continue practising.' *British Medical Journal 340*, 2 February, p.619.

of Mrs Addis not cooperating with the nurses to change her clothing, and her head not having been washed because it was bleeding? The facts became irrelevant. No sooner had the allegation been made than heavy political guns were brought to bear and the whole world of health seemed to go to war.

The government played out a strategy of 'swift, aggressive, rebuttal'. The medical director of the hospital, Professor James Malone-Lee, hotly denied the allegations, arguing that patients should not be used as cannon fodder. He was in turn labelled by the Conservatives as a government stooge because he was allegedly an active New Labour supporter.

The former Prime Minister, Tony Blair, took up the case in parliamentary debate; his office briefed about the case. The Conservative opposition, equally, sought to attack the government, arguing that the case of Mrs Addis was a microcosm of the NHS under New Labour. The Health Minister called for everybody to calm down, calling for facts not fiction; the woman's daughter took that to mean he was accusing her of lying. And so on. The essential point being that the truth – about this 94-year-old woman found crying in a cubicle in blood-stained clothes – 'was buried' in a political slanging match.[14]

This was a reminder of that great stoker of denial, genuine disbelief even in the face of the facts. For instance, in 2009, a Department of Health report about safeguarding vulnerable adults highlighted how the assumption – that, as a matter of course, NHS care must be safe – blinkers people to the obvious.[15]

Neglectful and inhumane care lends extra meaning to the word 'abuse' in the case of the NHS. When we are vulnerable through illness we have to place trust in those treating and caring for us, in whatever setting. But, in the case of the NHS, it is also an abuse of our trust in a major institution as a whole. The Public Inquiry into events at the Bristol Royal Infirmary, concerning heart surgery and the mortality rates of babies, noted that the NHS had been regarded as a beacon:

> A second influence of great importance on the culture of the NHS is that the NHS historically has been seen as more than a health service. It was seen as a national icon: a commitment to a particular set of values.[16]

---

14 Hinsliff, G., Harris, P. and Ahmed, K. (2002) 'The very public betrayal of Rose's private agony.' *The Observer*, 27 January.

15 DH (Department of Health) (2009) *Safeguarding Adults – Report on the consultation on the review of 'No secrets: Guidance on developing and implementing multi-agency policies and procedures to protect vulnerable adults from abuse'.* London: DH, p.39.

16 Kennedy, I. (Chair) (2001) *Learning from Bristol. The report of the Public Inquiry into children's heart surgery at the Bristol Royal Infirmary 1984–1995.* Cm 5207(1). London: The Stationery Office, p.265.

In 2009, the Independent Inquiry into events at Mid Staffordshire NHS Foundation Trust put its finger exactly on this hurdle of doubt. It referred to the refusal to accept, on the part of some staff and managers within the hospital, the 'enormity' of what had taken place, a scepticism that could be displaced only by the 'appalling experiences suffered by such a large number of people'.[17]

Such scepticism is unhelpful when flying in the face of the evidence. But it is understandable. Time and time again, in accounts given by relatives of the poor and neglectful care of patients, expressions of disbelief emerge. Until they see it for themselves, they cannot believe what sometimes happens in our health services.

When the penny drops, relatives express anger, fear, dismay, outrage, shock, disgust, depression and despair. And betrayal, as felt, for instance, by the wife of Mr David Perkins, whose care at Southend Hospital was referred to in Chapter 3 of this book:

> David worked his entire life, he was still working at 71 when he went into hospital. He had not been in hospital since he was 11 to have his tonsils out, but when he needed the NHS it, it failed him. I wanted to bring him home, if he was going to die I wanted him to have his family around him as I no longer had trust in the hospitals. He trusted me, I trusted him. I regret not taking him out. Had it been the other way round he could've picked me up and taken me out but I couldn't. I had to leave him in their hands.[18]

FLAT DENIAL OF anything wrong – even when plainly it is – is the defence of choice. It is as prevalent as the neglect and abuse it seeks to downplay. It runs throughout the NHS hierarchy, from the Department of Health down through the regional health bureaucracy (strategic health authorities [SHAs]), NHS trust boards, senior management and some staff. It amounts to a collective denial – political, professional and legal – at every level, about what are clearly serious problems.

Central government leads the way. In particular, the Department of Health has a strong incentive. As already emphasised, the health service is a hierarchical system run on a command and control basis. Concede systemic failure with systemic causes, and too easily the finger points

---

17 Francis, R. (Chair) (2010) *Independent Inquiry into care provided by Mid Staffordshire NHS Foundation Trust January 2005–March 2009*. London: The Stationery Office, p.4.

18 Patients' Association (2010) *Listen to patients, speak up for change*. London: Patients' Association, p.40.

at the chief executive of the NHS and above to government ministers. Inescapably, the NHS is a political animal, a plaything, idolised or dragged in the mud: portrayed in all her finery by the incumbent government and in her rags by the opposition.

Central government either denies a problem or dismisses it as isolated and local. More than this, it is active in making sure that nobody digs too deep to expose the opposite. For instance, in 2009, the Secretary of State for Health had steadfastly resisted calls for an independent inquiry following the Healthcare Commission's revelatory report into events at Mid Staffordshire NHS Foundation Trust. He wanted to draw the veil at that point. He was forced, however, by threat of legal challenge, into appointing an Independent Inquiry.[19]

The government still, however, made sure that the Inquiry would be prevented from investigating factors external to the NHS Trust – factors which could have implicated central government. The Inquiry itself explained this:

> It is clear from evidence given to the Inquiry that the public and the Trust's staff lack confidence in the ability of external organisations to effectively regulate and manage health services. It is clear there is more still to do to restore confidence. There is a widespread view that the system failed to detect and act upon the deficiencies of the Trust in a timely and effective manner. There is a genuine public concern that the present system of regulation cannot ensure that no such situations re-occur. It is clear from this evidence that neither the reviews commissioned to date by the Government, nor this Inquiry, given its terms of reference, are capable of allaying those concerns.[20]

The Inquiry needed both a magnifying glass and a telescope, it was given only the former. Thus, whatever the Inquiry's findings, the Health Minister, Andy Burnham, was always going to be able to state that Mid Staffordshire represented principally a local failure. Which is exactly what he did, instantly the Inquiry had reported. The Prime Minister chimed in and firmly blamed the local NHS managers.[21] Central government had taken great care not to be dragged into a midden, significantly of its own making and in its very own backyard.

---

19 Leigh Day & Co. (2010) 'Mid Staffordshire report leads to further partial inquiry, 26 February 2010.' Accessed on 12 July 2010 at: www.leighday.co.uk/news/news-archive-2010/mid-staffordshire-report-leads-to-further-partial.

20 Francis, R. (Chair) (2010) *Independent Inquiry into care provided by Mid Staffordshire NHS Foundation Trust January 2005–March 2009*. London: The Stationery Office, p.391.

21 Boseley, S. (2010) 'Mid Staffordshire managers must answer for hospital failures – Brown.' *The Guardian*, 24 February.

A full Public Inquiry was finally ordered in July 2010, with a much wider remit and with a view to reporting in early 2011.[22] However, we should not conclude that this meant the new government was less politically sensitive and defensive than the old; only that it knew it could blame its predecessor.

And it was only when he was out of office and after a general election that his party lost that the former Secretary of State for Health felt able to let slip that 'events at the hospital between 2006 and 2008 represent one of the darkest chapters in our national health service'.[23]

There is a further irony in the reference to 'dark times'. Back in 1994, Mrs Grace Huxstep, a 73-year-old nursing home resident, died in Dulwich Hospital. She had been living in the Greystone Nursing Home in that area of London. Her legs were covered with ulcers infested with maggots, with a blow fly in one leg. Her tendons were exposed. The Labour Opposition's health spokesman, David Blunkett, complained about the then government's system of regulation which was allowing a 'return to the Dark Ages'.[24] Little would he have foreseen that his own party, when in power, would plunge us all into the blackness still further.

DENIAL BY CENTRAL government has formed a predictable pattern. In 2007, the Healthcare Commission reported rampant infection, scores of deaths and very poor standards of care at Maidstone and Tunbridge Wells NHS Trust. The events were linked by the Commission to government policy in terms of financial and performance targets. The Health Minister referred at the time to the Commission's report as a 'truly shocking document' before reeling off the standard denial that it was not representative of NHS care elsewhere.[25]

Toward the end of 2009, the Department of Health issued a similar knee-jerk denial in response to the Patients' Association's *Patients not numbers, people not statistics*.[26] This report had detailed episodes of 'care' in other hospitals anticipating those revealed a few months later by the Mid Staffordshire Independent Inquiry.

---

22 'Health Secretary launches full public inquiry into failings at Mid-Staffordshire NHS Foundation Trust.' Department of Health Press Release. Accessed on 12 July 2010 at: www.dh.gov.uk/en/MediaCentre/Pressreleases/DH_116650.

23 Burnham, A. (MP for Leigh) (2010) *Hansard*. House of Commons Debates, 9 June, col. 335.

24 Kelsey, T. (1994) 'Pensioner suffered "Dark Ages neglect": maggots ate away woman's flesh in nursing home, inquest told.' *The Independent*, 9 April.

25 Rose, D. (2007) 'Hospital deaths scandal claims new victim as trust chief quits.' *The Times*, 16 October.

26 Patients' Association (2009) *Patients not numbers, people not statistics*. London: Patients' Association.

The government's rebuttal, as ever, was to the effect that the care revealed by the Patients' Association was not representative of what went on in the NHS.[27] This was despite the fact that, within a few days of publishing the report, the Association was inundated by hundreds of emails and telephone calls from people with their own stories of poor care.[28]

The Department of Health's response smacks of startling complacency; the Association's judgement as closer to the mark, balanced and realistic, when it referred to substandard care representing a small proportion of NHS care but affecting large numbers of people each year.[29]

And denial at national level is inevitably mirrored by the same at local level. Inevitable, because the Department of Health leads by example and, behind the scenes, imposes one politically-motivated diktat after another. Above all is the principle that NHS chief executives at local level must toe the line, stick together and preserve at all costs the reputation of the health service. The simplest way to achieve this, and to act in good faith, is to develop the mental skill of filtering and of shutting out the unwelcome. Then the denial, outlandish though it may be, is on one level perfectly genuine.

Not so far, in fact, from George Orwell's 'doublethink'. That is, the ability to play tricks with reality, to do it consciously enough so as to succeed with the chicanery – but also sufficiently unconsciously so as to avoid feelings of guilt and to believe genuinely that reality has not been compromised. At its very heart, it is about marrying conscious deception to a strength of purpose normally associated with total honesty. In essence, a monstrous system of mental cheating.[30]

In Cornwall, where people with learning disabilities were abused and neglected at the hands of the NHS, the investigating commissions noted that the NHS Trust viewed the problems as a result of the individual deviant behaviour of staff. It had no insight into the underlying culture, policies and practice that had created the climate for such abuse.[31]

---

27 Smith, R. (2009) '"Cruel and neglectful" care of one million NHS patients exposed.' *Daily Telegraph*, 27 August.

28 'Patients' Association receives overwhelming public response.' Press Release. Patients' Association, 27 August 2009. Accessed on 2 August 2010 at: www.patients-association.org.uk/News/289.

29 'Patients' Association receives overwhelming public response.' Press Release. Patients' Association, 27 August 2009. Accessed on 2 August 2010 at: www.patients-association.org.uk/News/289.

30 Orwell, G. (2003) *Nineteen Eighty Four*. London: Penguin Books, p.244. (First published in 1949.)

31 Healthcare Commission and CSCI (Commission for Social Care Inspection) (2006) *Joint investigation into the provision of services for people with learning disabilities at Cornwall Partnership NHS Trust, July 2006*. London: Healthcare Commission and CSCI, p.60.

In response to statistics apparently showing high mortality rates at the hospital, Mid Staffordshire NHS Foundation Trust – automatically it seems – had accounted for these as a problem of gathering statistics. Not for a moment did it seem to consider that the statistics might have actually been indicating that too many people were dying in the hospital. The Healthcare Commission observed that there was a reluctance even to contemplate, let alone acknowledge, that patient care might have been poor.[32]

A common refrain of staff who spoke to the Mid Staffordshire Independent Inquiry was that claims of poor care had been exaggerated and taken out of context; the picture was not as bad as had been made out. But the Inquiry heard from so many people about so many incidents of poor care that it could only conclude the opposite. It further pointed out that by publishing detailed written accounts of the evidence given by relatives and patients, staff would individually and collectively be able to acknowledge (and presumably take some responsibility for) the unacceptable level of care provided.[33]

> It is striking that in the face of a highly critical Healthcare Commission report, and the Colin-Thomé and Alberti reviews, so many former directors, senior managers and other staff appear to be unable to accept that the service provided by the Trust has been as bad as has been portrayed. This denial takes a number of forms. One group suggests that complaints may have been exaggerated or inaccurate. Some rely on their belief that there is much good practice at Stafford. Yet others believe the investigation or the report to have been unfair. Most resent the nature of the media reporting.[34]

Thus, local NHS trust boards and senior managers all too easily adopt a stance of collective denial. They are under great pressure to deliver to performance and financial priorities. They are wont to shut their ears and eyes, and then claim in good faith that all is well.

IF DENIAL FAILS, and the cat scrambles out of the bag, evading blame and accountability becomes the name of the game. There are three main levels, with many intermediate landings in between: central government, hospital board level and front-line staff.

---

32 Healthcare Commission (2009) *Investigation into Mid Staffordshire NHS Foundation Trust, March 2009*. London: Healthcare Commission, pp.3, 9.

33 Francis, R. (Chair) (2010) *Independent Inquiry into care provided by Mid Staffordshire NHS Foundation Trust January 2005–March 2009*. London: The Stationery Office, pp.49–50.

34 Francis, R. (Chair) (2010) *Independent Inquiry into care provided by Mid Staffordshire NHS Foundation Trust January 2005–March 2009*. London: The Stationery Office, p.180.

We have already seen how central government, despite keeping the NHS within an iron grip through the apparatus of the Department of Health, does not take responsibility for local catastrophes, even when it is deeply implicated. Nor is accountability imposed. Health ministers do not resign; neither do the chief executive and other key players at the Department of Health, when terrible things happen.

Yet, surely, Cure the NHS had a powerful argument when it stated that Andy Burnham, Secretary of State for Health, should have resigned when events at Mid Staffordshire became fully known.[35] The Secretary of State commands and interferes continually behind the scenes but then pleads detachment and ignorance. This is quite straightforwardly an exercise of power without responsibility. If Secretaries of State knew that they would be held accountable when patients were systematically neglected and abused, they would undoubtedly take greater care with their policies and political promises.

At the lowest level is the question of accountability of front-line health care professionals who have perpetrated or tolerated unacceptable practices and gone along with them. Being disciplined or sacked by their employers is unlikely to happen if the substandard care they are being forced to deliver is in line with that employer's financial and political priorities – which it often is. The further question of their accountability to professional, regulatory bodies – and their vulnerability, under 'vetting and barring' legislation, to being banned from working in health care – is explored in Chapter 24.

THIS LEAVES ACCOUNTABILITY at hospital board level. But when the finger does start to point at NHS chief executives and chairmen, they tend swiftly to slide away.

At Mid Staffordshire, the Independent Inquiry noted that the chair of the board was asked to resign (which he did) when the Healthcare Commission's report was published, but the subsequent Independent Inquiry commented that this meant that there was no process of accountability allowing for a fair determination of the chair's performance.

Likewise, the chief executive resigned before being suspended by the Board, which subsequently decided against disciplinary action on pragmatic and commercial grounds. So, again, there was no determination of the type of accountability that would have been expected, for example,

---

35 Smith, R. and Evans, M. (2010) 'Patients abused and neglected by hostile staff at scandal hospital: Inquiry.' *Daily Telegraph*, 24 February.

in the case of a doctor.[36] The chief executive subsequently avoided giving evidence to the Independent Inquiry.[37] He reportedly received a pay-off in the region of £400,000.[38] The director of nursing, who had presided over the disastrous scaling back of nursing resources at Stafford Hospital, had left the Trust by mutual agreement in June 2006; but within a year she was reported as employed by hospitals in Dudley to oversee cost cutting, ahead of an application for Foundation Trust status there.[39] (She was subsequently and belatedly given an interim suspension order by the Nursing and Midwifery Council in October 2010.)

Some years earlier, at Stoke Mandeville, the Healthcare Commission published its damning report into infection control and care standards on 24 July 2007. Shortly before it was published, the chief executive and the chair of Buckinghamshire Hospitals NHS Trust had suddenly resigned within ten days of each other. Both, ridiculously, denied that their resignations had anything to do with the Commission's impending report.[40] The chief executive received a £140,000 pay-off, despite the serious criticism of her management; she subsequently worked as an independent consultant to the NHS.[41]

At North Lakeland NHS Trust, where not just neglectful but plainly abusive and punitive care had flourished, tough action *was* taken. Three staff received disciplinary warnings, one was dismissed and one resigned. In addition, the Trust chairman was dismissed. The chief executive was suspended pending a disciplinary hearing and then dismissed. The director of personnel was dismissed. Other senior managers received disciplinary warnings.[42]

Pay-outs are not always the order of the day but redeployment within the NHS seems to be. At Manchester Mental Health and Social Care Trust, the abuse of elderly patients on Rowan Ward led to seven staff members being suspended. The chief executive resigned but, after initial

---

36 Francis, R. (Chair) (2010) *Independent Inquiry into care provided by Mid Staffordshire NHS Foundation Trust January 2005–March 2009.* London: The Stationery Office, p.23.

37 Francis, R. (Chair) (2010) *Independent Inquiry into care provided by Mid Staffordshire NHS Foundation Trust January 2005–March 2009.* London: The Stationery Office, p.8.

38 Rose, D. (2010) 'Stafford hospital caused "unimaginable suffering".' *The Times*, 25 February.

39 Sawer, P. and Donnelly, L. (2010) 'Nurses and doctors face being struck off for their part in the Stafford Hospital scandal.' *Daily Telegraph*, 13 November.

40 Green, T. (2007) 'Timeline: what happened and when.' *Bucks Herald*, 9 February.

41 de Bruxelles, S. (2010) 'NHS trust defends £2,500-a-day boss as value for money.' *The Times*, 29 July.

42 CHI (Commission for Health Improvement) (2000) *Investigation into the North Lakeland NHS Trust, November.* London: CHI, p.4.

negotiations for a pay-out, none was in the end forthcoming.[43] He was subsequently employed as a management consultant to the NHS.[44]

Similarly perhaps, yet another director of nursing at Mid Staffordshire NHS Foundation Trust, who had overseen such terrible care and reportedly left her position in 2009, was in 2010 still having her salary paid by the Trust; she was, however, working in the Directorate of Patient Care, part of the East Midlands SHA.[45]

THIS PATTERN SEEMS to indicate a tacit agreement between central government and, in particular, NHS chief executives and chairmen. The deal seems to be that chief executives will carry out, without question, orders from the Department of Health concerning finance and performance. They will also brazen out protests from clinicians and the public. In return they receive significant remuneration. For instance, at Mid Staffordshire, whilst care standards rapidly deteriorated and mortality rates rose, the Trust Board awarded itself very significant pay rises to celebrate achieving elite foundation trust status – on the back of a self-declared, though fictitious, high quality of care.[46]

Then, if necessary, there will be a closing of ranks all round and relative protection when things go wrong. Shelter will be afforded most of the time to chief executives and chairmen; equally, they should not break ranks by criticising their political masters. The agreement holds good by and large; chief executives and trust boards do what they are bid without asking too many questions, and when it all goes wrong – even very wrong with terrible consequences for patients – they generally escape with a reasonable amount of money, subject to a 'gagging' clause, and end up working still with the NHS in some capacity.

Sometimes, though, the accord frays.

SERIOUS STRAIN WAS placed on it following scandal and death at Maidstone and Tunbridge Wells NHS Trust. The events that followed the Healthcare Commission's report repay some study.

At Maidstone and Tunbridge Wells NHS Trust, the chief executive resigned in 2007 by mutual agreement with the Trust Board. This

43 Camber, R. (2004) 'Scandal ward boss leaves without a payoff.' *Manchester Evening News*, 2 April.

44 Linton, D. (2008) 'Scandal boss's new NHS job.' *Manchester Evening News*, 27 May.

45 Buss, C. (2010) 'Hospital scandal boss now trainer.' *Leicester Mercury*, 20 February.

46 Evans, M. (2010) 'Failed hospital bosses given pay rises while crisis unfolded: Senior managers who oversaw one of the worst scandals in the history of the NHS awarded themselves bumper pay increases at the same time as hundreds of patients were needlessly dying, it can be disclosed.' *Daily Telegraph*, 26 February.

followed the Healthcare Commission's investigation into the deaths of 90 patients. The agreement involved a sizeable pay-out which ultimately came to over £250,000. Then, instructed at the time by an embarrassed Secretary of State for Health to withhold the payment, the Trust did so. In 2010, the chief executive succeeded with a legal challenge in the Court of Appeal and received the full amount.[47]

So what was going on? The Secretary of State had weighed up the value of the compact of silence and complicity against the public outcry over so many deaths and such low standards of care. He decided that the chief executive would have to be thrown to the wolves. Showing the very determination that had made her hitherto so valued by the Department of Health, she believed she had been made a scapegoat. She was having none of it.[48]

Subject to a gagging clause when the pay-off was originally agreed, she did not defend herself in any detail at the time.[49] This came only later when the Secretary of State broke his part of the bargain. The legal case that followed and the arguments deployed in it are revealing. In agreeing the pay-out originally, the NHS Trust conceded that political expedience was in its mind. The High Court commented on this:

> By opting to seek to achieve a Compromise Agreement, the Trust plainly hoped to terminate Ms Gibb's employment cleanly, with a clean break and a confidentiality clause, making it easier to present a picture to the public of action taken in response to the report. I am sure the Trust had in mind that such an agreement would obviate a potential risk of a contest before the Employment Tribunal, which could serve to prolong the issues arising from the outbreak in the public domain, and distract the management from working to recover the position.[50]

Before agreeing to the pay-off, the Trust Board had questioned whether the chief executive's probity had been impugned by the Healthcare Commission report – given that the latter had identified a pattern of what appeared to be concealment of information about the outbreak of infection and associated deaths. A report produced by lawyers made no adverse findings on this score. In the absence of a lack of probity,

47 Jones, S. (2010) 'Ex-hospital chief wins £190,000 damages payout.' *The Guardian*, 24 June.
48 Hope, J. (2008) 'Family fury as report rules NHS will not be charged over 90 superbug deaths at hospital.' *Daily Mail*, 31 July.
49 Graham, M. (2009) 'Rose Gibb: I was victimised, demonised.' *Kent Online*, 27 January. Accessed on 5 August 2010 at: www.kentonline.co.uk/kentonline/newsarchive.aspx?articleid=55860.
50 *Rose Gibb v Maidstone and Tunbridge Wells NHS Trust* [2009] EWHC 862 (QB).

the Trust had concluded that there were no grounds for dismissing her; hence the generous pay-out initially agreed.[51]

This last point gives insight into how the health service sometimes thinks. In effect it is that terrible standards of care, under-staffing, over-occupancy of beds, broken-down and filthy equipment, lack of adequate infection control – and scores of associated deaths – all go with the territory. Somehow, they afford no grounds for holding chief executives accountable and for arguing that they have fundamentally breached their contract of employment.

The High Court ruled in favour of the NHS Trust's decision to withold the agreed payment. The Court of Appeal thought otherwise, basing its judgment essentially on the point that, as a matter of employment law, the Trust had itself decided that there was no probity issue and no grounds for dismissal. Thus, the original agreement to pay off the chief executive was not irrational and legally was well within the discretion of the Trust. Furthermore, the Trust had reneged on the agreement only because it was instructed to do so by David Flory, national director-general of NHS Finance, Performance and Operations.[52] In effect, on the instruction of central government.

The Court of Appeal was withering about the duplicitous nature of the game that had been played out:

> It seems that the making of a public sacrifice to deflect press and political obloquy, which is what happened to the appellant, remains an accepted expedient of public administration in this country.[53]

It continued, on the basis that it was dealing essentially with an employment law case (rather than a negligence or manslaughter case), to state that the Trust had been concerned only to placate the gods in Whitehall, even if this meant unlawful dismissal:

> The trustees took the view that one answer to such criticism, when the storm broke, would be that they had already taken remedial measures, and that the sacrifice most likely to propitiate the deities of Whitehall and the media was their chief executive officer, Ms Gibb. The fact that she personally had done nothing to merit dismissal was a problem, of course, but not an insuperable one. Provided the Trust was willing to pay the necessary price, she could be dismissed both unlawfully (that is to say, without

51   *Rose Gibb v Maidstone and Tunbridge Wells NHS Trust* [2009] EWHC 862 (QB).
52   *Rose Gibb v Maidstone and Tunbridge Wells NHS Trust* [2010] EWCA Civ 678.
53   *Rose Gibb v Maidstone and Tunbridge Wells NHS Trust* [2010] EWCA Civ 678.

notice) and unfairly (that is to say without any good cause). Both
of these were quantifiable in money.[54]

The chair of the Board also chose to break ranks. In a letter to the Secretary
of State for Health, the contents of which were widely published, he
was quite blunt in pointing the finger at central government, the grey
eminence. He related how the targets were applied by the Department of
Health inflexibly, meaning that the Trust's Board was forced to devote an
inordinate amount of time to them.[55]

WHEN RANKS ARE broken, one common refrain from departing chief
executives or chairmen is that they are being condemned to be the fall
guys for practices that are widespread; they have just had the misfortune
to have been caught and pushed into the public eye. For instance, in
1999, an Independent Inquiry into Eastbourne District General Hospital
identified a number of failings associated with poor patient care and
deaths. These included a senior management team described as autocratic,
centralist and unwilling to involve clinicians; unsympathetic attitudes
of nursing staff; excessive work pressures on nurses; and the skill mix,
management and supervision of nurses.[56] The Inquiry noted:

> There appears to be confusion in the minds of managers about
> the role of registered nurses and support staff. It seems that staff
> are considered to be interchangeable, and that pairs of hands
> rather than skills and qualifications are the priority. This gives
> rise to serious concerns about the consequences.[57]

The chief executive and chair resigned. The latter condemned the report
as inaccurate, that any problems stemmed from lack of funding and that
a similar review at other hospitals would reveal the same.[58]

They would say that, wouldn't they? Yet probably some substance
attaches to such protestations in general. Such is the prevalence of
problems in the health service, there is almost certainly an element of
'bad luck' in getting caught and pilloried publicly – whilst others, quietly
and unnoticed, go about their business and commit exactly the same sins
elsewhere.

---

54 *Rose Gibb v Maidstone and Tunbridge Wells NHS Trust* [2010] EWCA Civ 678.

55 Rose, D. (2007) 'Hospital deaths scandal claims new victim as trust chief quits.' *The Times*,
16 October.

56 NHS Executive South East (1999) *Report of the review of nursing at Eastbourne Hospitals NHS Trust*.
London: NHS Executive, pp.4–6.

57 NHS Executive South East (1999) *Report of the review of nursing at Eastbourne Hospitals NHS Trust*.
London: NHS Executive, p.8.

58 'They're not even sorry.' *The Argus*, 14 October 1999.

IN THE STORY *Heart of Darkness*, a Victorian seaman is gazing out over the great River Thames flowing at dusk to the sea and beyond to the overseas dominions. He narrates a tale to his companions about a distant continent and of slavery, racism, imperialism and a moral emptiness at the heart of empire. A company trader is dying; he has spectacularly hit quotas for collecting ivory but, in so doing, has come adrift. His entire constitution is wrecked. Dying, he refers to 'the horror, the horror' he has seen; and it is as much moral as physical.[59]

One can survey the splendid statements and claims flowing ceaselessly from Whitehall out into both the NHS and the world at large. Tracking them to their destination, we come across many good things but also an area of darkness. Including, as it happens, targets and other priorities pursued to astounding excess. Horror is in fact a word used by some relatives to describe experiences of their family members in hospital. We must be careful of extravagance and exaggeration in the use of language; but a reading of at least some of these accounts does not suggest that the word is ill chosen.

It is not just about what happens physically to patients, but about the moral implications. This is because nature, in the form of illness and the decay of the human body, is not necessarily kind and can be frightening, painful and hideous: in fact, precisely inhumane. So its physical ravages are unsurprising; they are indeed a law of nature. But we have great power, through medicine and health care, to alleviate the depredations of illness and to care for people in a humane way.[60] When those charged with such care do not provide it, we must ask how it is that they can stand back and allow such a state of affairs to arise and to persist. How can they regard it as nothing special, nothing out of the ordinary, indeed as simply the way of this modern world?

---

59   Conrad, J. (1973) *Heart of Darkness*. Harmondsworth: Penguin. (First published in 1902.)

60   See generally: Tallis, R. (2004) *Hippocratic oaths: Medicine and its discontents*. London: Atlantic Books, p.180.

19

Legal Implications of Neglect and Abuse

> My fourth, and final, heading relates to dignity in the day-to-day context, for example, caring for, feeding and toileting those who need assistance in these most mundane but also most intimate and sensitive activities. It is here, perhaps, that dignity has the most obvious role to play, just as it is, unhappily, precisely here that the dignity of the elderly and vulnerable is, too often and quite shamefully, ignored. One reads too often for comfort accounts of conditions in various institutional settings – hospitals and care homes – which are a disgrace to any country with pretentions to civilisation and which ought to shock the conscience of any decent minded person. (Lord Justice Munby, appeal court judge: on dignity, July 2010)[1]

It is with extreme reluctance that one turns to the law. It is not in the public interest to have health care professionals and managers running scared of lawyers, and resorting to ever more defensive practices. This is because it is not, ultimately, in the patient's interest. As Lord Justice Munby points out in the Foreword to this book, it should not be necessary for lawyers to spell out to the caring professions the fundamental nature of dignity, understanding, empathy and compassion.

Therefore, the overall solution to the neglect and abuse of vulnerable patients must primarily be a political and professional one. From above, politicians have to step up to the mark in highlighting the extent of the problem, and then making it a practical, rather than theoretical priority. At the very least, there needs to be a great deal more transparency, so that in a democratic system, voters understand better the issue – and, in particular, where current health policy and practices are threatening to lead us.

In addition, and from below, health care professionals must obviously begin to take more personal responsibility and action, rather than

---

1   Munby, Lord Justice (2010) 'What price dignity?' Speech at the Legal Action Group Conference, 14 July 2010. Accessed on 16 August 2010 at: www.lag.org.uk/Templates/Internal.asp?NodeID=93283.

remaining active in, complicit with or regular observers of undignified, inhumane and neglectful care.

But the law, too, has a role to play, if only, ultimately, as third fiddle. It is, or should be, a marker of what is acceptable in society. It is also a method of holding individuals or organisations to account, an important matter, given how elusive political and professional accountability has been in the case of neglectful care within our health services. If deployed effectively and publicly it may also be an effective deterrent. It is not desirable to over-legalise the health services, but it is equally unacceptable that patients should be subjected to degrading care when at their most vulnerable.

For instance, a genuine threat of individual or corporate manslaughter charges might concentrate the minds of National Health Service (NHS) chief executives and trust boards, with a view to a greater focus on patient welfare. Similarly, a few cases in which health care staff or managers in the health service were at least charged with the criminal offences of ill treatment or wilful neglect could have a much wider and beneficial effect. It would bring home to health care professionals how important it is not to become ensnared in not only unacceptable care practices but also criminality.

THERE IS NO shortage of law, civil and criminal, relevant to the neglect and abuse of health care patients although it is not used extensively or effectively against systemic breakdowns in health care, particularly in the health service. A summary of this law is as follows.

The *Human Rights Act 1998* is an obvious vehicle for protecting patients against neglectful and abusive care.

Ill treatment and wilful neglect are offences within the criminal law, situated within the *Mental Capacity Act 2005* and the *Mental Health Act 1983*. Further criminal legislation is enforceable by the Health and Safety Executive (HSE). A duty owed by NHS trusts to patients, under s.3 of the *Health and Safety Work Act 1974*, is of potentially wide application.

The Commission for Health Improvement (CHI), then the Healthcare Commission and now the Care Quality Commission (CQC), have been the regulatory bodies for health care providers. The last of these now has clear legal powers under the *Health and Social Care Act 2008* to enforce proper standards of health care. Additional and recently introduced regulatory legislation, the *Safeguarding Vulnerable Groups Act 2006*, bars workers, including health care staff, who have harmed vulnerable adults or at least poses a risk of harm to them. It contains criminal offences for breach of the rules it sets out. Likewise, further legislation exists, empowering professional bodies to impose sanctions against individual health professionals for professional misconduct.

In addition is government guidance called *No secrets*, about safeguarding vulnerable adults from abuse, which advises organisations, including the NHS, to work together at local level to protect vulnerable adults.[2]

Finally comes the civil tort of negligence, part of the common law. Negligence cases can be brought to seek financial compensation for pain and suffering and also to compensate for the costs involved of future care required as a result of negligent care and treatment.

A VERITABLE BEAN feast. One might ask, given that we are meant to be living in an over-regulated, litigious society, why there is so much law used to such little effect to protect people at their most vulnerable, when they are sick, confused, helpless and maybe dying. For some reason, from the lawyers and the judges one hears only a distant trumpet. They have not yet ridden to the rescue.

---

2   DH (Department of Health) (2000) *No secrets: Guidance on developing and implementing multi-agency policies and procedures to protect vulnerable adults from abuse.* London: DH.

20

Human Rights

> Where treatment humiliates or debases an individual, showing
> a lack of respect for, or diminishing, his or her human dignity,
> or arouses feelings of fear, anguish or inferiority capable of
> breaking an individual's moral and physical resistance, it may be
> characterised as degrading and also fall within the prohibition of
> Article 3 [of the European Convention on Human Rights].
>
> The suffering which flows from naturally occurring illness,
> physical or mental, may be covered by Article 3, where it is, or
> risks being, exacerbated by treatment, whether flowing from
> conditions of detention, expulsion or other measures, for which
> the authorities can be held responsible. (European Court of
> Human Rights: on degrading treatment, 2002)[1]

It seems odd that one should examine human rights legislation as it
applies to health care in a modern, wealthy, social democracy. This is
because the origins of the European Convention on Human Rights lie
in post-war Europe, in the years following 1945. The primary purpose
of the Convention was, and is, to protect the individual from the State.
Its drafters and proponents particularly had in mind certain regimes that
came to prominence in the 1920s and 1930s. There is no need to name
them.

It is a far cry from then to now, from that context to this – in fact,
to the local hospital down the road (or perhaps, increasingly, further
away) from you in 21st-century England. And that is why the Human
Rights Act should not be invoked lightly or trivially. It tends to receive
an unflattering Press in some quarters, but essentially the judiciary wields
it with a view to remaining vigilant. That is, alert to some of the abuses
of power that can tempt the State and its agents, unwittingly, down an
inviting path in the undergrowth of human affairs. A path that can lead
over a sheer and ugly precipice.

Are we to think that it is incongruous – and indeed disrespectful to
others who have suffered terribly in different times and places – to speak
of human rights when our father or mother, or indeed we ourselves, enter
a fine-looking new hospital for care and treatment? The response to this

---

1   *Pretty v United Kingdom* [2002] ECHR 427 (29 April 2002), Application 2346/02, para. 52.

question ought, in principle, to be in the affirmative. This would be to say that, yes, invocation of human rights represents a complete loss of perspective; surely nothing so awful can go on in our hospitals (or care homes) as to justify it. But this would not be the right answer.

THE *HUMAN RIGHTS Act 1998* brought into United Kingdom law the European Convention on Human Rights (ECHR). The Act applies by and large to public bodies only, because the Convention is generally about protecting individuals from the actions of the State – and sometimes about forcing the State to step in and protect people.

The Department of Health, National Health Service (NHS) primary care trusts (PCTs), NHS trusts and NHS foundation trusts all count as public bodies to which the Act applies. (As it does to independent nursing homes, also, but only in certain circumstances.)[2] The courts can hold that a public body is in contravention of the Act, force it to revisit a decision and to act otherwise in the future – and also impose financial compensation payment.

Not all politicians are in favour of the *Human Rights Act 1998*. But few would surely argue with human rights principles, in the context of health care, as set out by a cross-party Parliamentary Committee on Human Rights. In any case, this Committee pointed out that the legal implications of neglectful health care also go beyond the human rights legislation, to embrace common law and sometimes criminal law.

> Victimisation or neglect of older people within the health care system raises important issues of substantive human rights law under the *Human Rights Act 1998*, the ECHR and other international law obligations such as the prohibition of ill treatment, the right to respect for private and family life, physical and psychological integrity and the prohibition on discrimination (including the provision of health care on equal terms with the rest of the population). It is also potentially in breach of common law principles such as dignity, humanity and equality and, in particularly serious circumstances, criminal law. At their most severe, poor treatment could lead to an infringement of the right to life.[3]

In relation to neglect and abuse in health care, the obvious human rights in issue are article 2 of the Convention (right to life), article 3 (right

---

2   *Health and Social Care Act 2008*, s.145.

3   House of Lords and House of Commons Joint Committee on Human Rights (2007) *The human rights of older people in healthcare. Eighteenth Report of Session 2006–07.* HL 156-I, HC 378-I. London: The Stationery Office, p.5.

not to be subjected to, amongst other things, inhuman or degrading treatment), article 5 (right not to be arbitrarily deprived of one's liberty), article 8 (right to respect for home, private and family life) and article 14 (discrimination). The last includes a person's physical and psychological integrity.[4]

The Committee received evidence from inspectorates, providers and organisations supporting older people – all expressing concern about continuing poor treatment of older people in health care. The following list juxtaposed such care and treatment with the articles of the Convention:

- malnutrition and dehydration (articles 2, 3 and 8 ECHR)
- abuse and rough treatment (articles 3 and 8)
- lack of privacy in mixed sex wards (article 8)
- lack of dignity especially for personal care needs (article 8)
- insufficient attention paid to confidentiality (article 8)
- neglect, carelessness and poor hygiene (articles 3 and 8)
- inappropriate medication and use of physical restraint (article 8)
- inadequate assessment of a person's needs (articles 2, 3 and 8)
- too hasty discharge from hospital (article 8)
- bullying, patronising and infantilising attitudes towards older people (articles 3 and 8)
- discriminatory treatment of patients and care home residents on grounds of age, disability and race (article 14)
- communication difficulties, particularly for people with dementia or people who cannot speak English (articles 8 and 14)
- fear among older people of making complaints (article 8)
- eviction from care homes (article 8).[5]

The Committee stated that the Act gave legal force to concepts of dignity and respect:

> The *Human Rights Act* gives legal force to the concepts of dignity, respect, equality and fairness. It therefore has more teeth than any

---

4   *R (A&B, X&Y) v East Sussex County Council* (no. 2) [2003] EWHC Admin 167.

5   House of Lords and House of Commons Joint Committee on Human Rights (2007) *The human rights of older people in healthcare. Eighteenth Report of Session 2006–07.* HL 156-I, HC 378-I. London: The Stationery Office, p.9.

governmental initiative focusing on the need for dignity in care. The *Act's* functions are to provide a legal framework for service providers to abide by and to empower service users to demand that they be treated with respect for their dignity.[6]

The Mid Staffordshire Independent Inquiry, chaired by a barrister, noted that patients have a right not to be subjected to degrading treatment because of the *Human Rights Act*, and that in any case it was surely part of good hospital care not to be.[7]

Despite all this, significant numbers of patients have had their dignity seriously undermined over the last decade since the *Human Rights Act* came into force in 2000. The Committee may have made the point that as law, it has real teeth compared to non-statutory government initiatives, but no NHS trust has been found to have breached human rights through a failure to provide the most basic care, even when this absence has been associated with pain, suffering, total loss of dignity and death. In fact, no such case seems to have even been heard (or at least reported) in the English law courts.

This is a curious gap. Cases have been brought under the *Human Rights Act* on other matters, including treatment and detention under the *Mental Health Act 1983*,[8] the 'deprivation of liberty' of people lacking capacity,[9] the manual handling of people with learning disabilities[10] – and the degrading treatment of asylum seekers left destitute on our streets.[11]

The courts have even ruled that the Crown Prosecution Service (CPS) inflicted degrading treatment on a man with mental health problems, because it failed to take a prosecution against a man accused of biting off part of the complainant's ear.[12] Somehow, despite equal or far worse suffering, hospital patients have been left out; for them human rights law appears to be theoretical only.

The case about the manual handling of two adult sisters with learning disabilities in their own home did touch on matters relevant to hospital

---

6   House of Lords and House of Commons Joint Committee on Human Rights (2007) *The human rights of older people in healthcare. Eighteenth Report of Session 2006–07*. HL 156-I, HC 378-I. London: The Stationery Office, p.33.

7   Francis, R. (Chair) (2010) *Independent Inquiry into care provided by Mid Staffordshire NHS Foundation Trust January 2005–March 2009*. London: The Stationery Office, p.114.

8   *R (H) v Mental Health Review Tribunal, North and East London Region and the Secretary of State for Health* [2001] EWCA Civ 415.

9   *G v E* [2010] EWCA Civ 822, Court of Appeal.

10 *R (A&B, X&Y) v East Sussex County Council* [2003] EWHC 167 (Admin).

11 *R v Secretary of State for the Home Department, ex p Adam, Limbuela, Tesema* [2005] UKHL 66, House of Lords.

12 *R (B) v DPP* [2009] EWHC 106 (Admin).

care. The court reasoned that a question of inhuman or degrading treatment might arise in the following circumstances:

> Article 3 might well be engaged, for example, in circumstances where the consequences of failing to lift A or B manually might result in them remaining sitting in bodily waste or on the lavatory for hours, unable to be moved.[13]

Notwithstanding this dearth of full legal hearing and judgments, it was reported in 2010 that Mid Staffordshire NHS Foundation Trust was settling cases brought by patients on human rights grounds. The lawyers involved reported that they had:

> achieved a settlement on behalf of clients whose family members experienced ill-treatment at Stafford Hospital. The claims were all argued under the Human Rights Act and alleged that the poor treatment that the mostly elderly people received at Stafford Hospital directly caused, or hastened their deaths, or hastened their deaths through gross and degrading treatment. Leigh Day lawyers have settled 97 individual claims for just over £1.1 million.[14]

The same solicitors had, over a year before, threatened the government with a legal challenge based on article 2 of the Convention – about the need for a proper, independent inquiry to be held into events at Mid Staffordshire. The government had refused. The challenge was brought on behalf of the group of relatives, called Cure the NHS. It was on the basis that the European Convention required that the State properly investigate, with public involvement, deaths (under article 2) or inhumane treatment (article 3) occurring in NHS hospitals. Before the action was actually brought, the Secretary of State conceded the claim in part and agreed, in July 2009, to an independent inquiry.[15]

ASIDE FROM THE *Human Rights Act 1998*, is the *Equality Act 2010*, which came into force in October 2010. In so far as neglectful health care arises from discrimination against older people, there has in the past been no domestic legislation in force making this unlawful. (The *Human Rights Act 1998* covers discrimination generally in article 14.) This is because, in the

---

13 *R (A&B, X&Y) v East Sussex County Council* [2003] EWHC 167 (Admin).

14 Leigh Day & Co. (2010) *All Stafford hospital claims accepted.* 17 November. Accessed on 20 December 2010 at: www.leighday.co.uk/news/news-archive-2010/stafford-hospital-claims-all-accepted.

15 Leigh Day & Co. (2010) 'Judicial reviews and the Mid Staffordshire inquiries.' *News*, 12 May 2010. Accessed on 5 August 2010 at: www.leighday.co.uk/our-expertise/human-rights/mid-staffordshire-inquiry-1/judicial-reviews-and-the-mid-staffordshire.

provision of goods and services, domestic law has covered discrimination on grounds of race, sex and disability but not age.[16] However, the *Equality Act 2010*, when fully brought into force, will cover age discrimination involving the provision of goods and services, including health care. It remains to be seen if it is capable of making a difference.

IN SUMMARY, THE position is paradoxical, the message ambivalent. A formidable piece of human rights legislation exists which is meant to protect patients from neglect and seriously undignified treatment. It should be integral to government policy on the health service and to everyday hospital practice. It is not. Further, given how often it has arguably been contravened in the past decade, one would have expected the law courts to be awash with cases. They haven't been and they aren't.

---

16   *Race Relations Act 1976; Sex Discrimination Act 1975; Disability Discrimination Act 1995.*

21

Criminal Offences of Ill Treatment or Wilful Neglect

For some time before his death he had accordingly needed for all or part of the time one-to-one attention... Bit by bit the period of the one-to-one attention had been raised from a few hours to more hours and eventually, about 10 days before his death, it had been extended to 24 hours per day. That had been judged necessary by, amongst others, the manager of the home...and the care manager. They had described what would otherwise be the situation as "an intolerable risk to [the patient] and other residents". At about 4 o'clock or just after in the early hours of the morning of 27th September 2004 a call to the ambulance service was made from the care home. The patient was reported dead in his bed. The ambulance attended within a short time. Some two years after that, a police enquiry was launched and eventually in November 2008 some eight defendants were brought to trial. The kernel of the Crown's case was that the evidence strongly suggested that the one-to-one system of attendance had broken down and that the poor patient had died unattended. (Wilful neglect: legal case, 2009)[1]

The repugnant marks of neglect and ill treatment are evident in the health care practices cited in this book. Wilful neglect and ill treatment are criminal offences. Nonetheless, charges seem not to be taken against the health service for levels of care which in other contexts would be regarded as a crime and be prosecuted as such. This chapter considers what these offences look like, where and how prosecutions take place and why it is that hospital health care appears to form a separate and, to some extent, immune category.

CRIMINAL OFFENCES OF ill treatment or wilful neglect apply to people who lack mental capacity or have a mental disorder. These offences apply in any setting, in hospital or otherwise. They come under the *Mental Capacity Act 2005* and *Mental Health Act 1983* respectively.

---

1   *R v Salisu* [2009] EWCA Crim 2702.

The offences have been prosecuted on a significant number of occasions, particularly in relation to people in care homes; none seems to have been reported in connection with failure to provide basic hospital care, certainly not in the context of systemic neglect of vulnerable patients. It does not follow that this is because care in the health service has not sometimes sunk sufficiently low.

The potential application of the offences is clearly limited but, at the same time, also wider than might be supposed. A limitation is obviously that there must be a lack of mental capacity or a mental disorder. There is indeed no equivalent offence in the criminal law for people who do not lack capacity or who do not have a mental disorder, no matter how ill, vulnerable or helpless those people may be. This makes no sense and is a serious loophole in the law.

Another limitation is therefore that in addition to proving the circumstances of the neglect, lack of capacity or mental disorder at the relevant time also has to be proved. This might be problematic if a formal diagnosis or judgement about this was not made and recorded at the relevant time. Another obvious difficulty is that the patient might now be dead. For instance, at the Briars residential home in Southampton, the police investigation into the terrible conditions – and the pressure sores – of residents was made more difficult by the fact that many of the victims, nine in number, had died. Convictions for wilful neglect did eventually follow in 2010 but only after an 18-month investigation.[2]

That said, the existing offences may be of wider import than is sometimes appreciated. Under s.127 of the *Mental Health Act 1983*, it is enough that a person has a mental disorder and is in the care of somebody else – including in a hospital. Under s.44 of the *Mental Capacity Act 2005*, it is likewise sufficient that the person lacks capacity and is in somebody else's care, including in a hospital.

Furthermore, an elderly person in hospital may develop depression (even as a result of poor care), in which case he or she will have a mental disorder, now defined broadly in s.1 of the amended *Mental Health Act 1983*. Equally, a person may go into hospital with full mental capacity but – owing to infection, dehydration, malnourishment or serious constipation – become sufficiently confused so as to lack capacity at the time of the neglect or ill treatment.

---

2   Bennett, R. (2010) 'Women convicted of wilful neglect at filthy care home for elderly.' *The Times*, 7 August.

And if, under s.44 of the *Mental Capacity Act 2005* a person does not lack capacity, but the perpetrator believed that he or she did lack capacity, then a prosecution can still take place.[3]

THE TERMS 'ILL treatment' or 'wilful neglect' are not defined in either piece of legislation, the *Mental Health Act 1983* or the *Mental Capacity Act 2005*. The *Mental Capacity Act 2005 Code of Practice* notes that the offences are separate; that ill treatment involves deliberation or recklessness; and that wilful neglect usually means deliberate failure to do something that was a duty. In fact, recklessness will suffice in relation to wilful neglect as well.[4]

The courts have considered the meaning of ill treatment. They have stated that it involves:

- deliberate conduct which could be described as such, irrespective of whether it damages or threatens to damage the health of the victim, and

- involves a guilty mind (*mens rea*), namely an appreciation by the perpetrator either that he or she was inexcusably ill-treating a patient or was reckless as to whether he or she was acting in that way.[5]

On this definition of ill treatment, deliberate conduct is required, but not necessarily an explicit intention to ill treat; recklessness as to whether the conduct was ill treatment could be enough.

The courts have also contrasted the two offences. Wilful neglect is a failure to act – typically an omission – when a moral duty demands it, whereas ill treatment is a deliberate course of action.[6]

MANY OF THE reported cases, of convictions for ill treatment or wilful neglect, are not directly relevant to the systemic neglect and abuse of vulnerable hospital patients covered in this book. They are unedifying but give a flavour of how the offences have sometimes been prosecuted.

---

3 CPS (Crown Prosecution Service) (2008) *Guidance on prosecuting crimes against older people.* London: CPS, p.31.
4 *R v Salisu* [2009] EWCA Crim 2702.
5 *R v Newington* (1990) 91 Cr App R 247.
6 *R v Newington* (1990) 91 Cr App R 247.

Cases have included, for instance, locking people with learning disabilities for hours in motor vehicles,[7] distributing a photograph of a 92-year-old semi-naked care home resident,[8] hitting care home residents who had dementia and flicking food at them,[9] pushing, manhandling and swearing at a care home resident with mental health problems,[10] hair pulling and nose nipping of a person with learning disabilities with a development age of 12 months,[11] placing a bag over the head of an 88-year-old care home resident struggling to breathe[12] and encouraging care home residents to racially abuse and to kick each other.[13]

Such cases, and the above are but a few examples, are a reminder that, whilst this book has focused on the State-operated health service, the independent sector has its own struggles as well.

The neglect or ill treatment described in this type of case might touch on some of what happened at the North Lakeland National Health Service (NHS) Trust and on Rowan Ward at the Manchester Mental Health and Social Care Trust. That is, where the treatment is more deliberately abusive. Indeed, the police and Crown Prosecution Service (CPS) considered, but decided not to bring, charges under s.127 of the *Mental Health Act 1983* in relation to the events on Rowan Ward. The abuse that took place there included hitting patients, slapping them, stamping on them and twisting their thumbs.[14]

However, there are other reported convictions, again prosecuted in the context of care homes, which bring us considerably nearer to some of what has been occurring in the health service.

In 2001, two nursing home managers and a carer were convicted of a range of ill treatment under s.127 of the *Mental Health Act 1983*. This included administering sedatives to keep patients quiet, verbal

---

7   'Vulnerable patients locked in car for three hours while carers went to the bookies.' *Daily Mail*, 21 January 2008. And also: *Newton v Secretary of State for Health* [2009] UKFTT 19 (HESC) (details of conviction recounted in this Care Standards Tribunal case).

8   Cambridgeshire County Council (2009) 'UK nurse conviction makes legal history.' *News*, 24 August.

9   'Carer who abused elderly suffering with Alzheimer's and dementia avoids jail at Liverpool court.' *Liverpool News*, 13 February 2010. Also: 'Tammy Knox trial: care worker tells Liverpool crown court how he learned of patient abuse.' *Liverpool Echo*, 15 January 2010.

10   'Care home worker pushed patient.' *Billingham Evening Gazette*, 26 January 2010.

11   *R v Lennon* [2005] EWCA Crim 3530.

12   *R v Poderis* (2007) Chester Crown Court. See McKeever, K. (2007) 'Cruel carer is guilty in landmark court case.' *Wilmslow Express*, 15 August.

13   Gadelrab, R. (2006) 'Patients abused at care home.' *Islington Tribune*, 22 December.

14   CHI (Commission for Health Improvement) (2003) *Investigation into matters arising from care on Rowan Ward, Manchester Mental Health and Social Care Trust, September 2003*. London: CHI, p.9.

abuse, bullying, not taking people to the toilet when they asked, rough handling, kicking footballs at residents, throwing a resident across the room and leaving a resident naked and exposed by open windows and doors.[15] Some of the types of incident that led to conviction in this case are reported regularly of the health service – including, for example, not taking people to the toilet.

In this same case, a conviction of wilful neglect included delay in taking a resident with broken ribs to hospital for two days.[16] Presumably hospital staff not giving food and drink or essential medication (for pain relief) is just as potentially serious.

In 2008, a care home owner was convicted of the wilful neglect of Mr Peter Giles and sent to prison. In 2004, Mr Giles' brother had been on a ten-day holiday; on his return he visited the Abbeycroft care home, Blackpool, only to find Mr Giles unconscious, having lost two stone, with a black tongue, dehydrated and lying in faeces. He was admitted to hospital where the staff called the police. The Inquiry was drawn out over three-and-a-half years; the care home manager denied manslaughter but pleaded guilty to wilful neglect.[17] Again, in principle, this could all too easily have been a health service case.

ONE CASE, WITH distinct implications for the health service more generally, reached the Court of Appeal in 2009. An unnamed man died from natural causes in a nursing home on the night of 26 September 2004. The charge of wilful neglect, laid against a number of health care staff, was that he had died completely unattended, contrary to his care plan. He was 53 years old at the time and suffered from severe frontal lobe dementia sufficient to warrant detention under the *Mental Health Act 1983*. Having remained in a hospital bed for a year, he was then moved to a care home in which he lived for two years prior to his death.

Professional observers were unanimous that he had received a good standard of care over that period, and his family had wished for him to stay there. By the time of his death, he had lost the power of speech. He was not aggressive but lacked spatial awareness, bumped into things and people and might manhandle the latter out of the way. He was therefore

15 'Care home bosses guilty of abuse.' BBC News, 28 June 2001. Available at: http://news.bbc.co.uk/1/hi/wales/1412595.stm. Also: 'Patient abuse: Nurse struck off.' *BBC News*, 30 April 2003. Accessed on 20 September 2010 at: http://news.bbc.co.uk/1/hi/wales/2989241.stm.

16 'Care home bosses guilty of abuse.' BBC News, 28 June 2001. Available at: http://news.bbc.co.uk/1/hi/wales/1412595.stm.

17 Harrison, D. (2008) 'Care home death: "Nobody should die in such a terrible, cruel way".' *Daily Telegraph*, 24 May.

a risk both to himself and to others. About ten days before his death, his care plan had been amended to state that he required attention 24 hours a day; without this the risks would have become intolerable. Following his death, eight defendants were prosecuted, the essence of the case being that 'the one-to-one system of attendance had broken down and that the poor patient had died unattended'.

The identity of the first seven defendants repays analysis. They comprised four care assistants on duty that night, the staff nurse on duty that night, the general manager of the home and the care manager of the home. Convictions in the Crown Court were obtained against one of the care assistants, the staff nurse and the care manager (who had overall responsibility for the management of care and the one-to-one attendance of the deceased). The assistant did not appeal against conviction; the other two did. The Court of Appeal upheld the staff nurse's conviction but the overall care manager's conviction was overturned.[18]

This case is of particular note and relevance to other health care settings including health service hospitals. First, the wilful neglect complained of in this case on its face appears no worse – and is arguably, even, considerably less – than that suffered by many patients, as outlined in this book.

Second, there are many nurses – such as the staff nurse in this case – implicated in systems of neglect while on duty. The essential elements that led to his conviction were that the court found that there was both an 'objective' failure to meet standards and also 'subjective' recklessness on his part. This subjective failure included the fact that he had not given any instruction or briefing at the outset of the shift to ensure one-to-one attendance was maintained; he had simply left it all up to the carers. No one had been with the man when he died. And he maintained that he had carried out hourly checks but the evidence (including that relating to *rigor mortis*) suggested he was covering up his own failures, or those of other staff. Again, not of an order over and beyond that suffered sometimes by health service patients.

Third, the overall manager had been on holiday. This means that the courts are prepared in principle to consider whether absent managers – on holiday or indeed anywhere else – can be guilty of wilful neglect, not just the hands-on nurse in charge. True, the manager's conviction was overturned but not on the grounds that she was *in absentia*. Rather the evidence did not support the contention that she had either deliberately or recklessly set up a care regime, and in particular a rota system, which

---

18   *R v Salisu* [2009] EWCA Crim 2702.

was simply not good enough. In other words, had there been such evidence, not necessarily of intentionality but of a 'could not care less' attitude (as the court put it), then her conviction might have stood.

The implications of this case seem to be that where institutional neglect takes place – flowing not (just) from individual front-line staff but from a grossly flawed care system – then senior staff and managers could be at risk of being held liable for the offence of wilful neglect. This would be on the basis of, if not of deliberate intent, then recklessness. All depending.

A FURTHER PROSECUTION decided in August 2010 also points to the risk of prosecution against more senior members of the hierarchy in a health care setting. The owner and manager of the Briars care home in Southampton were convicted of wilful neglect under s.44 of the *Mental Capacity Act 2005*. The admission to hospital, and then death in August 2007, of a man with a large and badly infected bedsore was the trigger for a police investigation.

Residents were found malnourished and dehydrated, many had bedsores and ulcers and were in the wrong type of bed, residents were given inappropriate chewy food, floors were dirty, furniture heavily stained with faeces, broken and inappropriate lifting equipment was being used, dirty incontinence pads lay alongside clean clothing in the laundry room – and unqualified staff were routinely giving medication often to the wrong patients. The owner was given a suspended 30-week prison sentence and 200 hours' community service. The manager was given 200 hours' community service.[19]

A terrible case, but many of the characteristics of the care home could be seamlessly inserted into some of the descriptions of hospital care in the past decade.

IN SUMMARY, A significant amount of dreadful care provided within NHS hospitals is capable, in principle, of amounting to wilful neglect or even ill treatment. But prosecutions have not followed. The police and Crown Prosecution Service seem to have confined themselves to trawling for minnows outside of the health service.

The big fish, the great hospitals of the health service, appear too formidable to tackle, particularly if the neglect is institutional, embedded and not down to an individual. Almost certainly, if health service

---

19 Bennett, R. (2010) 'Women convicted of wilful neglect at filthy care home for elderly.' *The Times*, 7 August.

prosecutions do pick up in the near future, it will be in respect of the latter (the uncaring individual), rather than the former, type of neglect. This is simply because it is smaller scale, far easier to prosecute, less demanding of criminal justice resources and politically uncontroversial.

Such a state of affairs is understandable; it is clearly more difficult to pin down the essential *mens rea* (guilty mind) in criminal law if there are wider, systemic causes at work. Furthermore, nobody would want to see a hardworking nurse, health care assistant or medical consultant – dedicated but run off their feet – prosecuted for what essentially would be failings higher up the tree. Which might point to consideration, as in the case of *R v Salisbury*, of bringing managers – even senior – into the picture, who knowingly or recklessly bring about the conditions from which neglectful care is all but inevitable.

Manslaughter

> Following meetings with the HC [Healthcare Commission] and
> HSE [Health and Safety Executive], the police and CPS [Crown
> Prosecution Service] concluded that: the report did not contain
> sufficient evidence of a causal link between the actions of any
> individual and the deaths of the patients involved; and therefore, a
> police-led investigation on the grounds of possible manslaughter
> should not be initiated. (Statement about infection-related deaths
> at Stoke Mandeville Hospital, 2010)[1]

This book refers to many patient deaths associated with poor and
neglectful care. If a link can be shown between neglect and death, a
criminal manslaughter charge may lie. To be clear at the outset, no
such prosecutions have been brought when deaths have been many and
arguably caused by neglect and organisational recklessness. Manslaughter
prosecutions are, however, sometimes taken in the context of health
service hospitals, but against individuals for professional aberration.

A prosecution would need to show that neglect has caused death.
It is not enough if the neglect was awful but not, in the end, the killer.
This can be a difficult hurdle to get over; it may be that the patient
was dying anyway and the underlying condition was the primary killer.
Nonetheless, surveying prosecutions that do and don't take place, it
seems almost that the more lives that are lost in a hospital, the less likely
is a prosecution to take place.

Manslaughter is a terrible charge to bring against anybody. We do not
want a health care system in which dedicated professionals and managers
are running scared of the police and the Crown Prosecution Service.
Such a state of affairs would seriously impede the provision of health
care. The public good, and indeed the welfare of the population of NHS
patients, would be ill served.

But there comes a point when systematic recklessness with patients'
welfare and lives in a single hospital – such that tens, maybe hundreds
of lives are avoidably lost – raises the question of whether the public

---

1   HSE (Health and Safety Executive) (2010) 'HSE publishes investigation report into outbreaks
    of *Clostridium Difficile* at Stoke Mandeville Hospital.' *News*, 15 November. Accessed on 5 August
    2010 at: www.hse.gov.uk/press/2007/e07043.htm.

interest does sometimes demand serious consideration of this species of criminal law. And where legally villainous individuals cannot reasonably be located because of the systemic nature of the causes of the neglect – then the option of a corporate manslaughter charge beckons.

MANSLAUGHTER IS A common law offence that can be used to prosecute organisations or individuals. From 6 April 2008, organisations can be prosecuted under the *Corporate Manslaughter and Corporate Homicide Act 2007*.

One type of manslaughter in common law is known as involuntary manslaughter. This in turn divides into two categories: manslaughter by gross negligence or recklessness, or manslaughter by an unlawful act. Because gross negligence or recklessness is an ingredient of manslaughter, this offence is directly relevant to neglectful health care that results in death.

Gross negligence or recklessness does not precisely equate to deliberate intent; otherwise there would, of course, be a murder charge. On the other hand, manslaughter by gross negligence or recklessness is to be distinguished from ordinary negligence, which might give rise to a civil legal case for compensation. It is the 'gross' element of negligence that turns the death into a criminal matter.

Manslaughter prosecutions and convictions do sometimes take place in the context of the health service. They have involved severe lapses, in individual cases, of clinical judgements and interventions. For instance, 15 years ago an anaesthetist was convicted of gross negligence manslaughter. The offence occurred during an eye operation which involved paralysing the patient. A ventilator tube became disconnected; the patient had a heart attack and died.[2]

To date, there seems to have been no such prosecutions of either individual professionals, or National Health Service (NHS) trusts corporately, where patients have died following systemic neglect of basic care. However, the question of wider shortcomings in the system of work was acknowledged when two doctors were convicted and given suspended prison sentences in 2003 for failing to diagnose and treat a bacterial infection. The patient died; the episode had occurred after a routine knee operation.[3] The judge acknowledged that not all the circumstances were of the doctors' own making; defence counsel had

2   *R v Adomako* [1995] 1 AC 171, House of Lords.
3   Samanta, A. (2006) 'Charges of corporate manslaughter in the NHS.' *British Medical Journal*, 17 June, pp. 1404–5.

referred to under-staffing on the orthopaedic ward and to cumulative failure from top to bottom.[4] Nonetheless, the doctors were still convicted.

IT IS THE Crown Prosecution Service (CPS), following police investigation, which is responsible for taking decisions about prosecution; decisions not to do so are taken either for want of evidence or because it is deemed not to be in the public interest.[5]

In two particular cases involving systemic failings, consideration was given to prosecution: at Stoke Mandeville and then in Kent.

However, the reasons given for not taking forward a prosecution in these two scandals affecting the health service do not read wholly convincingly. This may just be because the statements made did not reflect the detailed reasoning, but if the statements are a reasonable reflection of the decision-making process, they are not reassuring. What is also unclear is how close, or not, the CPS came to launching proceedings.

First, consideration was reportedly given to prosecution of Maidstone and Tunbridge Wells NHS Trust – where up to 90 people died of *Clostridium difficile*, in association with shocking standards of care.[6] In the end, no prosecution occurred. The statement by Kent police did not refer – as might have been expected – to evidence being insufficient to prove that the poor standards of care were causative of any one individual patient death.

One reason why causation may represent a problem is that if you have a very ill patient, with other potential causes of death in waiting, who is to say whether the neglectful care killed them, let alone which bit of the neglectful care. But the statement did not seek to shelter in this particular lee. Instead it referred to there having been no grossly negligent act:

> Having reviewed the report and interviewed the author and the experts engaged by the Healthcare Commission, Kent Police has concluded that there is no information to indicate that any grossly negligent act has occurred.[7]

This is more surprising. The care standards at Maidstone and Tunbridge Wells NHS Trust were reported by the Healthcare Commission as appalling. They have been detailed elsewhere in this book. In addition,

4 Dyer, C. (2003) 'Doctors walk free after manslaughter conviction.' *British Medical Journal*, 19 April.
5 CPS (Crown Prosecution Service) (2010) *Code for Crown Prosecutors*. London: CPS, p.5.
6 Rose, D. (2007) 'Hospital ordered to halt pay off to chief after superbug scandal.' *The Times*, 12 October.
7 Hawkes, N. (2008) 'No-one to be prosecuted over 90 C-difficile deaths at Kent hospitals.' *The Times*, 30 July.

the NHS Trust had put targets before patient safety, resulting in suitable infection measures not being taken. If such an approach to the very lives of patients does not represent gross negligence, capable of potentially founding a corporate manslaughter charge, it is not clear what would.

Death from infection at Stoke Mandeville Hospital also gave rise to deliberation about manslaughter charges against the Trust Board. In this instance, the more obvious reason of causation was given as the reason not to prosecute, because no link could be made between the actions of any individual and patient deaths.[8]

This is more understandable, for the reasons already given. But even so, it begs questions. Even before the *Corporate Manslaughter and Homicide Act 2007*, it was possible to contemplate prosecution of the organisation if a senior mind could be implicated in what had occurred. The crux of the Healthcare Commission's report into events at Stoke Mandeville is that it pointed to the Trust Board's deliberate disregarding of infection control (and associated basic care) in the pursuit of other, essentially political, priorities and targets. This decision, in turn, led to the continuation of a whole range of poor practices associated with between 30 and 40 deaths. This might, one would have thought, have gone some way to serving up more than one 'senior mind' on a plate, enabling the organisation to be prosecuted corporately.

OTHER POSSIBLE PROSECUTIONS continue to be reported, but have so far not materialised. Inevitably, the events in Mid Staffordshire, revealed in March 2010, brought calls for a manslaughter investigation in relation to the many patients who might have died from grossly negligent care.[9] Specifically, when Mrs Gillian Astbury died in 2007 at the hospital after she had not been given her insulin, a police investigation was conducted into possible manslaughter charges against three nurses. In the event, in August 2010, the CPS decided there was insufficient evidence. Instead, two nurses were sacked and the third suspended.[10] A month after this decision, an inquest jury would find that Mrs Astbury's death was due to gross defects in care.[11]

8   HSE (Health and Safety Executive) (2006) *HSE investigation into outbreaks of* Clostridium difficile *at Stoke Mandeville Hospital, Buckinghamshire Hospitals NHS Trust.* London: HSE.

9   Davani, A. (2010) 'Police asked to consider corporate manslaughter charges at Stafford Hospital.' *Birmingham Post*, 9 March.

10 Corser, J. (2010) 'Two Stafford Hospital nurses sacked over patient death.' *Express and Star*, 30 August.

11 Grainger, L. (2010) '"Appalling" standards in care led to the death of Hednesford grandmother.' *Cannock Chase Post*, 16 September..

In 2010 also, it was reported that consideration was being given to a corporate manslaughter charge in relation to a younger adult who had reportedly the day before rung the police – because he could not get a drink in hospital, where he was being treated. The case had been referred to the police by Westminster Coroner's Court.[12]

Corporate manslaughter charges were also contemplated in 2009 against the Sussex Partnership NHS Trust, following several suicides at a mental hospital, the Woodlands Unit in Hastings.[13]

It is of course speculation only, but a suspicion must linger that an unspoken public interest test is being applied; prosecution in the case of systemic neglect in the health service – resulting from lack of staff, lack of beds and obsession with priorities other than patient welfare, and all connected to government policy – would prise open a can of highly unwelcome political worms.

THE APPARENT RELUCTANCE to try to prosecute corporately or otherwise in the context of the health service, even in the case of shocking standards of care and many deaths, does seem to contrast starkly with manslaughter prosecutions in other contexts, such as care homes and people's own homes.

In July 1999, Mrs Marion Dennis died from grossly negligent care of her pressure ulcers in Ballastowell Gardens nursing home on the Isle of Man. The manager and deputy manager of the home were both convicted. Mrs Dennis's pressure sores were as large as fists and gave off an overpowering smell of rotting flesh. The two nurses blamed the system, a defence rejected by the jury.[14] In another care home, two nurses were convicted of manslaughter for failing to give an epileptic resident her medication and then failing, during a period of two-and-a-half hours, to call an ambulance during a fit.[15] Neither of these cases, in principle, exceeds some of what is described in this book.

A council architect and Barrow Council were both prosecuted for manslaughter after a number of people died of Legionnaire's disease at a council arts centre. The architect had cancelled a maintenance and inspection contract for the air conditioning system. Five people died

---

12 Moore-Bridger, B. (2010) 'Hospital manslaughter inquiry after patient dies begging for water.' *Daily Mail*, 8 March.

13 Walker, E. (2010) 'Hastings hospital at centre of police inquiry will reopen.' *The Argus*, 10 April.

14 'Nurses guilty of neglect by death.' BBC News, 27 October 2003. Accessed on 19 January 2011 at: http://news.bbc.co.uk/1/hi/england/3218847.stm.

15 'Nurse guilty of gross negligence.' BBC News, 19 March 2008. Accessed on 5 August 2010 at: http://news.bbc.co.uk/1/hi/england/west_midlands/7305598.stm.

and another 172 were infected. The manslaughter case failed; both the architect and the Council were subsequently convicted of health and safety at work offences and fined.[16] One cannot but reflect that this short cut taken, in relation to maintenance of a piece of machinery, cannot be worse than the systematic neglect visited upon vulnerable patients in hospital – resulting in widespread infection associated with far more deaths than occurred in Barrow.

ALSO STRIKING IS the realisation that manslaughter cases are sometimes brought against people for failing reasonably to care for relatives in their own homes. This has occurred even when the defendant is less than equipped, psychologically and mentally, to supply the care and attention needed. It is almost as though a greater burden is being put on such people than on powerful managers and highly trained professionals in hospitals.

On 3 August, Ms Fanny Stone died. She was living at the time with her brother and his partner. They were both convicted of her manslaughter. She had come to stay with them three years before. She had lived in a room without ventilation, toilet or washing facilities and became very infirm, denying herself proper food. In the end, she died of toxaemia from infected bedsores, immobilisation and lack of food. Her brother and his partner made initial half-hearted, and then no, efforts to do anything about her deteriorating condition. They told neither the general practitioner (GP) nor the social worker who used to visit the man's 34-year-old, mentally impaired son. The couple were convicted of gross negligence manslaughter.

This was despite the fact that the brother, 67 years old, ex-miner and widower, was described as partially deaf, almost blind, of low intelligence and with no appreciable sense of smell. His partner, functioning as housekeeper and mistress, was characterised as ineffectual and inadequate.[17] The Court of Appeal, upholding the conviction but reducing the sentence, stated that the recklessness ingredient necessitated:

> ...reckless disregard of danger to the health and welfare of the infirm person...[with] the defendant being indifferent to an obvious risk of injury to health, or actually to have foreseen the risk but to have determined nevertheless to run it.[18]

---

16 Hogg, D. (2006) 'Architect fined over deadly outbreak of disease.' *Yorkshire Post*, 1 August.

17 *R v Stone* (1977) 64 Cr App R 186.

18 *R v Stone* (1977) 64 Cr App R 186.

This definition given by the Court of Appeal would appear to fit uncannily with what occurred, for example at Stoke Mandeville, at Maidstone and Tunbridge Wells NHS Trust – and at Mid Staffordshire NHS Foundation Trust. For instance, the indifference underlying the response given to doctors who had raised with the Trust's executives the risk to patients at Stoke Mandeville; namely, that nothing would change unless a disaster occurred.[19] Which it did.

Another domestic case involved the conviction of a man for the manslaughter of his mother. She was described as stubborn, domineering, hugely independent – and as someone who shunned help from doctors and home helps. Her son, in his fifties, had always lived with her. He had limited education and had worked as a labourer from the age of 15. He had never had a girlfriend. His sole friend was his aunt.

One January, he called an ambulance. His mother had severe bedsores all over her body. One, the size of two fists, had penetrated her sacrum. They were probably caused by lying in urine and faeces. She had been suffering from breast cancer. In the previous few months, as she had deteriorated, he had attended her bedsores, but not called a doctor. In the end, he had stopped looking after the wound on her back as it was too difficult to do so. He gave her drinks, hot meals and whisky. He was sentenced to four years in prison.[20]

In a third case, a man was convicted of the manslaughter of his wife. He had been her sole carer. She suffered from brittle bones; she fell and sustained a number of fractures. He failed to call an ambulance for three weeks; when he finally did so, she then died of pneumonia in hospital a few weeks later. She had not wanted to go to hospital and he could have called for assistance himself. His four-year sentence was subsequently reduced to 30 months.[21]

Such individuals are soft targets in that the perpetrator is easily identifiable with fewer variable and complicating factors involved. The hard, corporate targets go unhindered, despite some of their behaviour being arguably far more reprehensible than that depicted in these tragic, domestic cases. They are shielded by reams of protective documents, policies, risk assessments and procedures which may depict a fiction – but which nevertheless make it harder to prove reckless, gross negligence.

19 Healthcare Commission (2006) *Investigation into outbreaks of* Clostridium difficile *at Stoke Mandeville Hospital, Buckinghamshire Hospitals NHS Trust, July 2006.* London: Healthcare Commission, p.28.

20 *Land v Land* [2006] EWHC 2997 (Ch).

21 *R v Hood* [2003] EWCA Crim 2772.

So it is that senior management, the focus of a corporate manslaughter prosecution, can throw up a smokescreen. Behind which they would plead the sanctuary of ignorance and of having made reasonable efforts.

23

Health and Safety at Work Legislation

The Healthcare Commission report alleged a series of failings by the Trust and individuals. We have reviewed the report through a series of interviews with the Healthcare Commission's lead investigator and all the experts who considered the information gathered by the Healthcare Commission in compiling their report.

We share the police's conclusion that, from the information available, we cannot establish with certainty a causal link between failings to manage infection and the death of any particular person.

From the interviews with the experts who advised the Healthcare Commission we also concluded that there was insufficient information to link the actions of any individual with the spread of infection or to show that any senior managers within the Trust was personally responsible for any direct failure that led to infection. (Health and Safety Executive and police decide not to investigate the circumstances of 90 deaths at Maidstone and Tunbridge Wells NHS Trust, 2008)[1]

The background to the above statement involved events in Kent and any number of breaches of basic health and safety associated with a large number of deaths. The puzzling aspect to the statement is that harm, let alone death, is not a requirement for breach of health and safety at work legislation.

More generally, filthy environments, contaminated and faulty equipment, under-staffing, incompetent staff, starving patients of nutrition, avoidable development of pressure sores, soiled beds and clothing, sending confused and sick patients home in the middle of the night – all these and more point to unsafe systems of work directly responsible for harming, and placing at risk of harm, significant numbers of vulnerable patients.

---

1   HSE (Health and Safety Executive) (2008) 'HSE and Kent Police decide not to investigate Maidstone and Tunbridge Wells NHS Trust.' *News*, 30 July. Accessed on 5 August 2010 at: www.hse.gov.uk/press/2008/e08038.htm.

There is wide ranging health and safety at work legislation under which such grossly defective systems of work could constitute a criminal offence of which an organisation could be guilty. But the enforcement agency, the Health and Safety Executive, with the power to wield this legislation and to prosecute has decided not to do so. Instead, it has not only kept its powder largely dry, but has more or less retired from this particular field.

THE HEALTH AND Safety Executive (HSE) is responsible for prosecuting offences committed under the *Health and Safety at Work Act 1974*. It normally prosecutes organisations but is able to, and sometimes does, prosecute individuals.

There are various duties contained within the *1974 Act*. Under s.3, there is a duty on the employer to conduct its undertaking in such a way as to ensure, so far as is reasonably practicable, that non-employees who may be affected are not exposed to risks to their health and safety. In addition, under r.3 of the *Management of Health and Safety at Work Regulations 1999*, there is a duty to carry out a suitable and sufficient assessment of the risks to the health and safety of non-employees arising from, or connected with, the employer's undertaking.

Under s.7 of the *1974 Act*, individual employees have a duty to take reasonable care of their own health and safety and also that of other people who may be affected by the employee's acts or failure to act.

And under s.37 of the *1974 Act*, if an offence – such as under s.3 – is committed by the organisation, a director or manager will also be guilty individually, if it is proved that the offence was committed with their consent, their connivance or through their neglect.

ON THE FACE of it, the above duties are easily capable of covering systems of work in hospitals which directly lead to neglect – for example, grossly inadequate staffing levels, lack of hygiene, not helping people eat and drink, not taking people to the toilet, not managing pressure sores and not keeping equipment and the environment clean and in hygienic working order.

Furthermore and most importantly, actual harm does not have to be demonstrated, merely that reasonably practicable efforts have not been made to protect the health and safety of patients. This contrasts with a prosecution for manslaughter which needs to show not just grossly negligent care but also that this directly caused the death of one or more patients. This absence, of the requirement of causation of harm, would suggest that frequent prosecutions would have taken place in relation to systems of neglectful care reported in the health service over the last decade and more.

Not at all.

THIS TAKES A bit of disentangling. By and large, the HSE has shied away from prosecution for systemic, neglectful care. It works to a self-imposed restriction of excluding clinical matters. This is on the basis that standards of clinical governance, including systems of work, are the responsibility of the Department of Health and the Care Quality Commission (CQC). The HSE claims for its own 'non-clinical' risks to patients including trips, falls, scalding and some issues concerning health care-related infection.

The HSE does concede that the distinction between 'clinical risk management' and 'health and safety management' is not clear.[2] Well it might. For example, the HSE did consider whether a prosecution might be warranted when over 30 people died of *Clostridium difficile* at Stoke Mandeville hospital.[3] The reason for not proceeding was unconvincing: an unrealistic prospect of securing a conviction. The HSE did at least concede that an outbreak of infection, arising not from individual clinical judgement but instead, from an National Health Service (NHS) trust's system for managing infection, was within its purview.[4]

THIS CONCESSION IS significant because the systemic neglectful care described in this book is almost all the result of defective systems of work rather than individual clinical error or misjudgement. The logic of the concession made in this instance is that the HSE would and should look hard at systemic neglect. But it is not in practice doing so, even when the facts are staring it in the face.

Yet here was an NHS Trust that the Healthcare Commission had exposed as ignoring the advice of its own infection control team and failing to put in place basic precautionary measures. This was at least partly because to have done so would have jeopardised the hitting of finance and performance targets. As to whether such measures would have been reasonably practicable, the Trust changed its approach as soon

---

2   HSE (Health and Safety Executive) (2006) *Priorities for enforcement of Section 3 of the HSWA 1974 – July 2003* (rev. Oct 2006). Accessed on 19 January 2011 at: www.hse.gov.uk/enforce/hswact/priorities.htm#clinical.

3   HSE (Health and Safety Executive) (2006) *HSE investigation into outbreaks of* Clostridium difficile *at Stoke Mandeville Hospital, Buckinghamshire Hospitals NHS Trust.* London: HSE.

4   HSE (Health and Safety Executive) (2006) *HSE investigation into outbreaks of* Clostridium difficile *at Stoke Mandeville Hospital, Buckinghamshire Hospitals NHS Trust.* London: HSE, p.1.

as details of the infection and deaths were leaked to the national Press. Plainly, if such measures were reasonably practicable following the leak, they were so before. Why, then, was a prosecution not attempted?

The HSE did go into further detail; it listed the factors in favour of prosecution. These included the failure in clinical governance to ensure there were adequate criteria for declaring an outbreak of infection, absence of systems and procedures, failure to take sufficient steps to isolate patients and the paucity of recorded action and discussion which suggested that senior management did not appreciate how urgent the situation was.

Despite all this, the countervailing factors were deemed to be greater. The HSE pointed out that the *Clostridium* strain was particularly virulent and there was limited information about it; that other NHS trusts were having the same problem with *Clostridium* infection rates; that the buildings were not ideal for isolating patients; that there had been discussion at Trust Board level, albeit not recorded; and that the Trust had reasonably not decided to spend more money on isolation facilities after the first outbreak because it believed that the infection was under control.[5]

This reasoning is far from persuasive. It omits the overwhelming evidence that reasonably practicable isolation measures could have been taken; that the infection control team had explicitly and urgently advised these; and that the Board had equally explicitly rejected the advice, with wider performance and finance issues in mind.

It is not an exaggeration to suggest that the HSE effectively endorsed the priority given by this Trust – and in effect other trusts – to resources and targets over safety. Just as concerning was the reasoning that because other NHS trusts were also doing badly, this was not cause to single out Stoke Mandeville. Taken to its logical conclusion such reasoning would mean that the worse a problem is within the health service, and the more widespread the breaches of safe systems of patient care, so the less likely it is that the HSE will do anything about it. And systemic problems with infection control in the health service had already, in 2004, been reported on by the National Audit Office.[6]

The HSE may have had in mind a daunting vista of widespread prosecutions, for which it had neither the appetite nor the resources.

---

5   HSE (Health and Safety Executive) (2006) *HSE investigation into outbreaks of* Clostridium difficile *at Stoke Mandeville Hospital, Buckinghamshire Hospitals NHS Trust.* London: HSE, pp.14–15.

6   NAO (National Audit Office) (2004) *Improving patient care by reducing the risk of hospital acquired infection: A progress report.* London: NAO.

IF THE HSE's explanation for not prosecuting at Stoke Mandeville is unconvincing, the statement it made in respect of Maidstone and Tunbridge Wells NHS Trust is alarming. Quoted at the beginning of this chapter, it referred to lack of a causal link between management failings and the infection and deaths that were rampant within the hospital.[7]

Taken at face value, the statement betrays a misunderstanding of s.3 of the *Health and Safety at Work Act 1974*. This states that an employer must take reasonably practicable steps to ensure the health and safety of non-employees, amongst whom patients are numbered. There is no requirement that harm be caused. Arguably therefore, the HSE's statement, about lack of a causal link between the failings and death of an individual patient, is misconceived. The final sentence effectively dismisses the Healthcare Commission's report and findings, because the Commission had explicitly found a veritable host of practices exacerbating the spread of infection.

The Commission had identified a series of inadequacies in basic care given, or not given, to patients by nurses. Even if one concedes, according to the HSE's self-imposed policy of ignoring clinical issues, that eating and drinking and going to the toilet are 'clinical' (they are surely not), the HSE's approach does not add up. This is because, in addition, a shambolic system of work for maintaining hospital equipment was glaringly exposed by the Commission, affecting the fabric of the environment and hospital equipment.

The evidence for this conclusion included broken and worn equipment, furniture, fittings, dishwashers, showers, chair covers and curtains; dirty, rusty and leaking bedpan macerators; faulty bedpan washers leaving bedpans contaminated with faeces; shortages of commodes; over half of the commodes needing to be replaced; and overflowing sharps bins on the floors.[8] And these are but a few examples.

What makes the absence of prosecution even more notable is that the HSE is used to prosecuting for failures associated with equipment such as hoists and bed rails, *when individual patients meet with accidents*. It is therefore inexplicable that it should not have considered prosecuting for widespread failures in Kent – including those relating to equipment mentioned immediately above – which were clearly associated with infection that caused many deaths.

---

7   HSE (Health and Safety Executive) (2010) 'HSE and Kent Police decide not to investigate Maidstone and Tunbridge Wells NHS Trust.' *News*, 30 July. Accessed on 5 August 2010 at: www.hse.gov.uk/press/2008/e08038.htm.

8   Healthcare Commission (2007) *Investigation into outbreaks of* Clostridium difficile *at Maidstone and Tunbridge Wells NHS Trust, October 2007*. London: Healthcare Commission, pp.44–58.

An example of this inconsistency came in June 2010. Basildon University Hospital Trust was convicted and fined for the death of a man with learning disabilities who had died with his head caught in bed rails. Essentially, this was because of a lack of system to assess risk to particular patients on each ward.[9] It also prosecuted a local council for not maintaining properly an air conditioning system that led to deaths from infection at a leisure centre;[10] why then would it not prosecute for failure to maintain commodes and other equipment, essential to hygiene and infection control in a hospital?

Similarly, University College London Hospitals NHS Trust was prosecuted successfully in 2002, after it failed to control the risk of injury or infection. It had left a sharps bin in a place accessible to the public, including a 21-month-old child.[11]

One further example anyway casts doubt on the claim that clinical matters are beyond the HSE's remit. When two doctors were convicted of manslaughter for failing to diagnose and treat a fatal bacterial infection in a patient, Southampton University Hospitals NHS Trust pleaded guilty to inadequate management and supervision of the two doctors.[12] In other words, it was a defective system of clinical care. If the HSE could prosecute in this case, there is no reason it should not do so in numerous others described in this book.

IN SUM, WITHOUT wishing to be unduly critical, one concludes that the HSE's hands-off approach, to severe lapses of safety in the health service, appears defensible in neither principle nor practice. Its self-imposed no-go areas might be justifiable if successful prosecutions were taking place at the hands of other enforcement bodies, such as the CQC or the Crown Prosecution Service. But they are not. In effect then, it seems that the HSE has seen what is going on in the health service, doesn't like the look of the scale and the complexity of it all, and has shut up shop early.

9   Farmer, B. (2010) 'Basildon University Hospital trust fined £50,000 over patient's death.' *The Independent*, 8 June.

10   Hogg, D. (2006) 'Architect fined over deadly outbreak of disease.' *Yorkshire Post*, 1 August.

11   HSE (Health and Safety Executive) (2002) 'HSE successfully prosecutes University College London NHS Hospitals Trust.' Press release, 12 June. London: HSE.

12   'Trust guilty over death of doctors.' BBC News, 11 January 2006. Accessed on 7 September 2010 at: http://news.bbc.co.uk/1/hi/england/hampshire/4602228.stm.

24

Regulation of Health Care Providers and of Health Care Staff

> Failure to identify and/or meet care needs: untreated weight loss, failing to administer reasonable care resulting in pressure sores or uncharacteristic problems with continence. Poor hygiene, soiled clothes not changed, insufficient food or drink, ignoring resident's requests, unmet social or care needs. (Independent Safeguarding Authority: on harm to patients that could result in the barring from work of health care staff, 2009)[1]

Picture a cricket game on a long hot, summer's afternoon. The batting side is rampant. The pitch is giving the bowlers no spin or pace on the ball; the batsmen are seeing the cricket ball so well, it looks as big as a football. They are striking it to every corner of the ground, bisecting the fielders with well-placed ground shots or bypassing them altogether with lofted sixes over the boundary rope.

Aggressive field placings have long since been withdrawn; gone are the close-up fielders, such as the slips, the silly point, silly mid-off and silly mid-on (silly because it is so close to the batsman). Instead the fielders have been withdrawn to the boundary; the exhausted bowlers have more or less given up trying to bowl the batsmen out. It is just a question now of stemming the flow of runs, of damage limitation. Occasionally, a loose shot results in a catch on the boundary rope, but the batsmen are, on the whole, unchecked. The bowling and fielding side is made up of the regulators; and they are struggling.

Who are they? The Care Quality Commission (CQC) regulates health care providers. Individual health care staff, professional or assistants can be barred from working with patients by a body called the Independent Safeguarding Authority (ISA). And health care professionals can be removed from their professional register or have restrictions imposed

---

1 ISA (Independent Safeguarding Authority) (2009) *ISA referral guidance, September 2009*. London: ISA, p.10.

upon their practice by the Nursing and Midwifery Council (NMC), the General Medical Council (GMC) or the Health Professions Council (HPC).

The regulatory landscape would appear to show that the regulators do take some action against poor and neglectful care but, in relation to systemic problems in the health service, they have been fighting a losing battle. They are reactive and continually chasing the game. It is true that regulators cannot, as a previous chairman of the CQC rightly pointed out, be expected to prevent every fallen leaf.[2] But what about whole, blighted, oak trees?

It would be easy to blame them for doing a poor job. Maybe they are. But perhaps they have also effectively been set up to fail. That is, asked to grapple not just with occasional aberration or deviation, but with fundamental flaws within the system. In effect, defects due, at least in part, to the machinations of the very politicians by whom the regulatory bodies are controlled and directed.

THE REGULATION OF health care providers, including the National Health Service (NHS), is now the responsibility of the CQC. Previously, albeit with lesser powers, was the Healthcare Commission and, before it, the Commission for Health Improvement (CHI). The Commission registers, regulates and inspects health care providers. It is meant to prevent poor and neglectful care.

The Commission, in place since April 2009, is in fact an amalgam of the Healthcare Commission, the Commission for Social Care Inspection (CSCI) (previously responsible for regulating social care providers) and the Mental Health Act Commission. It is worth summarising the Commission's functions and powers because were the Commission (and its predecessors) fully effective, this book would not have been written.

The CQC's role under the *Health and Social Care Act 2008* is to register, review and investigate health (and social) care providers. It has the power to issue statutory warning notices, impose, vary or remove registration conditions, issue financial penalty notices, suspend or cancel registration, prosecute specified offences and issue simple cautions.[3] Urgent cancellation orders can be sought from a justice of the peace if there is a serious risk to a person's life, health or well-being.

---

2   Lister, S. and Baldwin, T. (2010) 'Ministers too sensitive to criticism, says regulator who resigned over healthcare.' *The Times*, 16 February.

3   CQC (Care Quality Commission) (2009) *Enforcement policy*. London: CQC.

The Commission can prosecute in some circumstances including for breach of specific regulations. The regulations about quality of services cover neglectful and abusive health care and specifically mention dignity, nutrition, hydration and infection control.[4] They also place a duty on care providers to operate systems to assess the risks of infection and to prevent, detect, treat and control its spread. Likewise standards of design, cleanliness and hygiene in relation to equipment and premises must be adhered to.[5]

Providers must make arrangements to ensure people's dignity, privacy and independence. There must be a proper system of record keeping to protect service users against the risk of inappropriate care or treatment; there must also be sufficient numbers of suitably qualified, skilled and experienced staff.[6] And service users must also be protected against the risks of unsuitable or unsafe premises, and against the risks of unsafe, unsuitable or lack of equipment.

In addition, there must be a complaints system geared toward assessing, preventing or reducing the impact of inappropriate care or treatment. It is a duty for the health care provider to report certain types of harm to the CQC (or National Patient Safety Agency [NPSA]) – including certain types of patient death, harm, injuries, abuse, police involvement, etc.[7] Health service reporting to the NPSA (reportedly due for abolition) is with a view to there being 'national learning'.[8]

THESE LEGAL REGULATIONS governing health care providers say, therefore, all the right things about safety, dignity, nutrition, infection and related matters. The CQC has the power to enforce them. However, the question is whether the legislation is effective, in particular whether the Commission has the will, resources, expertise and competence to root out systemic problems of neglect and abusive health care. The first chair of the Commission, Baroness Young, announced her resignation in December 2009; she explained that although central government knew it should have an independent regulator, it wasn't really very happy about it. It

4   SI 2010/781. *Health and Social Care Act 2008 (Regulated Activities) Regulations 2010.*

5   SI 2010/781. *Health and Social Care Act 2008 (Regulated Activities) Regulations 2010.*

6   SI 2010/781. *Health and Social Care Act 2008 (Regulated Activities) Regulations 2010.*

7   SI 2009/3112. *Care Quality Commission (Registration) Regulations 2009.*

8   NPSA (National Patient Safety Agency) (2010) *National Framework for reporting and learning from serious incidents requiring investigation.* London: NPSA.

didn't want a ruggedly independent regulator, but rather an emollient and collaborative one.[9]

In this sense, neither the Care Quality Commission nor its predecessors have been set up to function properly. The constant reorganisation of these commissions illustrates what an expert report prepared for the Mid Staffordshire Public Inquiry pointed out: they have been created by, directed by and beholden to the Department of Health. Their role has been more in the way of outsourced performance management than truly independent regulation.[10] When one considers that the Department of Health constitutes the senior management and political controller of the NHS, it is little wonder that the regulators are in tow to political whim and imperative.

The role of the Commission's predecessor, the Healthcare Commission, can be viewed in two ways. Some might claim it was a great success. It exposed events at Stoke Mandeville Hospital, at Maidstone and Tunbridge Wells NHS Trust and at Mid Staffordshire NHS Foundation Trust. Undoubtedly, behind the scenes, these inspections shook parts of the health service and concentrated minds on better infection control. And for those with a political penchant, the Commission also embarrassed central government at times.

Others might view the Commission very differently. They might claim that the scandals it reported should have been prevented in the first place. Worse, it did not uncover them through any laudable detective work of its own, but purely fortuitously. For instance, as already recounted, very poor care standards were exposed only because of leaks about patients dying at Stoke Mandeville or about patients being abused in North Lakeland; because of rising death counts in Kent or Mid Staffordshire; or because of the prosecution and conviction in Mid Cheshire, for attempted murder, of a nurse who had administered diamorphine to two patients.[11]

Worst of all, by the end of the Commission's watch in 2009, systemic, neglectful and abusive care was very much alive and well in the health service. It is hard not to see the Commission's function – and that of its successor, the CQC – as a continual, undignified pursuit, across an inhospitable health care terrain, chasing after horses that have long since bolted.

---

9   Lister, S. and Baldwin, T. (2010) 'Ministers too sensitive to criticism, says regulator who resigned over healthcare.' *The Times*, 16 February.

10 Walshe, K. (2010) *The development of health care regulation in England: A background paper for the Mid Staffordshire Public Inquiry*, p.18. Accessed on 20 December 2010 at: www.midstaffspublicinquiry.com/hearings/s/120/week-two-15-18-nov-2010.

11 Healthcare Commission (2006) *Investigation into Mid Cheshire Hospitals NHS Trust, January 2006*. London: Healthcare Commission, p.13.

An indicator of this state of affairs is the frequent and unfortunate disconnection between a care provider's official rating, according to the regulatory commission, and its actual performance. This concern applies, twofold, to both the CQC as well its predecessors. First, it is that the ratings given to providers are exposed with some frequency as being unreliable. Second, that these ratings have relied in the past, and continue to rely (though not wholly), on self-assessment and self-reporting.[12]

Thus, when Basildon and Thurrock University Hospitals NHS Foundation Trust was investigated by the CQC because of apparently excessive death rates, very poor standards of hygiene were found. The Trust was served with a warning notice. And yet it had recently scored 13 out of 14 for cleanliness.[13] The Mid Staffordshire NHS Foundation Trust had received a 'fair' rating for some years from the Healthcare Commission despite its high rates of mortality.[14] In its successful attempt to gain elite foundation trust status in February 2008, it had declared to the regulating body Monitor that it was delivering high quality care to patients – even though it was doing precisely the opposite.[15]

The Mental Health Act Commission reported a patient's evidence of infestations of mice and cockroaches, despite the Trust's own, declared approval of its standards of hygiene:

> ..."there are mice everywhere on the ward; in the bedroom, dining room, day room. They sometimes crawl up on the table when we have our meals." Although we had raised the issue of cleanliness and vermin infestation with the Trust, the hospital concerned had self-assessed itself as compliant with Healthcare Commission hygiene standards throughout this reporting period. Were it not for our visits to the hospital concerned this disparity would not have been evident.[16]

Similarly, at the Briars care home in Southampton, already mentioned, the owner and manager were convicted of wilful neglect, after the deaths of a number of residents between January 2007 and August 2008. Suspicion first arose in August 2007 following one resident's death in

12 'Spot checks reveal mistakes when hospitals self certify.' BBC News, 8 March 2010. Accessed on 5 August 2010 at: http://news.bbc.co.uk/1/hi/uk/8551668.stm.

13 Bowcott, O. (2009) 'Hygiene inquiry into deaths at Essex NHS trust.' *The Guardian*, 26 November.

14 Healthcare Commission (2009) *Investigation into Mid Staffordshire NHS Foundation Trust, March 2009*. London: Healthcare Commission, p.17.

15 Francis, R. (Chair) (2010) *Independent Inquiry into care provided by Mid Staffordshire NHS Foundation Trust January 2005–March 2009*. London: The Stationery Office, p.182.

16 Mental Health Act Commission (2008) *Risk, rights, recovery: Twelfth biennial report, 2005–2007*. London: Mental Health Act Commission, p.55.

hospital from a large pressure sore. And yet, no more than a few months earlier in May 2007, the CSCI – the then regulatory body for social care, now part of the CQC – had referred to the home as well maintained, bright and comfortable, as well as praising the commitment, attitude and professionalism of staff.[17]

The Eltandia Hall nursing home in Norbury, London, run by Southern Cross, also gained publicity for all the wrong reasons. An 85-year-old man was admitted in February 2009, from the care home to hospital, screaming with the pain of pressure sores and gangrene. The inquest found he died of heart failure precipitated by neglect. The coroner said it was one of the worst cases of nursing home care she had seen. The Inspectorate went in and began to enforce higher standards but only *after* the event, in April 2009.[18]

In Wales, the equivalent commission is the Care and Social Services Inspectorate; in September 2010 it confirmed that it was investigating possible breaches of care regulations by a registered (and therefore previously approved) care home, Highcroft Home in Prestatyn. Too late. A resident, Mrs Brenda Lucas, 78 years old, had been rushed to hospital in August 2009, where she died a month later. On admission, she was found to have 11 pressure sores; the worst, around her knee, measured 20 by 30 centimetres. She had been in great pain. The coroner gave a narrative verdict of death from respiratory infection, heart failure, severe problems in the blood supply to her legs and massive necrotic pressure ulcers.[19]

In 2009, a 37-year-old man with tetraplegia, Mr James Merrett, was living in his own home, where he received care and was dependent on a life support machine. Though physically paralysed, he could talk, use a wheelchair and operate a computer by means of voice activation. Responsibility for his care lay with Wiltshire NHS Primary Care Trust (PCT). The Trust contracted out his care to an agency. He was concerned about the standard of care, so much so that he complained by email to the NHS but received no answer. He had a web camera installed. The camera then caught a nurse switching off his life support machine inadvertently, and failing to switch it back on. Mr Merrett was aware of what was happening and urgently clicked his tongue, before he lost consciousness.

17   Martin, A. (2008) 'Everybody makes mistakes: Care home owner denies neglect following suspicious deaths of six elderly residents.' *Daily Mail*, 25 September.

18   Burnett, C. (2009) 'Norbury Eltandia care home resident died after neglect, coroner finds.' *Streatham Guardian*, 25 November.

19   Hughes, G. (2010) 'Woman, 78, died after suffering 11 bedsores in Prestatyn nursing home.' *Daily Post*, 18 September.

Deprived of oxygen for 20 minutes, he suffered brain damage which reduced his intellectual abilities to that of a young child.

The point of this story is that the agency, Ambition 24hours, to which the care had been contracted out, and for whom the nurse worked, had received the highest rating from the CSCI but three months before the incident. Furthermore, at the end of 2009, the CQC also gave it the maximum rating. However, the PCT's investigation revealed that the nurse involved was not qualified in the use of such ventilators, even though this was a requirement of the job. Furthermore, Ambition 24hours had inadequate systems for checking the training their staff had received.[20]

These are but a few examples. In fact, in every instance of 'scandal', of shocking care, of neglect, the Commission has almost by definition come on the scene too late. Up to that point, regulated and approved by the Commission, the provider would have been suitable, ready and open for business. To be fair, the odd case is inevitable, but what calls into question the regulators' effectiveness is the sheer number of instances in which very poor care has gone undetected.

THE LEGAL REGULATION of health care providers is only part of the picture; the other is the regulation of specific groups of health care professionals and other health care staff. And here there are two categories of legislation that come to the fore.

The first applies to all health care staff. From October 2010, an ISA has operated a barred list under a piece of legislation called the *Safeguarding Vulnerable Groups Act 2006*. This replaced a previous list, called the Protection of Vulnerable Adults (POVA) list, held by the Secretary of State for Health under the *Care Standards Act 2000*. The old list did not cover health care professionals working in the NHS although it did cover professionals working elsewhere, such as in nursing homes; the new list does, so we are moving into new territory in terms of the regulation of health service staff.

The new, barred list contains the names of people who are not allowed to work with vulnerable adults because of the risk they are deemed to pose. Guidance, produced by the ISA, about the sort of behaviour that could get people banned, includes neglectful care. The ramifications are therefore obvious; this legislation could affect very seriously health care staff involved in neglectful care of NHS patients. They could lose their job, their right to practise their profession and their livelihood.

---

20 Lister, S. and de Bruxelles, S. (2010) 'Nurse switched off life support by accident.' *The Times*, 26 October.

The legislation applies to workers involved in 'regulated activity', namely, hands-on work with vulnerable adults. However, it also includes day-to-day management or supervision of such work, and so has the potential, up to a point, to apply to managers as well. Vulnerable adults are defined to include anybody receiving any form of health care.

Grounds for employers to refer staff to the ISA include that the worker has endangered, or was likely to have endangered, a vulnerable adult. Guidance issued by the ISA – and to be used by its staff in making decisions about barring – gives examples of harm. One category stands out in the context of neglectful and abusive health care and includes untreated weight loss, failure to provide adequate care for pressure sores or incontinence, poor hygiene, soiled clothes not changed, insufficient food and drink – and not responding to requests for assistance.[21]

Taken at face value, and set against the evidence reviewed in this book, the implication of this guidance is that significant numbers of NHS staff could find themselves, in principle, the subject of referrals to the ISA. In practice, and ironically, this is less likely to happen when the problems of care in a hospital are systemic rather than isolated.

First, the main channel of referral to the ISA is the employer. (Although the ISA will consider referrals from other sources,[22] and certain other bodies have a duty of referral, including professional regulatory bodies such as the NMC, the GMC, the HPC, the CQC and local authorities.)[23]

It is plain that if systemic, neglectful care is a direct function of that employer's system of work, the employer is not, for obvious reasons, going to want to be making referrals. That said, it is an offence not to refer a worker if the criteria for doing so are made out, and if that non-referral takes place with the consent or connivance of a senior officer, such as a director or manager, that person can be held liable too.[24]

Second, if the evidence of poor care reveals anything, it is that significant numbers of managers and staff do not even recognise neglectful care when they see it. In which case, such care will not trigger referrals.

Third, even supposing that some referrals involving systemic, neglectful care are made, the ISA will face a dilemma; if the staff involved are not to blame because of under-staffing, should they be held

---

21 ISA (Independent Safeguarding Authority) (2009) *ISA referral guidance, September 2009*. London: ISA, p.10.

22 ISA (Independent Safeguarding Authority) (2009) *ISA referral guidance, September 2009*. London: ISA, p.2.

23 ISA (Independent Safeguarding Authority) (2009) *ISA referral guidance, September 2009*. London: ISA, p.10.

24 *Safeguarding Vulnerable Groups Act 2006*, s.18.

responsible for the care (or lack of it) of vulnerable patients in their care? Would a middle way be for the ISA to penalise staff if they had gone along with such neglectful care and not at the very least protested in some way? Alternatively, will the ISA demonstrate its toughness by going out of its way to make scapegoats of individuals, caught up in a mess not of their own making?

A further question is how the ISA will interpret the definition of regulated activity in so far as it includes day-to-day supervision and management; in other words, how far will it go in holding managers responsible? How high up the tree might it try to climb? Hazarding an informed guess, not very far; it is always easier to hold the hapless foot soldiers responsible.

THE RANKS OF the regulators are completed by professional bodies responsible for registering specific health care professionals and holding them accountable to codes of conduct, ethics and professional guidance.

What is the link between the barring scheme and this professional regulatory framework? A health care professional might be struck off his or her professional register but still work, in a non-professional capacity, with vulnerable people – but would not be able to do so if also placed on the barred list. In addition, a health care assistant, for instance, not coming under a professional body, could nevertheless be placed on the barred list.

For example, when five residents died in quick succession, following severe neglect at the Parkside House care home in Northampton, seven members of staff were reportedly referred by the CQC to the ISA and to the GMC.[25] This would be with a view, one way or another, to ensure that those staff would be working neither in a professional capacity nor in any other capacity with vulnerable adults.

As already noted above, in Chapter 5 on dignity and Chapter 17 on whistleblowing, various professional codes and guidance state that professionals must try to ensure safety and dignity of patients, and also raise concerns if things are going wrong. Relevant codes and guidance include the GMC's *Good medical care*,[26] the NMC's *The Code: Standards of conduct, performance and ethics for nurses and midwives*,[27] and the HPC's *Standards of conduct, performance and ethics*.[28]

---

25 '"Severe neglect" ruling on deaths at care home.' *Yorkshire Post*, 6 October 2010.

26 GMC (General Medical Council) (2006) *Good medical care*. London: GMC.

27 NMC (Nursing and Midwifery Council) (2008) *The Code: Standards of conduct, performance and ethics for nurses and midwives*. London: NMC.

28 HPC (Health Professions Council) (2008) *Standards of conduct, performance and ethics*. London: HPC.

Legislation allows these bodies to impose sanctions on professionals who contravene the relevant codes.[29] There is also a code of conduct for NHS managers, issued by the Department of Health.[30] However, unlike the codes of conduct for health care professionals, there is no explicit, legal mechanism by which this code can be enforced.

The GMC and NMC have not really got to grips with systemic, neglectful care. Typically, disciplinary proceedings tend to look at individuals with clearly suspect skills or attitude.

As with the ISA, the dilemma will be how far to consider penalising professionals caught up in systemic problems not of their own making. One must have some sympathy for the professional bodies in this respect; how absolute is a professional's responsibility to stay 'clean', despite overwhelming obstacles in their employing organisation?

SYMPATHY FOR THE regulators runs distinctly dry in cases such as that of Margaret Haywood, the details of which have already been described in Chapter 17. This was not the NMC's finest hour. It tried with might and main, albeit ultimately unsuccessfully, under the *Nursing and Midwifery Order 2001*, to strike off this nurse. She had exposed highly neglectful care at a health service hospital; the professional misconduct alleged was for unjustifiable breach of patient confidentiality. And yet it seems that no action was taken against the nurses actually delivering the care at the Royal Sussex Hospital. The Council had apparently levelled its heavy guns at the messenger.

In late 2009, following the exposure of high death rates at Basildon Hospital and Colchester General Hospital, the Nursing and Midwifery Council announced that it was considering action against nurses at both hospitals.[31] Subsequently, despite conducting a review which identified serious concerns at Basildon, the Council decided not to proceed against individual nurses. It levelled its criticism instead at the Trust Board.[32]

Systemic health service failings resurfaced with the Independent Inquiry into Mid Staffordshire NHS Foundation Trust. The Council

---

29 *Medical Act 1983* (for doctors). SI 2002/253. *Nursing and Midwifery Order* (for nurses). And: SI 2002/254. *Health Professions Order* (for allied health professionals). The latter two orders are made under the *Health Act 1999*.

30 DH (Department of Health) (2002) *Code of conduct for NHS managers*. London: DH.

31 Martin, D. (2009) 'Three thousand needless deaths every year in hospital as watchdog fails to spot poor standards.' *Daily Mail,* 28 November.

32 West, D. (2010) 'NMC will not take action against Basildon nurses.' *Nursing Times,* 16 March. And: NMC (Nursing and Midwifery Council) (2010) *Nursing and Midwifery Council report on the extraordinary review of pre-registration nursing (adult) education and the maternity services at Basildon and Thurrock NHS University Hospitals Foundation Trust.* London: NMC.

announced rather belatedly in 2010 – the Healthcare Commission had already reported on the issues a year before – that it was considering action against some nurses at the Trust. Of particular note is that it had the director of nursing at the hospital in its sights.[33]

The GMC also indicated that it would investigate doctors implicated in events at the Trust.[34] Its chief executive stated the potential consequences for doctors caught up in such terrible care:

> This is a distressing report that reveals significant failings at Mid-Staffordshire Trust. The report highlights a number of very serious issues about the quality of patient care, including concerns about the conduct and performance of some doctors working at the Trust. The Medical Director has referred several doctors to the GMC and we are working closely with the hospital to ensure that we have the information we require to investigate and, if necessary, to suspend or restrict their practice during the investigation. We will be in further discussions with the Trust in light of the recommendations made in today's report…
>
> If any doctor has reason to think that patient safety is, or may be, seriously compromised then they must take steps to put the matter right. If doctors have concerns that a member of the team may not be fit to practise they must take appropriate steps without delay. This includes raising concerns locally and, if there are still concerns about the safety of patients they should inform the relevant regulatory body. Doctors with management responsibility must make sure that there are systems in place through which colleagues can raise concerns about risks to patients.[35]

One suspects that both councils were dragged by the publicity into making such statements and investigations; it is far from clear what the outcome of the investigations will be and whether individual professionals will be held to account.

Nonetheless, hauled into taking action or not, it was reported in November 2010 that the two regulatory councils were investigating up to 57 doctors and nurses in Mid Staffordshire.[36] Such threatened large

---

33 Rose, D. (2010) 'Eight nurses may be charged over Mid Staffordshire hospital deaths.' *The Times*, 19 June.

34 Rose, D. (2010) 'Stafford hospital caused "unimaginable suffering".' *The Times*, 25 February.

35 GMC (General Medical Council) (2010) 'GMC responds to independent inquiry report into Mid-Staffordshire NHS Foundation Trust.' *News*, 24 February. Accessed on 5 August 2010 at: www.gmc-uk.org/news/5873.asp.

36 Sawer, P. and Donnelly, L. (2010) 'Nurses and doctors face being struck off for their part in the Stafford Hospital scandal.' *Daily Telegraph*, 13 November.

scale action would appear to be unprecedented. Suggesting that it might mean business, the Nursing and Midwifery Council had already in October made an interim suspension order against a director of nursing at Stafford Hospital, Mrs Jan Harry. The grounds related to allegations about the failure to maintain safe levels of nursing practice, infection control and patient care. The case against her was that they were serious allegations, there was a risk of repetition if she took on a similar, senior role elsewhere – and she evinced both denial and lack of insight into the alleged failings. An interim suspension order was justifiable for general protection of the public and also of the reputation of the profession and the Council.[37]

THE DIFFICULTY FOR the regulatory bodies in tackling systemic, neglectful care, as opposed to individual instances, is plain. Yet there is something singularly perverse about taking action against individuals but turning a blind eye to harmful care on a much larger scale.

Certainly, the rogues suffer sanctions. For instance, a nurse working at the Royal Victoria Infirmary, in Newcastle, was struck off the register of nurses. This was on a number of grounds including racist remarks about other nurses, falsification of patient records, rough treatment of patients, drawing a face on a patient's hernia and putting a patient's glass eye in a glass of cola.[38]

It is obviously so much easier for a regulator, in all its panoply, to pick on the malfunctioning individuals, notwithstanding that they may deserve it. Indeed, the NMC has produced separate guidance on the abuse of patients, the gist of which is to view abuse as a solitary practice of aberrant nurses. It does not even begin to deal explicitly with the implications of collective perpetration, or toleration, of neglect by nurses in health service settings.[39] Its almost scolding tone, that employers should report occurrences of professional misconduct to the Council, is irrelevant in the case of institutional neglect. No NHS trust is going to report to the Council swathes of its own nurses for neglectful care, when that care stems from the trust's very own policies and priorities.

---

37 NMC (Nursing and Midwifery Council) (2010) *Interim suspension order decision: Janice Margaret Harry, PIN 70I1747E, 25th October 2010*. London: NMC.

38 Phillips, R. (2006) 'Glass eye prank nurse struck off.' *The Journal (Newcastle)*, 17 February. Accessed on 8 September 2010 at: www.thefreelibrary.com/Glass+eye+prank+nurse+struck+off-a0142180313.

39 NMC (Nursing and Midwifery Council) (2006) *Registrant/client relationships and the prevention of abuse*. London: NMC, p.4.

The nub of the matter then is how far the regulators will fault professionals who, against their better judgement, are overwhelmed by systemic chaos, get sucked into poor and neglectful care and do not formally protest. Professionals may argue that it is unfair to place on them the burden to fight against a situation not of their own making. An alternative view would be that, if they do not do so, they are cowards. Unfair? Maybe not, if one considers the vulnerability of their patients. And that some of those elderly people, whom they end up neglecting, fought in the Second World War, risking their lives for those very health care professionals now meant to be caring for them.

On the other hand, how far should we expect a dedicated hospital consultant – juggling a next to impossible workload of patient care and management imposed bureaucracy – to speak out about the nursing care of patients? Especially because she knows that she will receive small thanks and may be earmarked as a troublemaker; and that the time she takes to raise the matter will be yet more time away from her patients.

On the whole, the regulators have not shown an eagerness to confront a culture of poor and neglectful care in particular hospitals, on particular wards; but professionals should not be complacent. A greater public awareness of such care may in future force the hand of the hitherto rather meek regulators. In which case the worm may turn, and professionals who have 'gone along' with really bad care practices may find themselves pilloried.

In September 2010, the NMC announced that it would look more actively at organisations; it would develop 'a critical standards intervention system to assist in the identification of possible systemic failure in an organisation'. How effective this will be is not clear, since the Council has no powers of intervention in relation to other organisations; primarily its role is in relation to individual nurses. Of some note is that the opening paragraph of the relevant Council paper does refer to safeguarding patients; but before even this is another telling reference. It is to concerns about 'public confidence' in the Council.[40] Which comes first?

So, HEALTH CARE professionals in hospitals should not assume that the Councils cannot or will not take action in relation in respect of systemic lapses in basic care – even if the track record of these regulatory bodies is less than convincing. It is possible that Mid Staffordshire may represent a turning point.

---

40 NMC (Nursing and Midwifery Council) (2010) *Critical standards intervention project: Final report, September 2010*. London: NMC.

The NMC has done so, for example, particularly in relation to nursing homes. Significantly, the Council has sometimes bitten the bullet and blamed the individual nurse, *even when wider systemic failings were present.* Crucially, one of the grounds for doing this lies in the professional code, which states:

> As a professional, you are personally accountable for actions and omissions in your practice and must always be able to justify your decisions.[41]

A systemic failure occurred in Birmingham. In 2002, a 77-year-old war veteran, Mr Leslie Vines, entered the Maypole Nursing Home. He suffered from Alzheimer's disease and Parkinson's disease, but was otherwise considered to be physically fit. Ten days later he was dead, having been sedated and placed in a bucket chair, which effectively immobilised him and may have restricted his ability to breathe when he contracted a chest infection. The inquest returned a verdict of death from natural causes.

This verdict did not mean that all had been well. By 2003, the home had been closed down because of concerns about the death of 15 other patients as well. As a result, in June 2008, three nurses – including a manager – responsible for the care of patients were struck off the nursing register by the NMC. Their professional misconduct included incorrect medication, inappropriate restraint, hygiene and personal care failings. All this had led to a lack of dignity for the elderly and vulnerable residents. In addition, the two general practitioners (GPs) who owned the home, husband and wife, were struck off the medical register by the GMC.[42]

In 2004, three nurses were struck off for their part in what must have been a systemic breakdown of care, in 2000, at the Wells Spring Nursing Home, Bradford. A fourth nurse received a caution. Mr Jack Portz was admitted to the home just for a week, while his wife underwent cataract surgery. He had longstanding Parkinson's disease but was otherwise described as strong and healthy. By the end of the week, he had developed multiple pressure sores so painful he cried if they were touched; he was admitted to hospital where he died three months later of bronchopneumonia. His wife had repeatedly asked the home that a pressure-relief mattress be supplied for her husband; it was not.

---

41   NMC (Nursing and Midwifery Council) (2008) *The Code: Standards of conduct, performance and ethics for nurses and midwives.* London: NMC, p.1.

42   Mitchell, I. (2010) 'Inquest returns verdict of natural causes in Maypole Nursing Home death.' *News,* 15 March. Accessed on 20 September 2010 at: www.irwinmitchell.com/news/Pages/InquestreturnsverdictofnaturalcausesinMaypoleNursingHomedeath.aspx.

In reaching its decision, the NMC's professional conduct committee stressed personal, professional responsibility: 'Each individual nurse had an obligation to champion the care of this patient, and failed.'[43]

In the following case, an argument put forward by a nurse, that her failure to attend to patients was part of the accepted system, failed. The allegation was that she had been the nurse in charge of three shifts in the working week over a long period of time, and had been negligent in her duty toward the residents in the care home. During these shifts, she did not care for all the needs of the patients, but referred pressure sore issues to the deputy manager. She explained that this was in accordance with an instruction from the management system in the home.

However, the NMC decided that irrespective of this point, she was responsible for meeting the care needs of the residents; they clearly had such needs, because a number of them had severe pressure sores. The NMC decided to impose interim conditions of practice, rather than to strike her off, particularly because she was now working in an occupational health setting.[44]

Likewise in another case, the senior nurse in a care home displayed failings in the treatment of pressure sores. Having been told by another nurse that a resident was suffering from a grade three pressure sore, she failed to inform the tissue viability nurse. She inaccurately dismissed the sore as superficial and failed to amend the resident's care plan. Two weeks later, when she was debriding tissue from around the sore and changing the dressing, she failed to use an aseptic technique. In mitigation, there was a lack of training provided in the care home as well as unclear lines of reporting. The nurse also conceded that she was inadequately supported and insufficiently trained for her role. But the panel emphasised that she had to be professionally accountable as an individual. It imposed a two-year caution order.[45]

A third instance also involved what seemed to be systemic lapses in the prevention and management of pressure sores. The allegations were against the registrant acting both as a registered nurse attending residents and as manager of the home; in particular, residents of the care home developed very severe pressure sores in the context of a care regime that was not directed toward this issue. This included a lack of appropriate

43 Patty, A. (2004) 'Nurses whose lack of care led to pensioner's death struck off.' *The Times*, 30 November.

44 NMC (Nursing and Midwifery Council) (2010) *Interim order decision: Girlie Franklin, PIN 73D0633E, 5th October 2010.* London: NMC.

45 NMC (Nursing and Midwifery Council) (2010) *Caution order: Lindelwa Mynaka, PIN 01Y0100, 8th September 2010.* London: NMC.

equipment and access to a nutritionist and tissue viability nurse. The NMC panel stated that it was not enough for the nurse to have said she had handed over responsibility to a deputy. It imposed an 18-month interim suspension order.[46]

THE FOLLOWING CASES involving the NMC may or may not – it is not always easy to tell from the reports – have involved systemic failures. Some of them may have been particular lapses by individuals, unrepresentative of the institution. Either way, they are about aspects of care which typically do surface in accounts of systemic failures in care. At the very least, therefore, these cases indicate that the Council can, and sometimes will, take action, in such circumstances.

For instance, not tending to patients, ignoring their needs and letting them die. In September 2010, a nurse working at the Queen Mary's Hospital, Sidcup, Kent was struck off the nursing register. The patient was Mr Derek Sauter, a retired administrator from the Healthcare Commission. He had been admitted ostensibly for treatment of a chest infection requiring antibiotics but died of pneumonia.

During the last night of his life, he rang his wife and she heard him ask for a glass of water; he was ignored. She then heard the nurse saying to her husband that he had been telling lies; the nurse then apparently confiscated the phone. He was removed to a side room because of the disturbance he was creating, but the nurse failed to carry out checks or to call a doctor when his oxygen levels sank. In addition, she did not inform Mr Sauter's wife about his deterioration until after he had died the next morning. When she arrived, the nurse showed no sympathy at all; this was in contrast to the behaviour of Mr Sauter who, as he lay dying, had apologised for his unruly behaviour of the previous night. The NMC concluded that she had not caused his death, but had not respected his dignity, had left him to die alone and not responded appropriately to his death.[47]

Call bells are a recurring matter in the neglect by nurses of patients' needs. In September 2010, a nurse working at West Suffolk Hospital in Bury St Edmunds had conditions placed on his work and registration. This was in relation to an incident in 2006 when, having connected antibiotics direct to a patient's heart, he failed to seek help for 20 minutes when the

46   NMC (Nursing and Midwifery Council) (2010) *Interim suspension order: Phyllis Marcelle Johnson, PIN 66J0816E, 5th October 2010*. London: NMC.

47   Fagge, N. (2010) 'Nurse refused dying man glass of water then took his mobile phone when he tried to call for help.' *Daily Mail*, 16 September. Also: Randhawa, K. (2010) 'Nurse who denied dying patient water is struck off.' *London Evening Standard*, 17 September.

flat-line alarm sounded.[48] Although apparently not a straightforward call bell case, involving overrun or lax nurses, but more about that particular nurse's failings, nonetheless it is clearly not unconnected to the leaving of patients untended when they are in need.

Another call bell case involved a nurse working at Darent Valley Hospital, Dartford. In 2005 and 2006, she silenced ventilator alarms on several occasions without investigating why the alarms were sounding and without calling for help. She also suctioned a patient's mouth instead of the lungs when it was the latter that required the process, and failed to give prescribed drugs to a patient.[49]

A nurse was suspended for 18 months following other misconduct, which included call bell related issues. This followed events at Stanley House care home in Herefordshire. On several occasions, she placed a call bell out of reach of an extremely vulnerable patient, who tended to use it a lot and disturb other residents. After he had settled down, she would return the bell to him. There were some mitigating circumstances because the nurse did not conceal her actions and recorded them in her nursing notes. In addition, management did not take steps to change her approach, nor did it consider a better solution to the particular resident's behaviour. Nevertheless, the nurse's actions constituted misconduct.[50]

In another such case, a nurse at Burton Hospital NHS Trust did not attend the patient until later one evening, during which time the patient had been left in pain. The nurse told the patient not to use the call bell, failed to check the notes to see what pain relief could be administered, did not realise until early the next morning that oramorph could be administered – and did not seek help from a doctor. Because of her hip and problems in moving, the patient was variously in discomfort, pain and complete agony. A suspension order was imposed.[51]

CALL BELL ANSWERING, or not, seems to be closely associated with people's needs to be assisted with bowel or bladder function, including being helped to the toilet. The evidence suggests some wards in some hospitals where patients are routinely ignored and staff appear not to care.

---

48   Thewlis, J. (2010) 'Nurse banned from critical care.' *Ipswich Evening Star*, 1 October.

49   NMC (Nursing and Midwifery Council) (2009) 'Nurse struck off for putting patients at risk.' *News*, 30 March. Accessed on 20 September 2010 at: www.nmc-uk.org/Press-and-media/ News-archive/Nurse-struck-off-for-putting-patients-at-risk.

50   NMC (Nursing and Midwifery Council) (2010) *Suspension order: Nicola Edwards, PIN 04L0490E, 5th, 6th and 7th October 2010.* London: NMC.

51   NMC (Nursing and Midwifery Council) (2010) *Suspension order: Susan Lesley Bloore, PIN 88A0628E, 26th May 2010.* London: NMC.

Such a general disregard of patients' needs can spill over into blatantly abusive treatment. As happened in the case of a nurse, working in a care home, who received a striking off order for various items of misconduct, including shouting at a resident with the words to the effect: 'disgusting woman pissing all over the floor, I am not here to wipe up piss'.[52]

In 2007, at the Worcestershire Royal Hospital, an elderly woman had wet herself. The nurse then shouted at her, stripped her naked in front of other patients and pushed her on to a commode, on which she was left sitting in full view whilst the nurse went to fetch a mop and bucket. When the woman asked to be washed before being given a clean nightdress, the nurse refused. The woman was left crying inconsolably.[53] The nurse was struck off.[54]

In principle, it is misconduct on the part of nurses to leave their patients lying in their own bodily waste. In May 2010, for example, a suspension order was imposed on a senior nurse, responsible for provision of care on a night shift. Another member of staff had discovered patients lying in their own excrement.[55]

ANOTHER THEME IN the case of systemic failures in basic care is the lack of monitoring and recording of patients' conditions.

At Paignton Hospital a nurse was struck off after a number of allegations were made against her in relation to the care she provided for a dying woman in 2006. Apart from giving antibiotics without medical authorisation, she did not carry out blood pressure and oxygen level observations, did not note the patient's deterioration and did not keep records (such as fluid balance charts). Nor did she instigate a medication review, despite the cocktail of drugs the woman was taking which might have been responsible for the patient's renal failure and also lowered her blood pressure.[56]

In the same vein, a nurse at Leeds General Infirmary in 2005 failed to record blood pressure, oxygen saturation, fluid balance and to ensure that a turning chart was kept. Following this, when the patient was found

52 NMC (Nursing and Midwifery Council) (2010) *Striking off order: Kanthee Devi Ramdhunee, PIN 68A0094W, 18th and 19th October.* London: NMC.

53 'Nurse "shouted at elderly woman and stripped her naked in full view of other patients because she'd wet herself".' *Daily Mail,* 25 June 2009.

54 'UK discharge heartless Zimbabwe nurse.' *Zimdiaspora,* 26 June 2009. Accessed on 20 September 2010 at: www.zimdiaspora.com/index.php?option=com_content&view=article&id=1466:a-zimbabwe-nurse-struck-off-register-in-uk&catid=38:travel-tips&Itemid=293.

55 NMC (Nursing and Midwifery Council) (2010) *Suspension order: Karen Louise Weatherhogg, PIN 00I1772E, 21st May 2010.* London: NMC.

56 Pope, S. (2008) 'Nurse struck off for care of patient.' *Express and Echo* (Exeter), 9 December.

unresponsive, she then failed to sound the emergency alarm, to apply basic airway management and to start basic life support. The nurse was a staff nurse, in charge of the ward on the night in question and with specific responsibility for the particular patient. This patient had supranuclear palsy, required monitoring and observation, was fed through a naso-gastric tube, could not move independently, needed regular turning in bed and had been subject to low oxygen saturation levels. The faults of the nurse amounted to misconduct and a three-year caution order was imposed.[57]

THE TOPIC OF falls has been covered in Chapter 10. Failure to assess for the risk of falls in hospitals, and to record and act on falls once they have happened, also form a pattern. In 2008, at Tor-na-dee nursing home in Aberdeen, a patient fell but the nurse neither assessed the patient's condition nor completed the appropriate paperwork. She then denied the patient had fallen; this dishonesty was fatal to her career and she was removed from the register of nurses, following an NMC hearing.[58]

At the Crown Nursing Home, Oxford, a nurse found a resident at the foot of the stairs with a cut head and bruised face. The resident was elderly, frail, suffering from Alzheimer's disease, with a tendency to 'wander'. The nurse failed to call the emergency services, to record neurological observations and to assess (both before and after she was moved) whether an internal head injury might have been sustained. The resident was taken back to her room. A few hours later, her head was bleeding profusely; she was taken to hospital where she died of a subarachnoid haemorrhage. A suspension order was imposed by the Council.[59]

At another care home, In 2006, a nurse failed to seek assistance from a doctor, another nurse or ambulance when a resident's behaviour changed, a bruise appeared on her leg and she screamed in pain. The nurse did not assess properly the manual handling technique to be used after the resident had fallen, and did not, on a subsequent occasion, seek help when the resident fell, sustained bruising and complained of pain. The panel noted that practice in the care home was lax, with little supervision or training; in fact a former manager described it as horrific. Nonetheless,

57 NMC (Nursing and Midwifery Council) (2010) *Caution order: Helen Garrand, PIN 86J049E, 14th April 2010.* London: NMC.
58 Davidson, R. (2010) 'Nurse struck off after lying about fall.' *The Press and Journal* (Aberdeen), 9 June.
59 NMC (Nursing and Midwifery Council) (2010) *Suspension order: Nonhlanhla Kubheka, PIN 04A0789O, 20th July 2010.* London: NMC.

...rse had to retain responsibility for her own professional conduct within the team. A suspension order was imposed.[60]

The following case, too, resulted in the striking from the register of a nurse for multiple individual failings in care in 2005, at the University Hospital of Wales, Cardiff. They included failure to take and to record a patient's blood pressure and oxygen levels, to record that a patient had sustained an injury falling from a commode – and to update that patient's risk assessment and care plan following the fall. In addition, whilst about to wash a patient who was in the bath, she received a call on her mobile phone; she turned away from the patient to take the call, leaving the patient lying there naked.[61]

In a further case involving falls, a nurse working at the Rydale Court Nursing Home had conditions of practice imposed on her following a hearing about conduct and competence. The patient involved was an 80-year-old lady. She was obese and immobile. She suffered from osteoporosis, arthritis, epilepsy and dementia. The misconduct proven was as follows.

First, the nurse was told that the patient was suffering from pains in her leg after the patient had fallen from a hoist; she said she would come to examine her but did not do so. Second, she was informed that the patient was now in pain and distress. Instead of taking any action, she instructed the care assistants to continue washing and dressing the woman. No alleviation or relief of the pain was provided. Third, over a five-hour period, the nurse was urged to call an ambulance given the swollen state of the patient's legs; she failed to do so. This meant the patient was left unnecessarily without pain relief for an extended period of time. The patient was finally taken to hospital; she had suffered multiple fractures to her legs.[62]

FAILING TO KEEP people warm, well groomed and clean can be misconduct. At Drey House nursing home, a nurse acting as clinical manager was found guilty in these respects and given a caution to last for five years. Particular misconduct included failure to keep the temperature at an appropriate level in a resident's room, to ensure the resident was dressed appropriately in relation to the temperature (the resident was cold to the touch on some occasions), to change regularly the resident's clothes

60 NMC (Nursing and Midwifery Council) (2010) *Suspension order: Meundju Hungi, PIN 03J00920, 21st–23rd April 2010.* London: NMC.

61 'Nurse watched porn on duty and put patients at risk.' *Wales on Sunday,* 11 November 2007.

62 NMC (Nursing and Midwifery Council) (2010) *Conditions of practice order: Philomena Omolade Owenkpa, PIN 04E09780.* London: NMC.

and to ensure that the resident's fingernails were properly or regularly cleaned.[63]

Lack of communication with patients, a frequent criticism made by health service patients, is also capable of founding misconduct. When a nurse checked patients for the infusions they were having in cubicles at the Royal Victoria Hospital, Newcastle-upon-Tyne, she did so without talking to the patients. She also did not check that patients understood their care plans. This was misconduct and, together with other failings, resulted in a suspension order of 12 months.[64]

And not helping patients generally. A nurse at Linlithgow Care Home was given a suspension order. The conduct and competence panel noted that she worked with elderly residents who needed good nursing care, including wound care and management, drug administration and responsiveness to their needs. Contrary to this, the nurse did not attempt to assist a patient calling for help. She also failed to administer eye ointment properly, to dress leg wounds correctly, to administer medication correctly and to report, at shift handover, what had happened to two of the residents.[65]

PLAINLY THEN, THE regulators can and sometimes do take action: the CQC, and the various professional regulatory bodies, particularly the NMC. Yet, between them, they have apparently failed to stem a flow of highly neglectful care in the health services that has serious consequences.

Which leaves the question as to why, between them, health care professionals and their regulatory bodies have not put their foot down more firmly, and why they have allowed professional integrity and patient dignity to be so thoroughly compromised in so many hospitals. Never mind the suffering patients, this state of affairs is capable of inflicting huge damage on the reputation of those professions involved – and of those bodies purportedly regulating them.

It would seem that the regulators need to set a more attacking field. Or maybe not. And this is the difficulty. Perhaps the impotence of the regulatory bodies comes precisely because they are now up against fundamental flaws within the world they are meant to regulate. After all, regulators are expected to maintain the integrity of a system, not

63 NMC (Nursing and Midwifery Council) (2010) *Caution order: John Mitchell-Whiteford, PIN 87A1871E, 17th February 2010.* London: NMC.
64 NMC (Nursing and Midwifery Council) (2010) *Suspension order: Morag Isobel Robson, PIN 9013697E, 29th March 2010.* London: NMC.
65 NMC (Nursing and Midwifery Council) (2010) *Suspension order: Beauty Basizeni Khumalo, PIN 04B09710, 19th April 2010.* London: NMC.

fight it. To expect them to do the latter is arguably unrealistic. Were they to try they would fail; their attempts would add still further to the bureaucracy, climate of fear, paperwork and defensive practice – all of which are detrimental to the business of health care.

It is the architect and perpetrator of such systemic flaws, effectively central government, which needs to seek to rectify them at source. Yet the very opposite appears to be the trend, with the Department of Health placing (in theory) an ever greater premium on regulation over the last decade. And this, in turn, is because it has aimed to exercise ever greater political control over health care professionals and providers. Perhaps it has even dimly recognised that the health care system is becoming a wilder and more dangerous place for some patients.

So, a more attacking field? Yes, whilst central government persists in ignoring serious defects. No, in the wider scheme of things. The stifling effect of excessive regulation in the NHS speaks against it. Even aside from this, it may in any case be an irrelevance; the regulators are, at least in some respects, up against such odds that not only has rain stopped play but it simply isn't cricket any more.

25

No Secrets: The Policy of Safeguarding Vulnerable Adults

> Health respondents said there was a widely held perception that care provided by healthcare professionals was "safe". This assumption of safety and good-will and the assumption that everyone was doing their best – it was argued – meant it was difficult for staff at all levels to engage with the questions of abuse and safeguarding. Additionally, respondents thought the hierarchical culture in the NHS meant it was difficult to question staff practices, staff attitudes and patient outcomes. The result was a resistance to engage with safeguarding issues. (Department of Health, 2009)[1]

A quasi-legal strand of policy exists that should in principle protect patients from neglectful and abusive care.

It comes in the form of a piece of government guidance published in 2000 and called *No secrets*, designed to protect vulnerable adults generally from abuse, including neglect, omissions in care and institutional abuse.[2] It was aimed primarily at local social services authorities (local councils), who were given the lead coordinating role in what is now called 'adult safeguarding'. Councils were given no new legal powers to do this because the guidance was not accompanied by any new legislation.

As far as the health service goes, there are at least five key points to make about this guidance and the context in which it sits.

First, the guidance states that National Health Service (NHS) bodies should be involved in local safeguarding. Second, however, the guidance is of negligible legal weight in relation to the NHS. Third, neither the

---

1   DH (Department of Health) (2009) *Safeguarding adults – Report on the consultation on the review of 'No secrets: Guidance on developing and implementing multi-agency policies and procedures to protect vulnerable adults from abuse'.* London: DH, p.39.

2   DH (Department of Health) (2000) *No secrets: Guidance on developing and implementing multi-agency policies and procedures to protect vulnerable adults from abuse.* London: DH.

guidance nor any other legislation authorises or empowers local councils to investigate or take action against systemic neglect of NHS patients.

Fourth, local councils are charged with working cooperatively with the NHS and have a track record of nervousness when challenging their health colleagues. This is so much so that, if a nurse were suspected of stealing from a patient, the local council and NHS would have no difficulty raising that as a safeguarding matter. If, on the other, that patient was not being helped to eat, was being left in pain and was being left in their own faeces and urine – then not only might nobody notice, but even if they did, it might well not be raised as a safeguarding matter.

Fifth, therefore, the NHS has generally not got to grips with the concept of safeguarding and, in particular, the safeguarding activity that is required to protect patients from the harm that the NHS itself perpetrates.

Sixth, additional guidance was issued by the Department of Health about serious incident reporting in the health service and the links with safeguarding activity. This guidance has been considered in Chapter 17, but in short, it carries little, if any, legal weight. It emphasises the process of reporting incidents, but is short on substance. It does not make clear the sort of thing that should be reported; crucially it omits to say that the health service faces systemic problems linked to its own policies; and it is even ambivalent, for instance, about whether pressure sores, caused by a shortage of beds and by patients being passed round wards like parcels, are a safeguarding matter at all.[3]

THE TOOTHLESSNESS OF local councils, the lead coordinating agency for safeguarding vulnerable adults, in relation to the NHS was exposed in the investigation into the care of people with learning disabilities in Cornwall. The two investigating commissions found that the local authority, as the lead agency for coordinating the protection of vulnerable adults, had failed in its role. It had not been sufficiently active. Crucially, they found that social workers had been too ready to accept, without challenge, the opinion of the very NHS staff implicated in the abuse, neglect and poor care of adults with learning disabilities.[4]

---

3   DH (Department of Health) (2010) *Clinical governance and adult safeguarding: An integrated process.* London: DH.

4   Healthcare Commission and CSCI (Commission for Social Care Inspection) (2006) *Joint investigation into the provision of services for people with learning disabilities at Cornwall Partnership NHS Trust, July 2006.* London: Healthcare Commission and CSCI, p.60.

At the Mid Staffordshire NHS Foundation Trust, the Independent Inquiry was not reticent when pointing out that some of what went on constituted abuse:

> It has been submitted that some of what occurred at Stafford amounts to abuse of vulnerable adults. The broad definition of this term…includes…neglect and acts of omission, including ignoring medical or physical care needs, failure to provide access to appropriate health, social care or educational services, the withholding of the necessities of life, such as medication, adequate nutrition and heating. It would be wrong to suggest that such abuse has occurred in every case, but in some of the cases that have been recounted in oral evidence it would be right to say that it has. Whether or not patients were abused in terms of the Protection of Vulnerable Adults definition, many were subjected to treatment that cannot be justified. The Trust needs to look carefully at the way it provides care for the elderly, infirm and vulnerable on its acute admission wards.[5]

Yet the Inquiry did not mention the local council in relation to the safeguarding of patients, even though its hospital social workers must have been observers of what was going on at that Trust for many years. The council, in its safeguarding role, was apparently nowhere to be seen.

THIS IS A short chapter for a simple reason. Its size reflects the impact the *No secrets* policy and guidance has had on tackling institutional neglect in the health service. Local councils have, on the whole, passively looked on or, in some cases, more actively looked other way. They should not be wholly blamed for this. As already pointed out, they have been given no explicit legislation empowering them to investigate and intervene to safeguard vulnerable adults. In law, when they investigate so-called safeguarding issues, they are doing no more than carrying out community care assessment of people's needs for community care services. Community care services are by definition not health services; the local council's writ does not therefore run in hospitals.

In summary and from a legal point of view, local authorities have been given, by central government, no more than a toy water pistol with which to safeguard vulnerable adults in the community. In relation to safeguarding hospital patients, they have been afforded not even that.

---

5   Francis, R. (Chair) (2010) *Independent Inquiry into care provided by Mid Staffordshire NHS Foundation Trust January 2005–March 2009*. London: The Stationery Office, p.401.

26

Negligence

The law of negligence is about people seeking financial compensation for harm suffered. It is called a civil tort, meaning a wrong. In the context of this book it is about health service hospitals and professionals having a duty of care toward their patients. If they breach that duty by falling beneath a reasonable standard of care, and that breach causes harm, then they are potentially liable. Compensation is payable, amongst other things, for distress and suffering.

The law of negligence seems not to have played a major role in holding the National Health Service (NHS) to account for neglect and abuse of vulnerable patients. There seem to be no major reported cases involving the type of care described in this book. This contrasts with the many negligence cases brought against the NHS in general – for example, over injuries at birth, or surgical procedures that have gone wrong.

However, there is evidence of a significant number of cases being settled out of court, for instance, in relation to pressure sore care. A few such cases have been mentioned already in previous chapters. Whilst this may be a good result for the claimant, the disadvantage is that first, the wider public do not become aware of the prevalence of negligent care. Second, no legal precedents are set. Third, this pattern may suggest that NHS trusts find it cheaper to pay out the odd legal settlement for those patients or families persistent enough to go to solicitors. Cheaper than paying upfront for more and more competent staff, to ensure that neglectful care is not provided in the first place.

Last, and perhaps most importantly, negligence cases about neglectful care are ultimately, in the wider scheme of things, beside the point. Once patients or relatives get around to bringing them, it means the harm has already been done. The patient has already suffered or even died. For this reason, this area of law is not considered in any further detail.

Concluding Postscript

This book has charted the course, over a 14-year period, of an affliction in our health services. It is blight not blemish, but equally not yet a plague. But the signs of a possible, incipient plague are present:

> "Well, doctor", he said, while the injection was being made, "they're coming out good and proper, have you noticed?" "The rats, he means", his wife explained. "The man next door found three on his doorstep."[1]

The rats coming out to die were a precursor to the bubonic plague in Algiers jumping from the rodent to the human population. The analogy is that the last decade and more has seen increasingly serious reports of poor, neglectful and abusive care emerge. And behind these are the conditions in which they breed; hospitals, or wards within hospitals, with too few beds and staff to provide basic care for some patients, particularly older people; and an increasing obsession with matters other than patient care.

Let us be clear. The subject is not about the politics, the ideology and the bureaucracy of the health service. It is not another grey, besuited argument about structures, targets, aims, objectives, statistics, paperwork. These all may be virtuous, or at least useful, if they judiciously supplement basic patient care, rather than dispel it. The subject is instead about a particular aspect of the health service that is red raw; a vivid panorama of not just sight but also sound and smell.

Of sight: the bold colours of grade four pressure sores to the bone, the sunken patients deprived of nutrition and hydration, the food gone cold out of reach, the medication untouched, the grime of unwashed patients, the fallen patient in a heap on the floor, the naked patients on view to others and covered only in dried faeces or an incontinence pad, the dying patient nursed in a dining room next to the diners — and the sick stowed away to be treated in the windowless storerooms of new, shiny hospitals.

Of sound: the screams of pain from those suffering pressure sores or otherwise deprived of pain relief, the unanswered call buttons buzzing and buzzing, the crying of those untended patients, the nurses giggling as a patient dies out of sight, the thump of ignored patients as they hit the floor — and the silence of the nurses as they simply fail to talk to patients.

---

1   Camus, A. (1960) *The plague.* Harmondsworth: Penguin Books, p.10.

And of smell: the pungent, reeking odours of faeces, urine, infection and sometimes rotting flesh.

And, behind all this, in great contrast, the quiet of the board room, the smooth financial and political machinations reaching up to central government, the quietly doctored information, the smart public relations statements, the civilised covering up of the seething scenes beneath – and the euphemism, so unctuous as sometimes to be sickening.

And vanishing fast from this world is the white milk of human kindness and compassion – the sight, sound, smell and texture of it – all spilt and fast flowing away.

If only this were sensationalist hyperbole and ludicrous licence. But in fact, it is not quite this, as the evidence reveals. So what is the extent of the affliction, why does it exist and persist, what might be done about it and how likely is a remedy?

Briefly, a number of key points emerge as to its nature, extent and causes. These are that it is systemic and crucially is perpetrated, rather than merely tolerated, by the State. It is on a large enough scale as to deter, entirely perversely, remedial action and to encourage disbelief and denial that there is even a significant problem.

At best, half-hearted policy measures are announced and implemented with ambivalence but tend to remain superficial and disconnected from the underlying political, ideological and financial drivers of the health service. Responsibility and accountability are in short supply. And the obstacles standing in the way of quick and effective solution are many.

These points want teasing out.

BUT BEFORE ANALYSING these key points, we should summarise the wider battlefield, as it were, on which the conflicts and tragedies in hospital health care have been played out. And this takes us inevitably to the key ingredients of any hospital: the story of beds and of their associated hands-on, professional staff. The scarcity of these is a toxic solvent – though not the only one – implicated in the erosion of dignified, professional care for patients. And how their demise (that is, the beds, but sometimes the patients as well) together with other factors – unevidenced decision making, wastage of resources on managers and management consultants, resulting managerialism and bureaucracy, the taking of professionals away from patient care – lay down a seed bed of poor care, which grows into neglect and abuse.

We have seen in earlier chapters how, in 2000, the government spoke in *The NHS Plan* of a health service needing more acute hospital beds, as well as more beds in community hospitals or in specialised care homes – and, where possible, more care in people's own homes. Development of these *additional*, community services was to be called intermediate care. Older people were to be provided with what they needed and to be treated with dignity. Special guidance was issued, the *National Service Framework for Older People.*

Let us consider what has actually happened in a typical health area in England – it could be anywhere – and contrary to the official policy. During the decade following 2000, the local acute hospital shuts scores – whole wards – of elderly and rehabilitation beds, and sheds many staff posts at the same time. The remaining staff are sometimes too few in number and competencies even for the reduced number of beds. Community hospital beds in the area are also lost; this is despite widespread local opposition including tens of thousands of names on petitions. Managers, acting supposedly in the name of the patient voice but in fact on ruthless political orders, close them anyway. By the end of the decade, the area has lost 20 per cent of its health service beds.

These fast and ill-conceived closures result locally in huge pressure on those acute hospital beds and staff remaining. Wards are over occupied, staff are rushed off their feet, and patients, especially the elderly, do not receive adequate treatment or care. The idea that somehow so many patients can be treated, nursed and rehabilitated in their own homes, instead of in hospital, is revealed as pure fiction; and even for the subset of patients who can be, it is not cheap. Yet the community teams are not resourced adequately. When challenged as to the rationale of such hasty and drastic actions, the chief executive recites the words 'intermediate care', even though what is happening is inconsistent with that policy. It was meant to provide care and rehabilitation over and above people's hospital needs, not to deprive them of proper hospital care. The real reason for the closures, hasty financial and ideological orders from the Department of Health, is not mentioned.

The chief executive, when further challenged to provide an evidential basis, simply retorts that people should not worry. Everybody will have the right care in the right place at the right time. It is all about modernisation; people just need to be more trusting. In the face of reasoned, evidenced, professional and clinical objection, the chief executive even resorts to telling people that they must have faith. Unaware, presumably, of just how inimical the word 'faith' is to scientific, rational and evidenced health care.

Making the best of limited resources is also cited as a reason for these changes. During this decade, however, management posts locally double in number (nationally, the figure is an 84 per cent increase),[2] whilst the nursing posts and beds are decreased. As a result new, office premises have to be bought for the swollen management team at considerable cost. Even then, astonishingly, when major decisions have to be made, the managers seem unable to take decisions and implement change themselves. They have to call in management consultants, at further great expense, to manage the change as well as to advise them how to save even more money. (For example, as reported in Leeds in January 2011, £500,000 – the equivalent of employing 16 nurses – was being spent on management consultants to help cut up to 1000 health service posts in the city.)[3]

When local people write to the Secretary of State, civil servants reply on her behalf that it is all for the best. It turns out in fact that the Department of Health has been advised by the very same management consultants. Likewise at great expense.[4]

During this decade, local staff find themselves subjected to a constant barrage of new targets, aims, objectives, projects, working groups, mantras – and the gathering of more and more management statistics. Half the statistics never get used because the administrative staff are so far behind inputting the data. The reduced numbers of care staff are subjected to ever more pressure and productivity demands, spend increasingly less time with their patients, and become correspondingly demoralised and stressed. Staff sickness levels rise, thus placing even more pressure on those still standing.

Immense amounts of time, effort, energy and resources are wasted on endless restructuring. In our sample locality, between 2004 and 2012, primary care trust staff (responsible for providing the community services meant to be relieving the pressure on the acute hospitals) will have been doing the same job in the same place. However, they will have had *six different employers in eight years*; first an acute NHS trust, then two different primary care trusts, followed by the provider arm of the second primary care trust, then a completely different, third, primary care trust – and, finally, envisaged in 2012, an independent provider to whom the NHS

2   Kaffash, J. (2010) 'NHS managers increase by 84 per cent in a decade.' *Public Finance*, 26 March. Also: Ramesh, R. (2010) 'NHS management increasing five times faster than number of nurses.' *The Guardian*, 25 March.

3   'NHS Trust spending £500,000 to save cash.' *Yorkshire Post*, 4 January 2011. And: 'NHS spends £1 billion on management consultants.' *Daily Mail*, 7 June 2006.

4   Craig, D. (with Brooks, R.) (2006) *Plundering the public sector*. London: Constable.

staff will be transferred, leaving behind them the National Health Service forever.

As we already have noted, health care professionals locally are spending increasingly less time with patients; not only are they distrusted by management to provide the right the sort of care but increasingly they are prevented from providing care at all. So much so that, by 2011, local staff are told they have to sign up to a new project. It is called *Releasing time to care: The productive ward*, dreamt up by the NHS Institute for Innovation and Improvement. The ideas have come from the car manufacturing and aviation industries; it is all about time, motion and productivity.[5] Perhaps only in health service management circles could this be suggested with a straight face. Any other observer would greet with incredulity a policy, the very existence of which concedes how – over the last decade and more – health care staff have been sidelined from doing the very job they are employed to do: look after patients.

Officially, the only problem at our local hospital, which is preventing its becoming a foundation trust, is financial. It has largely assessed itself as providing good care; indeed, the Care Quality Commission and Monitor, the two regulatory bodies, accept this self assessment. However, in order to put its finances in order, and satisfy Monitor, the hospital plans further cuts to qualified nursing and therapy staff, as well as to medical consultant sessions, and an even further reduction in bed numbers.

We could go on. The above, typically anywhere in England, might read like a march of pure folly involving not just a waste of money but diminution of patient care. And we would be right in so reading it. But it is much worse than this. Over this decade, our local acute hospital has increasingly adopted practices that are detrimental to inpatient care, with elderly people inevitably the worst affected. It has done so because of the pressure it is under – self-imposed or inflicted by politicians, whichever way you wish to look at this. It is a hospital that has not made its way yet into a major reported scandal of neglect and abuse. But the conditions for these are in place, because this short story of what has been happening in our typical locality means that significant strains of poor care are unmistakably present.

Stepping back and considering the position nationally across all hospitals generally, the strength and visibility of these strains will be more or less, depending on the particular hospital or indeed the particular

---

5   NHS Institute for Innovation and Improvement (2011) *Releasing time to care: The productive ward*. Accessed on 20 January 2011 at: www.institute.nhs.uk/quality_and_value/productivity_series/ productive_ward.html.

ward. And their virulence will vary also from time to time, as a function of fluctuating pressures and staffing levels, for example. But they are widespread.

AND SO BACK to our key points. The evidence discloses overwhelmingly a systemic blight in the health service, as opposed to a series of local random failures. Recognition of this fact is crucial to political, or any other, priority being given to a remedy.

It can be judged to be systemic not only because of the prevalence of poor care but also for another reason. The National Health Service (NHS) is run on a command and control basis. The policies and major actions of NHS trusts at local level are governed by nationally set policies, priorities and targets. They are overseen and effectively enforced internally, hierarchically and sometimes ruthlessly from the Department of Health downward.

In other words, if a pattern of local failure emerges and continues over many years, then as a matter of course there will be a link with the central controller. In any case, there is no need to rely only on this logical inference of a significant link. Repeatedly and for many years now, respectable bodies – such as the National Audit Office, the House of Commons Health Committee and Healthcare Commission – have fingered aspects of government policy as contributing directly to serious deficiencies in the very basics of health care.

A systemic strain of bad practice does not preclude the existence of widespread good practice; and it is precisely the existence of the latter that sometimes leads people, erroneously and illogically, to deny the existence of the former. Likewise, guidance and statements about good practice do not automatically translate into the real world; yet, too often, policymakers and senior management in the health service appear to believe that they do.

THE PROBLEM IS concentrated in a *State-run* health system, namely the NHS. In other words, the neglectful and degrading treatment visited upon people is, by definition, *actively* perpetrated by the State. This raises the stakes when it comes to matters of responsibility, accountability and blame.

It is certainly true that neglectful care in health and nursing care is by no means confined to the NHS; abuses are reported from independent, private care homes and hospitals. But even here, the State has a significant role to play. This is because it, through both the NHS and local councils, contractually places many people in nursing homes and private hospitals. As commissioners of these placements, using public money, these public bodies bear a responsibility when things go systematically wrong. In addition, the health care regulatory body, the Care Quality Commission (CQC), is in effect controlled by the government, albeit that it is a notionally independent regulator.

IT SEEMS PRECISELY because the problem is so extensive that full recognition and action have not followed. This might seem odd. But it is to do with the crucial difference between publicly acknowledging systemic, as opposed to a little local, difficulty. Cleaving to the latter is simply not enough to jolt anybody into serious action.

Central government has been happy to publish general guidance on improving care for older patients in hospital. But when confronted with unpleasant and disturbing reports from regulatory commissions and other bodies, it has tended to acknowledge, grudgingly, local but not systemic shortcomings. To own up to anything other would be to concede the enormity of what is going on, to necessitate a shake-up of priorities and to pose political, financial and practical difficulties.

There appears in fact to be a law of disproportionality at work. The bigger the issue, the less drastic the remedial action. This is so for a number of reasons: it is difficult to grapple with, involves too many entrenched interests and requires uncomfortable introspection.

A further factor is at play. An intuitive sense of scepticism prevails about the neglect and ill treatment of NHS patients; the same sense of doubt tends not to be applied, for instance, to nursing homes. The health service has for many years been regarded as a fundamental and greatly trusted national institution. It is therefore more difficult for people both within and without it to grasp the gravity of what is going on. This has contributed to the continuing denial, evidenced in this book, that the ills are systemic as opposed to mere local aberration. It has had a paralysing effect. The rooting out of neglectful health care remains, even now, a sideshow.

A CULTURE OF denial, sophisticated and multi-faceted, has developed to gloss over unpalatable facts. In addition, information gets concealed or released in highly selective fashion. NHS trust boards are starved, or conveniently starve themselves, of relevant information. Regulatory bodies look the other way in the case of all but the most serious or inescapable lapses.

And highly euphemistic language, bordering on Orwellian doublethink, is used extensively, whilst mantras masquerade as rational thinking. Arguably, the greater the problem, the more absurd and parodic is the language used to describe it.

We must not forget the absurd excesses of language: the 'world class' commissioning of neglect, of cupboards renamed 'treatment rooms', of empty 'guarantees' fronting up dehydration and malnutrition. Nor the 'clinical sustainability' ('less is more') of staffing and bed cuts leading to inadequate capacity to care and to lethal pressure sores. And of wholly vacuous mantras, such as the stultifying 'right care in the right place at the right time', which suppress both rational analysis and clinical evidence.

Nor should we underestimate the immense harm inflicted by the deniers, the concealers of facts, the spinners of tall tales and of seductive words – and, sometimes, the outright deceivers. If you deny a problem you cannot talk about it; if you do not talk about it you cannot even begin to solve it.

This cocktail becomes more unhealthy still when we add in the arrogance, the unshakeable belief that we inevitably are making civilised progress – and a corresponding disbelief that we have anything to learn from history or even the relatively recent past. On the one hand, this encompasses an inability to acknowledge the importance of compassionate, humane care, albeit less technologically and medicinally equipped. If it is old and past, it must be bad. On the other hand, still less is there an ability to entertain the possibility that certain 'modern' policies and practices are casting us backward in time to other aspects of health care – the dangerous and dirty – which we would like to condemn as the province of benighted custom and error.

Scientific medicine has undoubtedly, as Raymond Tallis has so clearly pointed out, relatively recently transformed our very notion of the nature and efficacy of medicine. It has performed, from the perspective of even the recent past, miracles. And in this country, the National Health Service has, for the past 70 years, been the vehicle for its successful application to the population.[6] But it is being undermined, for some patients, by its less glamorous, but equally essential sidekick – basic nursing care. Nobody wants to admit this. Yet such an undermining is not only harmful to patients, but also a waste of money. Like the child with a splendid new toy, which is then carelessly left out in the rain to rust, rack and ruin.

The fiction that *all* is well must be dispelled. Joseph Conrad once wrote strikingly of a ship called the *Narcissus* and that 'on her lived timid

---

6   Tallis, R. (2004) *Hippocratic oaths: Medicine and its discontents*. London: Atlantic Books, Chapter 2.

truth and audacious lies'. In the context of the abandonment of older patients to poor care and worse, and of this being hushed up, both the phrase and the name of the ship suit well the health service. They befit too many of its managers and policymakers, inward looking and caught up in distorted reflections of their own making.

UNSUPRISINGLY, THEN, RESPONSIBILITY and accountability are in short supply when things go badly wrong. It is plain who the key players are. Starting at the top, they include politicians, senior civil servants at the Department of Health (a government department), regional health bureaucracies, local NHS trust boards, senior management, middle management and front-line health care staff. All are implicated.

Despite the obvious identity of the perpetrators and the equally evident detriment to patients, few hold their hand up to own responsibility. Worse, relatively little action is taken against the perpetrators in order to hold them accountable.

Sometimes, if a local scandal has blown up, senior managers may pay with their jobs – as often as not though, departing with significant pay-offs and resurfacing elsewhere in the health service. It is hard not to conclude that, at a deeper level, the real sin committed in these high profile cases – at least in the eyes of central government and higher echelons of the NHS – is not so much the maltreatment of patients but the political embarrassment of getting caught.

Likewise, professional regulatory bodies governing the conduct of doctors, nurses and allied health professionals seem to have taken relatively little action against professionals involved in systemic neglect and abuse of patients in the health service.

Such bodies are far readier and more able to move against individual bad eggs, but unprepared or perhaps unable to tackle significant numbers of professional staff who are complicit with – that is, more or less active in, or passive, tolerant observers of – the most terrible health care. Perhaps we should not blame them. They appear to have been set up to fail in current circumstances; taking on fundamental cracks in the system is not their role. Excusably or not, these regulatory bodies have, on any view, failed to turn the tide.

Even law – which at least has the virtue of pinning legal and sometimes effectively moral responsibility on individuals and organisations – has been relatively little used to tackle systemic neglect in the health service. Whether this is due to the content of the law, or the way in which it is being applied, it is clearly failing to protect highly vulnerable people from care which we would surely wish to say is not only morally but also legally indefensible. The legislation has turned limp and wilted in the hands of the regular enforcers, the Care Quality Commission and Health and Safety Executive. And if ever those unpredictable but powerful irregular forces, the lawyers and judges, were to be regarded as the cavalry, it is high time they left their chambers and barracks, mounted up and did battle on what is turning out to be a bloody field. Not, counter-productively, to terrify and cow the health service with the law for the sake of it, but to put a stop to some of its worst and uncontrolled excesses.

An impression emerges that, somehow in practice, the health service is to an extent untouchable and vested with some sort of immunity. This is difficult to understand; it is clearly not for want of the gravity of what is happening within our hospitals. If you do not give vulnerable patients food and drink, this entails recklessness as to whether they recover or linger in sickness, whether they live or die. How much more serious can it get?

THERE IS A tendency to point to the 'system', thus absolving individuals of any blame. If everybody is guilty, then nobody is guilty: *tutti colpevoli, nessuno colpevole*, as the Italian expression goes.

The danger of this passive, fatalistic and arguably amoral approach is that neglectful and inhumane care, especially of older people, comes to be regarded as akin to a law of physics such as gravity. Scientific laws are not about human agency; they are thus outside of morality, which concerns judgements about human actions and affairs. For such immutable phenomena, nobody can be morally, politically, professionally or legally blamed; even worse, nothing can be done about them. Superficially comforting and conscience salving, such thinking can lead down dark roads.

We have been blown a long way off course, almost without qualm. We are talking of real people and of human perpetration and agency, not of an impersonal spanner dropped accidentally into a mechanical set of works. It is not just a game of pounds, pence, statistics and political points.

The patients are real as is their suffering and, all importantly, the perpetrators. That is, the politicians making their way wilfully oblivious to the collateral damage of their opportunistic and ideological policies; NHS trust chief executives working hard but disastrously obedient to political whim no matter the consequence; senior health professional managers who have sacrificed ethical and professional principle; and front-line health care staff, who have become numb to it all or simply hardened their hearts. These last witness, and sometimes get dragged into, shocking scenes played out daily – morning, afternoon, evening and night performances.

Baroness Neuberger has asked generally how we, as a society, have come to treat the elderly so badly, as to amount to the infliction of 'punishment and neglect for being old'.[7] It appears that kindness and compassion are in retreat before an unspoken savagery. As a society we have sleep walked into this. Where, we might ask, are the lay gods of our social democracy; the equivalent of Juno's sacred geese raising the alarm when ancient Rome was threatened? In fact, the analogy is not quite right, because we are talking about State-perpetrated action and omission. The barbarians are not so much at the gates as already within.

THE OBSTACLES IN the way of remedy are formidable. They are not immovable but are resilient because of an absence of political, professional and moral will. After all, it cannot be beyond the wit of competent politicians, managers and front-line staff to ensure that patients are helped with food and drink, with getting to the toilet and with keeping clean.

A state of affairs confronts us, in which increased awareness of neglectful care has been around since at least 1997. Fourteen years on, it would appear that little progress has been made; for all the superficial protestations about dignity and compassion, an underlying inertia prevails. Some might even argue that we have gone backward and that things have got worse. Acceptance or imposition of responsibility and accountability remain conspicuous by their absence.

Iron-fisted implementation of government targets, priorities and financial imperatives have played their part, as has inadequate staffing in terms of numbers and competencies and very obvious hospital bed shortages.

Targets in principle might have been useful but only where they improved health care, not where they have been used to enhance one aspect of the health service at the cost of undermining another. In other words, to claim on paper success for meeting financial and performance targets, but to keep quiet about the other aspects left to rack and ruin – such as the safety and dignity of patients – is just disingenuous. And where such claims have been made by central government, chief executives and NHS trust boards, it is therefore akin to cheating; a triumph of unbalanced managerialism, bureaucracy and spin over basic care and the real world.

---

7   Neuberger, J. (2009) *Not yet dead: A manifesto for old age.* London: Harper Collins, pp.269, 272.

Professional, clinical and ethical judgements are sometimes undermined; staff who do protest at being forced to provide poor and neglectful care do so fearfully and may not be listened to. Whistleblowing staff are not welcomed and, in terms of their future employment prospects, play a dangerous game. Perhaps more health care staff than we would care to admit have become inured to unacceptable care practices; this, in turn, can only happen if management is tacitly encouraging, cognisant, tolerant or unconcerned.

Furthermore, it appears that health service hospitals are being run in a way that is not attuned to the needs of many older people, notwithstanding that they are the main users. Policies of the moment such as 'choosing and booking' elective treatment, care pathways and 'payment by results' (pricing up interventions and treatments) are not well suited to older people with complex and overlapping needs resulting from multiple pathology. Such patients are not the happy, active shoppers, apparently envisaged by central government, operating in a health care market.

For example, an acute episode lands them in hospital as a matter of urgency, but the current system too often militates against the extra time, trouble, expertise and staffing resources required for proper diagnosis, treatment, care and rehabilitation of such patients. The consequence of this is that not only are patients with greater and more complex needs less likely to have them met, but also that a fertile soil for neglect and abuse is laid down. There is, it seems, a terrible, if unspoken, fear in the health service of older people with more complex needs.

HAVING OUTLINED THE present position, the following are some of the obvious steps that might be taken.

First, it would be beneficial if central government were to stop issuing reams of ineffective and aspirational guidance about dignity and appropriate care, which many people anyway ignore, and instead were to adjust underlying mechanisms, which frequently are grinding away in exactly the opposite direction to that of the guidance and of good practice.

There is of course no reason, in principle, why guidance should be so ineffective. But in the context of this book, we need to picture just how it is failing. One way would be take a great ship, dual powered by sail and by steam. The guidance flutters like small, handsome topsails unfurled by earnest crew members in the rigging, to drift the ship slowly and safely into port on a gentle breeze. But out of sight of the passengers and of the onlookers on shore, down in the engine room of power, the stokers and engineers are frenziedly working, under the gaze of the captain. The latter, in turn, is being guided by well-dressed, land-going advisers who know little about the sea; and he in any case barely goes up on deck to survey the scene. Far from going into port, the ship is in fact propelled at speed in precisely the opposite direction out into an open and rough sea.

Second, politicians need to be transparent with the public about the implications, explaining that health care is not just about 'high-tech' interventions for the young but also the unglamorous basics for the elderly too. This does mean explaining that it is not acceptable, morally or indeed legally, to sacrifice humane care on the altar of other clinical and political priorities.

Most of all, government has to tackle the hospital care of older people, particularly the increasing numbers with multiple pathology or co-morbidities. This is the crux of the matter: if basic, good care and treatment were assured for these patients with more complex needs, so would it be for others with simpler requirements. It entails also recognising the link between poor, neglectful and abusive care. A seed bed of poor care develops when hospital services are not run with older people in mind, beds are far too few in number and staffing levels and staffing competencies are inadequate. From these spring neglect and abuse.

This will of course require political courage, rather than wishful thinking, empty gesture and denial. Otherwise the elderly – and sometimes younger patients as well – will continue to be at risk of being treated as problematic and unwanted statistics, rather than as human beings.

Third, the Health Minister of the moment, in his or her role as the chief executive of the NHS, should be held directly and politically accountable for the suffering of patients when the causes are clearly systemic and the effects serious.

Equal with the third point, NHS senior management should be held accountable for poor and neglectful care and this should trump failure to meet performance and financial priorities and targets. And whilst significant amounts of poor and neglectful care persist, the CQC should be resourced and supported by central government to enforce far more rigorously decent care, rather than be constrained, as at present, by both financial and political restrictions. Used as a truly independent regulator rather than a performance management tool on behalf of politicians, it might work better. However, equally, its limitations should be recognised;

it cannot be expected to fight against flaws in the health care system itself, perpetuated or allowed to flourish by government.

Fifth, from another direction, professional regulatory bodies could put their heads over the parapet and spell out the implications for health care professionals on the front line. This would be to the effect that not only must professionals personally not provide poor and neglectful care, but that, at the very least, they must be seen to be raising formal, effective objections to it.

These regulatory bodies should set up mechanisms to facilitate this; these must link surely to a much more effective system of whistleblowing. Even if professionals are not the architects of this care, but merely passively involved or just regular observers at their place of work, they must still speak up. If they do not, they should be made aware that, at least in some circumstances, they may suffer sanctions from their regulatory body.

It might impress upon individual health care professionals the importance of their moving away from what could be regarded as a cowardly stance, given the vulnerability of some of their patients; that is, passing by in silence the suffering of those they are meant to be caring for. Equally, however, we – and government – should not await great things from whistleblowing; its role is well suited to exposing isolated instances of bad practice, but not to combating a general malaise. How far is it reasonable to expect, as a matter of course, hard-working, altruistic professionals to risk their jobs and their careers, when they are subsequently victimised for voicing their concerns?

Sixth, on the criminal law side of things, the Health and Safety Executive (HSE) could come out of the comfortable and highly artificial compound it seems to have constructed around itself and start to tackle some of the grossly defective systems of work in our hospitals which are highly detrimental to the health and safety of patients, sometimes on a large scale.

Seventh, in similar, criminal vein, the police and Crown Prosecution Service (CPS) could consider more carefully why it is that prosecutions involving independent sector care homes for offences such as wilful neglect or even manslaughter seem not to be reflected in the context of health service hospitals. A few well-placed prosecutions could have a positive and galvanising effect on policymakers, management and staff in the health service.

If, in some circumstances, there is hesitation about bringing cases against individuals caught up in systemic malaise, then prosecutions could be brought against the organisation. For instance, organisations can be prosecuted by the CPS for corporate manslaughter, by the HSE for health and safety at work offences and by the CQC for care standards offences.

Last, the glaring loophole in the criminal law, relating to wilful neglect and ill treatment, should be closed by the government. Such a change would mean that these offences would no longer be confined, as at present, to victims with diagnosed mental incapacity or mental disorder, but could be applied to protect other highly vulnerable people albeit without such a diagnosis.

IT IS OF course all very well to pontificate about what could or should be done, and there may indeed be other, far more effective measures to be taken than those outlined immediately above. However, the last major question is whether effective remedial steps, of whatever type, are likely to be taken. It is possible to form two different views about this, one optimistic, the other less so.

Surveyed from one vantage point, the signs are promising.

When, in *The War of the Worlds*, the Martians landed first on Horsell Common, near Woking, and then elsewhere in Surrey, there was panic and terror. Nobody knew what they were up against or what to do; so much so that, in the end, it was not human agency that defeated the invaders but bacteria.[8] But within our health services, we are dealing not with an alien, but with a known, phenomenon. The evidence is abundant and incontrovertible that a strain of poor, neglectful and abusive care is on the loose. And we know what it is, where it is, the causes and who is responsible for it.

Our subject matter is therefore of a different order. It is man-made and much of it lies within a largely State-operated system of health care. And the solution is simple. It is not, after all, about training up a new generation of highly skilled heart surgeons; it is only about reminding managers and staff of the most fundamental tenets of care, such as keeping people nourished, hydrated, taken to the toilet, monitored, spared agonising pressure ulcers, clean and in a state of dignity.

Even better than this, because such fundamentals have continued to elude too many managers and health care staff, all the good practice guidance has already been written. So that if for some perverse reason health care providers have forgotten about what health care is, it is all in

---

8   Wells, H.G. (1946) *The War of the Worlds*. Harmondsworth: Penguin Books. (Originally published in 1897.)

print. And if the guidance fails, there lies behind it a range of legislation that can be used as a buffer to keep everybody on the rails.

The picture gets rosier still. Providing basic care is not one of those controversial issues about which there is disagreement, political or professional. Government ministers, regulatory bodies governing health care providers and health care professionals, parliamentary committees, voluntary bodies, relatives' groups such as Cure the NHS – all are in unison that undignified, degrading and neglectful care is completely unacceptable.

Even the media, across the political spectrum, speaks with one voice; for instance, *The Observer*'s Dignity on the Ward campaign starting back in 1997 and the *Daily Mail*'s Dignity for the Elderly, begun in 2002 and ongoing. Contrasting newspapers, but a common stance.

As far as health care in the NHS goes, central government does not have to grapple with external factors over which it has limited control, as it actually runs the system. It is the perpetrator and has the power to change things, to apply the brakes. This is in contrast to many other social ills, over which it holds less sway and little or no control.

We also know that good care can be achieved, because as emphasised in this book, there is plenty of good, compassionate and attentive practice within the health service. It is doable.

Last, at the time of writing, a golden opportunity exists to crystallise the issue in the public mind and to do something decisively about it. This comes in the form of a statutory public inquiry into the events at Stafford Hospital, held under the *Inquiries Act 2005*.[9] Its report, due in the latter part of 2011, could be used by both central government and regulatory bodies as a catalyst to deal with the problem seriously, politically, professionally and legally. Politicians even have the opportunity to garner votes, if only they made common humanity a priority, rather than an afterthought trailing behind ideology, bureaucracy and endless structural change to the health service.

In short, in sporting terms, it is an open goal. And yet, as followers of football know too well, open goals are regularly missed.

WHICH BRINGS US to a less optimistic point of view. Fourteen years' worth of compelling evidence has stacked up. Little has been done. Scandalous and shaming reports and accounts seem almost to lower, rather than raise,

---

9   *The Mid Staffordshire NHS Foundation Trust Public Inquiry.* Details of inquiry progress. Accessed on 28 October 2010 at: www.midstaffspublicinquiry.com.

the bar; perversely, they set a benchmark of entirely the wrong sort. Inertia and inaction have largely been the order of the day.

Central government and the politicians are deeply implicated in this continuing state of affairs. Either they deliberately wish not to upset the applecart, for fear of where it would lead. This may even involve a cold calculation that the interests of more vulnerable patients, often the elderly, requiring basic care, will have to be sacrificed. Or they genuinely believe that all is well with only the odd rotten fruit to worry about. If this is so, it calls into question their competence and that of their advisers. Whichever explanation is correct, it is unpalatable.

The late Claire Rayner's near final words, just before she died, are unlikely to be enough: 'Tell David Cameron that if he screws up my beloved NHS I'll come back and bloody haunt him.'[10]

Two months after her death, a Patients' Association report had been published about the plight of the elderly in hospital. Claire Rayner's husband commented in November 2010 that the haunting should begin.[11] By now it was clear that the new coalition government was seemingly as preoccupied as its predecessor not with basic care, but with yet further structural and bureaucratic change, with ideology (of a free market in health), and with essentially empty incantation about patient care (such as 'nothing about me without me').

Regulatory bodies continue on the defensive. The CQC, for instance, continues to arrive too late on the scene; the carnage, literally sometimes, has already taken place in hospital or care home. Some health care professionals themselves appear, pusillanimously, to have given up the fight, plummeting the depths of poor care, tolerating or even joining in, with indifference.

Well-meaning, earnest guidance continues to be issued in one form or another, without underlying mechanisms being altered or modified in order to ensure its efficacy. This is a bit like floating a pilotless, rudderless dinghy against a rising flood tide.

Even the forthcoming report of the Public Inquiry into the events at Mid Staffordshire may have been set up with various ends in mind. For instance, it is about keeping electoral promises; in opposition both Conservatives and Liberal Democrats had urged a public inquiry. And any adverse findings of the Inquiry can be laid at the door of the former Labour government.

---

10 Turner, L. (2010) 'Last words for David Cameron as agony aunt Claire Rayner dies.' *The Independent*, 12 October.

11 Martin, D. (2010) 'Scandal that shames Britain: Join our campaign to end appalling treatment of the elderly on NHS wards as complaints reach record high.' *Daily Mail*, 2 December.

More worryingly, the Inquiry, strange though it may seem, may turn out to be a way of kicking the whole matter into the long grass – by looking specifically at Mid Staffordshire, rather than what has been going on in the health service as a whole. This may give more room for the government, hedged around by financial restrictions, to minimise the implications of the Inquiry's findings, to escape some of the awkward questions about the care of older people and to avoid getting dragged in out of its depth. The Inquiry's findings may even be hijacked, opportunistically, to support further the drive toward a market in health care and the breaking up of the NHS. Whatever one's view of this policy development, it would be singularly unfortunate if the Inquiry came to serve such ends; it would divert attention away from root problems and causes.

In any case there is already ample evidence as to what has been going wrong in the health service generally, which led to Stafford Hospital in particular; on this pessimistic note at least, there is a risk that the Public Inquiry, the recommendations it makes and the discussion about implementing those recommendations will be but another vehicle for obfuscation and delay.

In addition to the Public Inquiry, one might look to the new coalition government's White Paper, the equivalent of New Labour's *The NHS Plan* back in 2000. Published in July 2010, it is entitled *Equity and excellence: Liberating the NHS*. It fails to mention the word 'neglect' and refers to older people only once, when stating that they will not be forgotten when criteria are formulated for measuring quality. It includes the word 'dignity' only once and then in relation to social, not health, care.[12]

The White Paper refers also to the need for increased 'productivity', a word associated with the efficient grinding out of consumer goods; such a reference to the financial bottom line does not bode well for humane and dignified care. There is talk elsewhere of the importance of the 'patient experience' and that some, but not all, targets will be removed, to be replaced by outcome measures.[13]

Prevention and reporting of harm is also covered in terms of safety and pressure sores, falls, infections and so on.[14] But in essence, it has been said before; if anything, *The NHS Plan* in 2000 promised rather more in

---

12 Secretary of State for Health (2010) *Equity and excellence: Liberating the NHS*. Cm 7881. London: The Stationery Office.

13 DH (Department of Health) (2010) *Liberating the NHS: Transparency in outcomes, a framework for the NHS*. London: DH, p.31.

14 DH (Department of Health) (2010) *Liberating the NHS: Transparency in outcomes, a framework for the NHS*. London: DH, pp.37–40.

terms of dignity, particularly for older people, than *Equity and excellence.* The world has been promised to patients on many occasions.

The effect of all this on priorities, and on how they affect neglectful care, will not necessarily be straightforward. The misuse of targets may have exacerbated, but was not the sole cause of, neglectful care; indeed such care existed before the target culture became all consuming over the last ten years. It is financial and performance priorities that call the shots and will inevitably continue to do so.

The coalition government confirmed, in its spending review of October 2010, the need for £20 billion of efficiency savings over a period of four years.[15] That is, cuts in ordinary language; such as the 250 nursing posts, 100 inpatient beds, 550 consultant sessions, 83 clinical and diagnostic posts and 220 administrative staff – all due to be lost at Barts and the London NHS Trust, as revealed by documents leaked in February 2011. In the cause of saving £56 million.[16] In any case, although targets are meant to be giving way, the NHS Operating Framework still contains some 100 indicators, including targets, outcomes and other matters – not least financial – to be measured.[17]

The words from politicians and health service trust boards come easily, but the one thing that the last 14 years have taught us is to look behind the words, to what is actually going on. And such is the degree of ingrained poor practice, and failure to do anything about it, that optimism must be tempered with caution.

Indeed, groundless optimism, expressed even by health campaigners, can be equally as damaging as the empty words of those who would, from different motives, conceal and deny what is happening.

Into the long grass? Tucked away in the coalition government's proposals on health care outcomes is reference to 'complex and multiple service use (for example, mental health, frail and older people with complex co-morbidities)'. This might seem promising; but the document refers only to 'future' (not present) thought being given to this group.[18] That is, the very group of patients which, far more than any other, lies at the heart of poor, compassionless and neglectful care in our hospitals.

15 Chancellor of the Exchequer (2010) *Spending review of 2010.* Cm 7492. London: The Stationery Office, p.43.

16 Cecil, N. (2011) 'Barts and the London set to lose 250 nurses as part of budget cuts.' *Evening Standard,* 3 February.

17 DH (Department of Health) (2011) *Technical Guidance for the 2011/12 Operating Framework.* London: DH.

18 DH (Department of Health) (2010) *Liberating the NHS: Transparency in outcomes, a framework for the NHS.* London: DH, p.37.

Thus is the very nub of the matter – and of the care described in this book – nonchalantly brushed away.

THUS, WHILE IT would be tempting to finish on a high note, a reading of the runes suggests this would be a rash thing to do. The underlying characters have not yet changed. It is far from clear that those in political power have really learned anything from the last 14 years and equally doubtful whether the regulators and professions are ready – or even equipped – to take up the force of arms needed.

In recent times, it all started with that Dignity on the Ward campaign in 1997; the end is certainly not yet in sight. Things are, on balance, likely to become worse. This will be through a combination of financial cuts and the throwing open of the health service to competition. Whatever the ideological arguments generally, for and against, on which this book does not presume to pronounce, this move to a free market – as currently conceived and being executed – will almost certainly work against the elderly and vulnerable patient with more complex needs. They will inevitably be commercially unattractive, as explained in Chapter 13. To the extent that they are packaged, costed up and tendered out to other providers, it will inevitably be at a cut price because nobody wants to pick up the expense of their proper care – neither the commissioners (presently primary care trusts and, in future, general practitioner consortia) nor the providers.

And so the great game seems set to roll on – of politics, hospital patient throughput, statistics, targets, priorities, outcomes, money and, above all, of inconvenient numbers of older people with complex needs. And neglect. We must hope this melancholy note proves, sooner rather than later, to be out of tune, that the care described in this book becomes a thing of the past and the book itself a curious and anachronistic relic. But the note should, in the meantime, not be played with a mute in place.

THE ROAD TO hell, they say, is paved with good intentions. And much has been argued in the last 14 years about improvement in the health service and the ulterior, beneficent motives of all those involved.

We should finish therefore with Judith Allen, a nurse for 36 years and also adviser to the Royal College of Nursing. In 2006, her 87-year-old mother went into hospital with a urinary infection and kidney failure; she kept a diary.

Her mother stayed five months before dying. In between, she contracted *Clostridium difficile,* hygiene measures were ignored, nutrition and hydration charts were not kept and she complained of being handled roughly. She would be left lying in diarrhoea, tablets were left on the locker even though she could not take them herself and she was not helped to drink; the family had to help her. The family also cleaned her dentures, put in her eye drops, cut her fingernails and cleaned her spectacles. The nurses didn't do these things.

One day her daughter arrived to find her mother crying, with the door closed. The room was hot, smelling of faeces; she had also been sick. The alarm on her infusion drip was bleeping. The call bell was tied to the cot side on the other side of the bed. Nobody was attending. And so on, eventually to pain relief being denied by a nurse as she lay dying, chest bubbling, until a doctor intervened.

The daughter noted the 'mission statements and philosophies of care' proudly displayed within the hospital. At some point, in the middle of all this, her mother said to her daughter: 'Don't let anyone tell you there's no Hell – there is – I've been there.'[19]

---

19 'The NHS put my mother through hell, says a former nurse.' *Daily Mail*, 21 August 2007.

Subject Index

Author Index